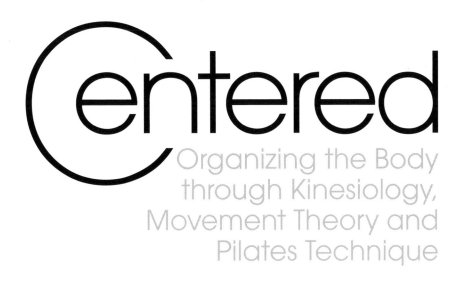

Centered

Organizing the Body
through Kinesiology,
Movement Theory and
Pilates Technique

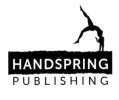

HANDSPRING
PUBLISHING

EDINBURGH

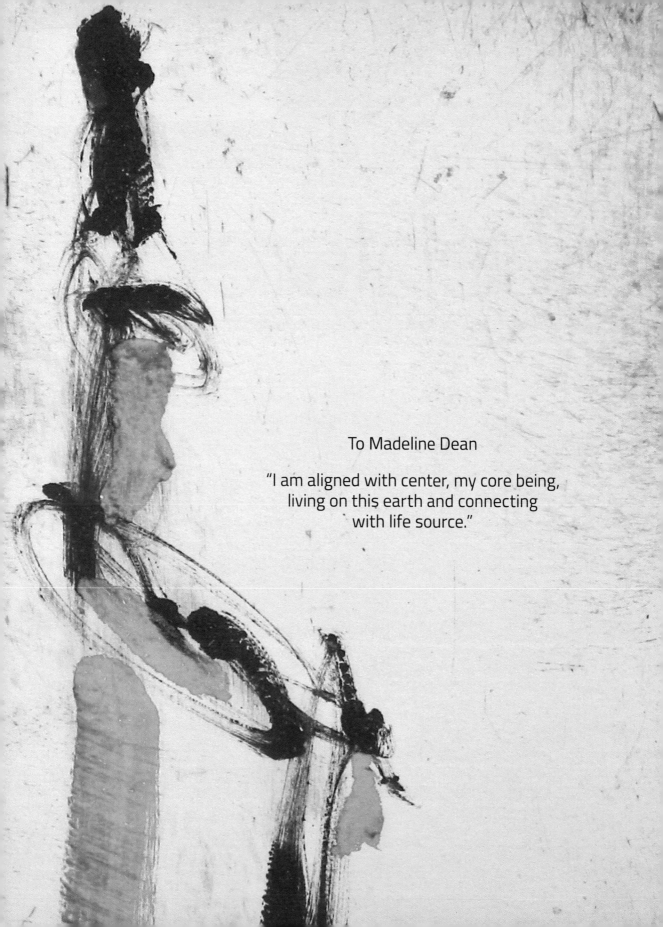

To Madeline Dean

"I am aligned with center, my core being,
living on this earth and connecting
with life source."

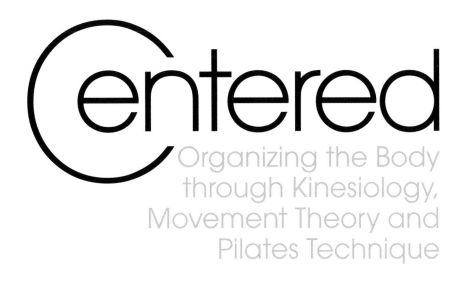

Centered

Organizing the Body
through Kinesiology,
Movement Theory and
Pilates Technique

Madeline Black

Forewords
Blandine Calais-Germain and Andry Vleeming

HANDSPRING PUBLISHING LIMITED
The Old Manse, Fountainhall,
Pencaitland, East Lothian
EH34 5EY, Scotland
Tel: +44 1875 341 859
www.handspringpublishing.com

First published 2015 in the United Kingdom by Handspring Publishing
Reprinted 2017

ISBN 978-1-909141-15-5

British Library Cataloguing in Publication Data
A catalogue record for this book is available from the British Library

Library of Congress Cataloguing in Publication Data
A catalog record for this book is available from the Library of Congress

Commissioning Editor Sarena Wolfaard
Design direction, cover design and illustrations by Bruce Hogarth, kinesis creative.com
Cover artwork by Brigitta McReynolds
Photographs by Cathy Stancil, www.cathystancilphotography.com
Index by Laurence Errington
Typeset by DSM Soft
Printed and bound in Great Britain by Bell and Bain Ltd, Glasgow

The
Publisher's
policy is to use
paper manufactured
from sustainable forests

CONTENTS

Madeline Black has filmed a workshop that complements this book. The online video workshop contains 32 short videos that further explore the material. To gain access to the free videos, scan the QR codes in the book with your smart phone, or go to PilatesAnytime.com/centered, and use the coupon code "CENTERED". By watching the videos and passing the online quiz it is possible to earn three Pilates Method Alliance CECs.

REVIEWS

"Madeline has elegantly accomplished the complex task of creating the book we need and always wanted. A book for teaching and understanding what we teach and a comprehensive guide for 'doing', understanding why we do it. . . . I highly recommend this book for all of us who teach movement, therapeutic or otherwise. It may just become your best guide in practice. Thank you Madeline."

Marie-José Blom, CPMT; Pilates Master Teacher, Movement Educator, Lecturer and Int. Presenter/Consultant; PMA Gold Certified; Creator/Educator of SmartSpine™ System; CEO, SomaSom, Inc.; www.smartspine.com

"Madeline's book 'Centered' is an amazing experience and exploration of qualitative movement, a must have for all who consider themselves movement practitioners. I believe it will become a classic tool for our profession."

Brent Anderson, PhD, PT, OCS, PMA(r)-CPT; Founder, Polestar Pilates, Florida, USA

"Madeline aims to make one more durable and utilitarian, fit for the needs of life. You will move with more ease and grace by both listening and then doing this deeply informed bodywork."

Phillip Beach, DO, DAc; author of *Muscles and Meridians: The Manipulation of Shape*, Churchill Livingstone, 2010

"A comprehensive and practical book that combines science, movement education, and self-awareness from a master teacher and practitioner. I highly recommend it."

Tom Hendrickson, DC; author of *Massage and Manual Therapy for Orthopedic Conditions*, Lippincott, Williams & Wilkins, 2009

"Exploration of the gray area between science and exercise, which falls under the umbrella of Pre-Pilates, serves to improve balance and function so that exercise will reinforce good movement patterns. Madeline approaches movement from a foundation of dynamic anatomy. ... 'Centered' is full of insight and accessible, practical information for movement teachers."

Deborah Lessen, PMA-CPT

"An essential read for students and practitioners of the movement arts; wonderfully descriptive and clearly illustrated! My favorite is Chapter 5, about the importance of the diaphragm – read it first, and then again. Madeline has synchronized all her studies and knowledge into a valuable gift for those of us who love to learn. Your efforts are truly appreciated!"

Marika Molnar, PT, LAc; Director, Westside Dance Physical Therapy; Director of Physical Therapy Services to New York City Ballet

"The implications of this book are far-reaching. I believe that it has significance across all disciplines of traditional behavioral medicine as we know it today. The mind initiates movement. Is it possible that movement in turn manifests creative thought? Madeline's expertise in this area is well defined in this book."

Dr JC Bobo, MD, psychoneuroimmunologist

"Having attended Madeline's lectures and workshops over the year, I welcome her first book. It will be an important addition to my Pilates reference library."

Alan Herdman, author of *The Pilates Directory* (2004), *The Gaia Busy Person's Guide to Pilates* (2003), *Pilates for Men* (2007) and *The Complete Pilates Tutor* (2014)

FOREWORD

I am honored to be invited to make a small contribution to the book I see before me. The author's ambition in writing it is to give a clear insight into therapeutic methodologies, and to support an established field of movement together with the practitioners and therapists who apply these innovative manual and movement skills in practice. In this manner, they effectively create a positive functional change for their clients.

The author began her career as a dancer and choreographer and she writes that choreography is the process of translating feelings and ideas, ideally leading up to a flawless execution of movement. Her book is ultimately based on a whole body approach, addressing its kinematics for optimal function, using insights gained from her background, as a dancer, choreographer, movement and integrative orthopedic massage therapist, Pilates teacher, and now also an excellent writer.

Madeline Black has combined her years of self-reflection in the movement and dance field with an earnest intention of taking care of the proper execution of movement and finding balance. Creating this sensibly arranged book required the confluence of her 25 years' experience in movement and therapy and her seriousness of purpose is clearly reflected in it.

It is both pleasant and logical that the author, coming from a dance and movement background, uses the most effective name for this book by entitling it *Centered.* The concept of *Centered* is artistically captured in a striking logo, showing exactly what the book is all about. The content encompasses properly applied motor control, body alignment, and sharing the load: using neither too much nor too little force – just enough, precisely balanced, to synchronize forces throughout the body. It employs a combination of movements based on kinesiology, manual techniques, strengthening, and proper muscle recruitment.

The text is organized sequentially, starting from the feet and working upwards through the body, while each subject chapter also interrelates with the whole body. Chapters commence with a contemplative introduction to help to stimulate intuition. They are based on Pilates methodologies but also on other techniques and studies, to clarify principles of movement.

Centered is about the body's potential working on maladaptive patterns after trauma in an integrative way (both physiologically and psychologically). It is both impressively structured and excellently written. There are clear overviews in each chapter, embedded between attractive and expertly created photos, drawings and artwork. These give instant clarity about the expected correct execution of movement. *Centered* could be considered to be conjointly a book of movement and a pleasant touch of art. When you read it, you may feel the urge to emerge into the beautifully arranged pages to become part of the actual exercises.

This script presents a captivating guide and effective resource to develop skilled movement in practice. Its goal is clear: becoming an effective practitioner of movement to regain a functioning whole body, especially at times when it is malfunctioning.

I would advise that after having had the pleasure of reading this beautifully composed book, you spread the word amongst your colleagues. It is an excellent opportunity to enrich your (and their) clinical skills.

Prof. Dr. Andry Vleeming
2015

Department of Anatomy, Medical College of the University of New England, Maine USA

Department of Rehabilitation Sciences and Physiotherapy, Faculty of Medicine and Health Sciences, Ghent University, Belgium

FOREWORD

Madeline Black is known as a teacher who integrates science, movement, and Pilates into the osteopathic tradition. Throughout this book we encounter familiar Pilates themes and equipment such as the Reformer, the Cadillac, the Magic Circle, the Wunda Chair and others, as well as exercises. But we are invited to revisit these in depth: region by region, her work itemizes and focuses in on refinements of practice which will enhance the subtlety of approach of both students and teachers. Step by step, the author invites us to observe how the body combines various kinds of movement, particularly those frequently overlooked micro- or mini-movements concealed within the larger and more visible movements which are obvious to anyone at first inspection. These refinements of method may serve to prevent unwanted and avoidable tiredness and even injury, especially in the case of intensive practice.

The book's organizational structure is based on an exploration of the regions of the body. Each region is introduced by a quotation from the literature, which not only locates it in the overall structure of the body, identifying its local function, but also makes clear its specific contribution to the overall process of body movement and balance.

The exploration begins with the feet. The work thus constitutes a preparation for enabling patients to stand firmly on their feet, even if this involves lengthy preliminary sequences of lying down, sitting, or supported positions as a means to that end. It shows the importance of meticulous attention to the anchorage of the feet to the ground, by exploiting a wide range of plantar exercises as well as the adaptability of the ankle.

This is followed by numerous observations on the principles of movement of the lower limbs, which facilitate adjustment of the thigh and the lower leg and the three major weight-bearing articulations of the ankle, knee, and hip. The author reminds us, quite rightly, of the abundance of connective tissue around the hips. The exploration then moves upward, where it naturally arrives at the foundation of the spinal column, the pelvis. Here, the author offers numerous observations and suggestions, particularly regarding spinal stabilization and the provision of a solid support to allow the trunk to project itself from the spine. The pelvis is presented as a central point of coordination for the legs and the trunk. In order to assume this role, the hips must be more mobile than the sacroiliac joints, and when that is the case the four articulations perform correctly.

Chapter 4 brings us to the trunk, where we reacquaint ourselves with the fundamental insight of Pilates, embodied in the description of the trunk as the powerhouse of all movement, or the "core". The author invites us to locate the "pivot point" where the ribs meet the lower vertebral column. Detailed investigations are proposed for the different layers of fascia, which represent separate organizational levels of the many and varied strategies of movement and balance unique to every individual. The following chapter describes many sorts of breathing exercise, without which the central body exercises cannot work.

In Part 3 we reach the stage of the upper limbs, where the author suggests numerous procedures to improve suppleness and coordination. This brings us finally to the neck and the head, the centre for "non-verbal communication."

Throughout my reading of this book I was impressed by the author's long experience of movement teaching, which has given her heightened powers of observation. Our thanks are due to her for sharing the results with us with such precision.

Blandine Calais-Germain
2015

Author of: *Anatomy of Breathing; Anatomy of Movement; Anatomy of Movement: exercises; The Female Pelvis: Anatomy and Exercises*

PREFACE

Centered is written for those who wish to learn more about the body, whether you are a practitioner or a person desiring a new discovery about their own body. *Centered* is the confluence of my 25 years in the separate body-based worlds. I have written many training manuals and handouts and I was encouraged by many colleagues, teachers, friends, and family to write what I have formulated about the body in movement, the body for healing, and the body for gaining strength. Through my synthesis of these worlds, I processed and integrated the work into my teaching of movement educators. I offer the professional movement practitioner more skills to educate the client about their body strategies and how to improve function. The worlds of bodywork, movement education, and fitness are merging toward a point where the goal is to optimize a person's physical nature to live in this life fully.

As I sit here and contemplate writing this preface, I am struck by the process of creating *Centered* and am reminded of a similar feeling in my life as a choreographer, when completing a new work and about to see it on stage. Creation for me is unstructured until the form begins to take its own shape and flow. It starts with an idea, a seed, then flow begins to develop the basis for the work. The form becomes the structure for the work. It feels like a metaphor for how the body moves and how a movement practitioner notices, touches, and uses the structured knowledge of science to coach a client toward better health and improved movement. The body is a beautiful representation of art and science. Achieving physical fitness requires one's training to be this combination. All bodies have the potential to improve and maintain the body for a lifetime. Joseph Pilates states: "Our interpretation of physical fitness is the attainment and maintenance of a uniformly developed body with a sound mind fully capable of naturally, easily and satisfactorily performing our many and varied daily tasks with spontaneous zest and pleasure" (Pilates, 1945). To move functionally well serves our structure's ability to sustain healthy movement over a longer period of time, making living life more pleasurable, and follow our path.

The passionate Pilates teachers and other movement educators are in the never-ending process of perpetual learning. It is my intention that you, the reader, will use *Centered* as a study guide, reference book and practice manual using the video links provided as well as the descriptions and photographs. To experience and improve upon the body's movement potential is to understand its design and sensing (seeing, feeling, touching) function so that you may change the dysfunctional conditioning of the body. We truly can heal our bodies through movement

Madeline Black
2015

ACKNOWLEDGEMENTS

I am so fortunate to have the people in my life who through their passion, knowledge and vibrant life forces inspired me to search, question, expand and be supportive in my life, all through a body–mind connection. I acknowledge Jean Claude West, a man who in my opinion began the expansion of the Pilates Method into the realm of science. He has inspired me from the first time we met in the late 1980s in New York through today. Jean Claude is my friend and colleague who has been part of my development of this book. His references, endless conversations, and support helped me continue working toward my vision of *Centered*. And at the last moment, a pre-eminent guardian angel, Tom Hendrickson, contributed his vast knowledge of the body and his superb editing skills which helped me fine tune the final proof.

The seed for publication came from Handspring Publishing, especially Sarena Wolfaard, who has been by my side through the entire process, and Andrew Stevenson, with his savvy ways of making connections. Thank you to Stephanie Pickering, my editor, who helped me find my blind spots. I appreciate greatly the openness and problem solving skills of John Marston of Pilates Anytime to stretch beyond the business model and provide video footage for *Centered*. Seeing live action of the important hands-on movements and coaching was so important to me to convey what and how to perform the techniques. I wish to thank Kristi Cooper for being persistent and gracious over our first meeting and now subsequent professional and friend relationship. Cathy Stancil, the photographer, and Brigetta McReynolds, the artist whose work inspires beauty and motion, are women I first connected with through our children. I am honored to have both of these talented women contribute to *Centered*. Gratitude is a word and feeling I have for my husband, Bill Doty, who lived with me throughout this process, and for his gift of words.

Last but not least, this book also acknowledges all the teachers and body centered people who came before me.

INTRODUCTION

"The body's continuous attempts to find the original center creates shifts in the structural midline, which will, in turn, produce accommodations that change the body's entire structure and function for the better or worse."

Charles Ridley, *Stillness*

Inspiration: coming full circle

One of my earliest dance memories was watching the kaleidoscope of movement patterns created by the June Taylor dancers on an old black and white television. The synchronized precision of movement performed on the floor awakened a passion for dance in me. As a child, I was in constant motion until I realized I could direct my energy into performances. My family sat through hours of shows in the basement that I choreographed to the music we listened to on our 78 rpm record collection. No one in my world conceived of a career involving movement. I loved science too. In 1974, the world of science had not yet met the movement world. A high school advisor, who helped me choose colleges, asked what interested me. I said I wanted to study science and dance. According to the advisor, that was not an option. I had to choose one or the other. So, I chose dance.

I attended a college where a renowned New York City Ballet dancer spearheaded a new dance major. Here, I was required to study anatomy, physiology, and kinesiology. My interest in science helped me focus on becoming a better dancer, being stronger, jumping higher, and being more flexible. I found it interesting studying the muscles and their function and how the different lines pull on our structure, which in turn influence our movement. Beyond the dance training, I wanted to put this information into practice.

This led me to the gym, which was then an old fashioned weightlifters' world. Here, I began the journey into traditional weightlifting. In my day, dancers did not work with weights unless they were injured and working with a physical therapist. Personal training was not an industry like it is today. The men in the gym had fun showing this skinny dancer how to lift. Under their guidance, I learned how to weight lift in a systematic, progressive way. However, I was so invested in good form that observing the movement habits of the people in the gym gave me concern. I was seeing how the imbalances in the body were actively being strengthened through repetition and how awkward body mechanics were compounded by the mentality of lifting at all cost. Does this truly develop strength in terms of real life needs and goals? My goal was to be a stronger dancer and performer. I realized weightlifting wasn't serving me. I experienced spinal tensions and decreased range of motion in my hips and shoulders that were hindering my ability to continue on my path in dance.

Back in the studio, I was inspired by Hanya Holm, who taught a vigorous and intelligent way of moving. She challenged not only the body but also the mind, demanding both a letting go and critical thinking. When I met Eve Gentry, an original teacher of Pilates and a former dancer with Hanya Holm, I learned that Hanya's technique included the Pilates mat movements. To discover how Pilates was integrated into my dance training prior to my transition from performer to Pilates teacher was a full circle moment for me.

Pilates methodology: more questions

Pilates became my answer to a movement methodology by incorporating a full range of movement using resistance to develop an evenly strong body. The versatility of Pilates was enormous, matching many levels of training intensities or healing approach. I would jump into my science brain and ask why and how this method was working. I continued my search for answers by aligning myself with brilliant practitioners who instilled a wisdom and passion for reaching beyond the routine system being taught. My understanding expanded, leaving me with more questions.

So, I ventured into the bodywork world. I was exposed to Rolfing, craniosacral therapy, visceral work, orthopedic massage, muscle energy techniques, and neuromuscular facilitation, both as a client and as a student attending many workshops. I committed to a full training program of orthopedic massage and spent over 10 years studying and practicing Integrated Manual Therapy (IMT). I now regularly attend workshops led by Canadian or English Osteopaths to gain the additional kinesiology knowledge along with manual techniques for restoring misalignment and dysfunctional movement. I integrate this information and these techniques into client sessions and teach my methodology primarily to Pilates teachers who desire to achieve better results for their clients.

Over 25 years, I have worked on myself and with clients to bring the body back to a functioning whole, especially at times when the body is malfunctioning. In my opinion, the combination of manual techniques, movement based on kinesiology, and strengthening with an eye towards muscle recruitment is the most effective way to move a body from dysfunction into a strong functioning one.

What I expect from a healthy and strong functioning body is:

- durability: to remain in good condition for a lifetime

- utility: to train the body so that it is suitable for the purpose for which it is intended

- beauty: to move with grace and ease for any body type or age.

Smart movement matters

A smart body is moving through its architecture as it has been designed with balance and strength. And the smart body has reached the point where the ability to perform a given task, as in a squat, or naturally walking down the street in good movement patterning comes without over-effort of thought, with an unconscious consciousness of movement. Today,

there is a greater need to increase the "body I.Q." to decrease dysfunction and pain.

Science shows us another perspective that gives solidity to the theories presently being taught, either confirming or clarifying a myth. Keep an open mind to the idea that training a body is a continual and evolving process. In addition to the science, the experience of self-discovery based on smart movement mechanics is just as important for expanding our movement capabilities. Having been a student of the old school, and continuing to be a student of current information, shapes my perspective on the ever-evolving field of body training.

During my years of teaching, I have often been asked if I have a book of my practice. I would recommend the long list of books by others that I continue to reference and re-read before eventually deciding it was time for me to write my own, *Centered*, to provide an integrated source for my multidisciplinary approach to working with the body.

Integrative movement practitioner

Centered sets out to define a scope of practice – the integrative movement practitioner. The practice encompasses:

- an understanding of the body's movement potential

- analysis of the available movement in the body by identifying holding patterns caused by dysfunctional movement in the individual

- changing restrictions through techniques such as muscle energy, innovative Pilates set-ups on the apparatus and hands-on work

- developing a whole body approach for strengthening and brain imprinting exercises to reinforce a new way of moving

- self-practice and continued education.

Centered is a sequentially written account of the body, starting at the feet and progressing upward. Each chapter focuses specifically on a single area, such as the foot, and also examines its relation to the whole body. The most current and significant scientific findings are presented supporting movement theory. Movement theory defines how the body moves from the micro to the macro and in combination. Exercises (both Pilates and non-Pilates) are presented to support the whole body approach to training. I offer alternative techniques using physioballs, rollers, mats, and more for those who do not have access to Pilates equipment. Clear and concise cueing tips are written with each exercise section. Personal and client stories are shared to demonstrate the process chosen and the effectiveness of working in this method. There are "try it" moments throughout the book so you can experience and sense what is being described. Practitioner notes have more detail, interesting facts, sources for the various techniques described and helpful tips to take your practice to a new level.

Each chapter in *Centered* begins with a contemplative awareness to bring about your thoughts, emotions, and awareness, to help stimulate your intuition as you work. Working with the body is a process requiring a range of skills, critical thinking, and intuition. As an integrative movement practitioner following my methodology, being present and aware of oneself and the person or people working with you requires assessment of the whole person, not just their physicality. The mind and body work together and at times disassociation of the two can occur, which creates a disconnect with life events, emotions, and other energetic factors. This disconnect can cause physical discomfort or dysfunction.

Staying current in our field of physical training is important to deliver the best and most efficient way to teach people to move well. Eve Gentry, known for her eye to detail of movement, is quoted in her documentary as saying "are you a conveyor belt or a teacher?" I wish to recognize the field of integrative movement practitioners beyond the teacher, so I go further than Ms. Gentry and ask "Are you a teacher or a practitioner?" A practitioner, as defined by Merriam-Webster, is one who brings an art or science to full realization. My intention is to help develop a field of movement practitioners who work with people from science-based groundwork, with innovative manual and movement skills for structural and functional change of bodies. *Centered* is a guide and resource to develop your practice into a new level, a practitioner of movement. In addition to the book, continuous study through mentoring and hands-on guidance is recommended for receiving feedback, support for growth and exploration of questions, observations and challenges.

May *Centered* serve you well in your path, in whatever movement model or discipline you practice.

Part 1

Starting at the base:
sole to spine

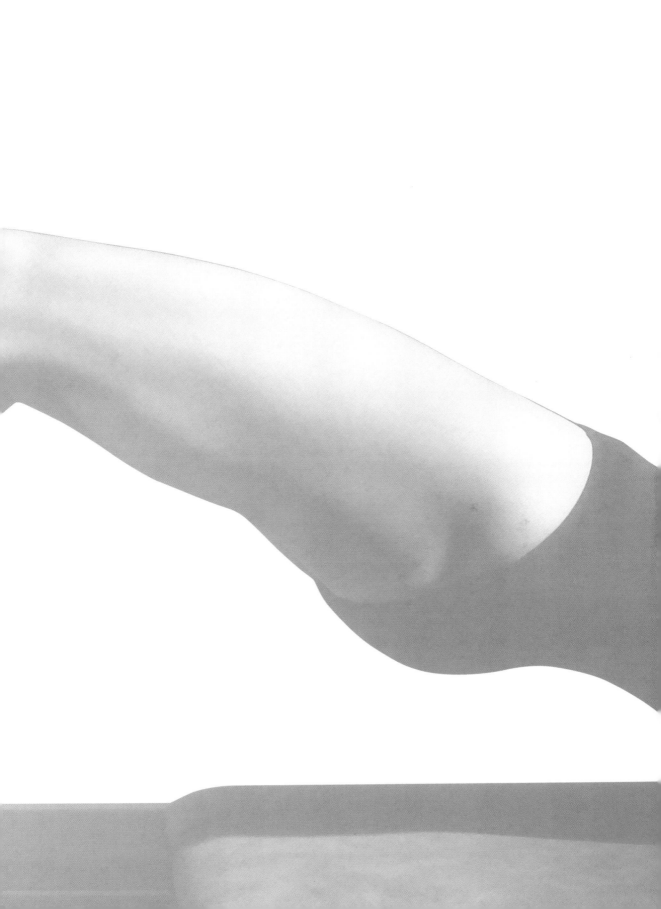

Our base

> "The sole of each foot functions like a retina that grows developmentally outward from the pelvis, central core structure of the body, down through the leg to spread the bottom surface of the foot in an ever-widening base of support is looking down and out into the ground."
>
> Irene Dowd, *Taking Root to Fly*

Contemplative awareness: grounded

Feet guide and center the body in so many ways. The soles of the feet touch the ground; functioning feet move the body along the ground; and the feet are a grounding source for the body. To "feel grounded" in oneself is to be standing on a solid foundation. The body experiences a sense of connection to the earth and the self when organized around its center of gravity. This sense begins at the feet, traveling through the many layers of the body and ultimately reaching the crown of the head.

The feet are one of the most highly innervated parts of the body, possessing sensory and fine motor capabilities, and can be both expressive and sensual. This means that the experience of human touch through the foot is as profound as being touched by the hand. Indeed, in some ways, the foot's gesture and touch are softer than those of a hand. Without healthy and functioning feet, physical movement is limited and overall health is compromised, while many aspects of the feet connect the body into its whole dynamic movement and sensory experience.

Despite the importance of the feet to our whole state of being, they are rarely given much attention unless there is discomfort or pain. When the feet are injured or not functioning properly, each movement becomes a source of constant irritation. Even when there is no pain, if the feet are not functioning well this may contribute to pain elsewhere in the body, for example pain in the knees, hips, lower spine, or neck. Working to improve the health of the feet improves the movement potential of the entire body, right

from the soles of the feet upward through the legs and all the way up the spine to the head. The agent of this powerful connection is an intricate body-wide system known as the fascia. Fascia forms a continuous tensile connective tissue throughout the body, covering and connecting every part, from the major organs to the tiniest nerve and fiber of each cell. It is considered both an organ in itself and a vehicle for communication to pass from the feet to the brain and back again.

Plantar fascia

The best known fascia of the foot is the plantar fascia. Injury to the plantar fascia (called plantar fasciitis) may cause significant pain and inability to bear weight on the feet. Plantar fascia pain is typically described as heel pain on the bottom of the foot. The role of the plantar fascia is to support the medial longitudinal arch (between the big toe and inner heel) of the foot along with the intrinsic muscles of the foot, specifically the flexor muscles (Wearing, 2012). Any reduction in strength of the intrinsic foot and lower leg muscles predisposes one to develop plantar fasciitis. The movement mechanics of the lower limb also play a vital factor in the stress placed on the arch. The condition of the foot myofascia and how the weight is distributed on the feet is easily seen in length differences of the legs, arms, and trunk.

Without the proper strength and movement mechanics, the plantar fascia bears an increased proportion of the body's weight, thus creating strain, tightness, and possible tearing of the fascial fibers. In addition to the local issue, the body's inability to sustain the spine in an elongated way adds to the amount of pressure on the arch of the foot.

Influence on overall alignment

The body moves as an integrated whole made up of multiple bodily systems interacting with each other. How movement is organized affects the body's structure and function. The feet have a direct influence on movement since anything that affects the highly innervated soles of the feet can find a swift response in the whole body – step on an unsuspected object, for example, and the whole body reacts.

Movement has a universal spiral pattern throughout the body, even within the feet.

> ### Try it!
>
> To sense the continuous line from the feet to the head, first stand up tall. Slowly begin to roll the head forward with the arms dangling and relaxed down, as if reaching to touch the toes. Continue to roll slowly and smoothly toward the floor, dripping down like a melting candle. Stop at the point where the hands are hanging over the knees.
>
> Notice whether one arm is hanging down longer than the other. If there is a difference in length (which there often is), take note of which arm appears shorter. Slowly roll back up to standing. It is common to have an apparent arm length discrepancy due to the tightness that spirals throughout the body (Fig. 1.1). Try the "Small Ball Foot Exercises" below and feel how the resilience returns and balances.

Small Ball Foot exercise

The ball series is excellent for realigning the foot through release of the fascia and muscles within the foot. It helps correct foot cramping and shortened toes, and restores the arches of the feet. Be mindful of the amount of pressure the foot applies to the ball. Harder is not better! The points may feel tender but should not make you jump. Remember to breathe evenly throughout the exercises. Practice the "Small Ball Foot" exercise three or four times a week to improve the mobility of the foot through stimulation

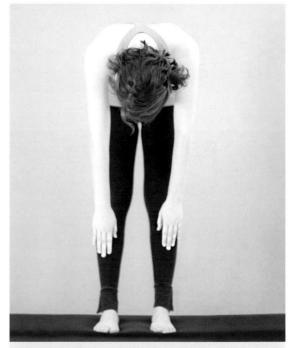

Figure 1.1
Try it! Noticing apparent arm length

of the muscles, fascia, and the micromovements of the bones of the foot.

Ball tool

Use a 1–2 inch (3–5 cm) soft rubber ball, such as the kind tied with a string to a paddle and ball toy. For more sensitive feet, use a larger softer ball. Do not use a hard ball – it may cause irritation or tear fibers, especially at the number 1 point. If inflammation is present, do not use the ball. Consult a professional for advice prior to using the ball technique.

Starting position

Begin on the side of the apparent shorter arm. Stand with the feet parallel, facing forward as if standing on cross-country skis. For people who have sensitive and highly dysfunctional feet, it is recommended to perform these movements seated in a chair as sitting lessens the pressure of the foot on the ball. Be sure at each point that the feet are parallel, so that the force moves through the body directly onto the ball (Fig. 1.2).

Point 1

This is at the heel (called the calcaneus).

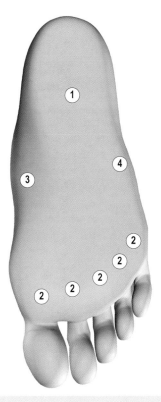

Figure 1.2
Foot map

- Place the rubber ball in the center at the front edge of the heel (Fig. 1.3); a tender point may be felt where the arch of the foot fascia meets at the heel.
- Step gently onto the point. Repeat 3 times.

Using the foot, roll the ball to the first toe ball for point 2 (Fig. 1.4).

Point 2

This point has five places for each toe along the knuckles of the toes (the metatarsal bones). From toe one through toe five, the toe knuckles or ball of the foot make an arch transversely.

- Start working point 2 with the small ball underneath the first toe ball.
- Step gently onto the ball, and the toe will automatically lengthen.

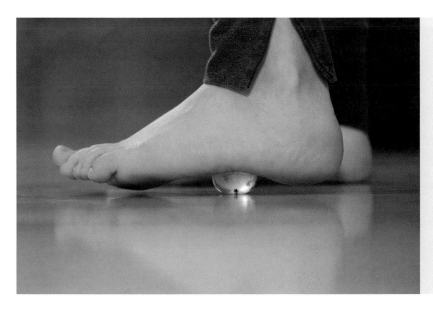

Figure 1.3
Point 1

- Imagine pressing on a cat's soft toe pad. As one presses on the pad, the cat's claw pops out; in the same way, as the ball presses on the metatarsal (cat's pad) the toe elongates (cat's claw).

- Step on the ball 3 times.

- Roll the ball to the second metatarsal and repeat for each toe.

- The arch of the toe balls is curved so be sure to roll the ball where the bone is located (the little toe is usually the shortest).

Points 3 and 4

Inner and outer arches are the next points.

- Roll the ball from the fifth metatarsal to the mid-point of the inner arch, which is point number 3 (Fig. 1.5). Feel a tender point at this position; to know if the ball is truly in the right place, feel the tender point and see the ball partially exposed at the inner arch.

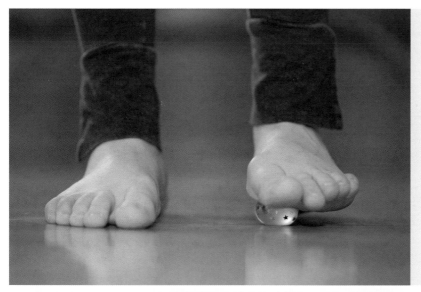

Figure 1.4
Point 2

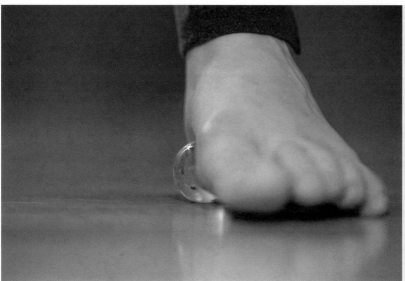

Figure 1.5
Point 3

- Press into the ball 3 times and roll the ball to the outer arch (point 4).

- The outer arch position is placed in a mid-point between the fifth toe and the heel (Fig. 1.6). Feel a tender point (it may be slightly closer to the heel).

- Place the ball at this point so that part of the ball is exposed on the outer edge.

- Press into this point 3 times.

Rolling the ball

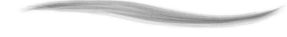

- Move the ball back to the first toe ball (the metatarsal).

- Roll the ball in an arcing way from the first toe ball along the transverse arch toward the fifth toe.

- Repeat the arcing of the ball several times; rolling across the arch by moving the forefoot (not the whole leg).

- Move the ball, rolling it to the first metatarsal again.

- Now roll it along the inner (medial) arch.

- Press into the ball as it moves from the first toe toward the heel.

- Reposition the ball without pressure back to the first metatarsal. Feel how the pressure is moving the fluids of the foot up the leg and toward the heart. There is no pressure repositioning the ball to avoid moving fluids toward the toes.

- Repeat the rolling with pressure toward the heel and no pressure back to repositioning the ball.

- Repeat this 3–5 times.

- Move the ball to the fifth metatarsal and roll the ball with pressure along the outer edge (lateral arch), with no pressure to reposition the ball.

- Repeat this 3–5 times.

- Randomly roll the ball throughout the entire bottom of the foot until you experience a warm feeling (the ball creates friction, increases circulation, and moves the fascia of the foot in multiple directions).

- Repeat for a count of 20 seconds – or longer if it feels good.

- Release the ball from underneath the foot and take a moment to stand.

- Feel the difference between the feet. The foot that was worked with the ball is more pliable and the ability to balance on that foot has improved.

After working on this foot, let us go back and see if it made a difference.

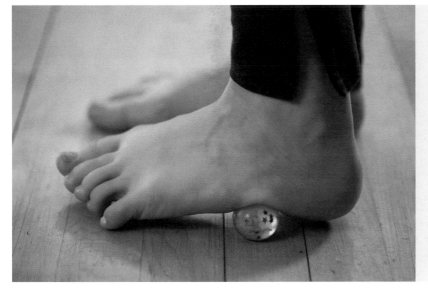

Figure 1.6
Point 4

Repeat the arm length test

(see Fig. 1.1)

Again, stand up tall and repeat the arm length test by slowly and smoothly rolling the spine from the head down toward the floor, arms dangling, and stop at the point when the hands are hanging over the knees. Notice if there is a change in the apparent arm length difference. If the arms are the same length, the work is finished. If the other arm is now shorter, repeat the exercise on the other foot, then retest the arm lengths. If the shorter arm is still shorter it most likely gained some length but not enough to match the other arm. This means that there is another force at play within the body that is preventing the lengthening. It may be addressed in the pelvic section (Ch. 3).

Working with the feet in Pilates

The feet play an essential role in the whole body philosophy of Pilates. In Pilates the feet are placed on the floor, on the bar, in the straps of the Reformer, or on the tower bar of the Cadillac. In mat work, the feet may be on the mat or hovering off the ground. Each of these surfaces (or the lack of a surface) enables the body to engage in different ways that train our connections between body and brain. It is the sensation of connecting feet to movement that engages body and mind. The soles of the feet are directly linked to L5/ S1 (the lower back) through the nerves that exit the lower spine and travel down the leg to the bottom of the foot. The bottom of the foot is continually sending data back to the spine so that the local stabilizers close to the spine turn on or off (Beach, 2010). When the feet are functional everything "clicks," feeling strong and connected.

A compromised foot structure may inhibit the training effect of an exercise, such as footwork on the Reformer, when dysfunctional feet are placed poorly on the foot bar. Or if one is performing a squat or standing pose and the weight is not distributed well on the foot, the body's effort hinders the movement intent. A clear understanding of the structure and function of the foot and its relation to the body's alignment is vital to achieving effective training.

Influences on foot function

The size of the trunk, the shape of the pelvis, and the distribution of weight all influence leg and foot function. Since the female pelvis is wider than the male pelvis, for example, a woman's thigh bones tend to be farther apart at the top, angling inward and drawing the knees closer so that the feet are in the best position to support the body. A man's narrower pelvis, in contrast, follows a straighter line from thigh bone to foot. The body weight may land more on the inside or outside of the foot.

Any rotation in the pelvis changes the length of the legs and subsequently the position of the feet (Fig. 1.7). When a rotation causes one leg to be longer than the other, the feet may adjust by dropping the arch, or by favoring the foot's lateral (outer) edge, causing imbalance in the stance and movement. Changing the alignment of the pelvis and spine with a focus on foot function will improve the body's overall potential for better function.

Foot dysfunction can be caused not only by the body's shape but also by external factors, such as improperly fitting shoes. "Shoes are sensory deprivation chambers," according to Dr. Phillip Beach (Beach, 2010). He encourages walking barefoot as much as possible, especially on a rock garden or other uneven surface to challenge the righting reflex of the body in response to the bottom of the foot.

Local view: feet and ankles

The foot plays an important role in taking a step, initiating a wave that spirals upward from the foot with each step. Let us start where the spiral begins, in the foot structure. Referring to the drawing of the bones of the foot (Fig. 1.8), notice the relationship of the small bones and how the articulating surfaces of the bones are able to move in coordination with one another. The movement relationship of the foot bones provides the flexible structure needed to meet and adjust to the ground's surface. When the foot adapts and moves the body toward the center, balance and stability are maintained. The body is propelled forward in a step, through the foot's rigid structure. At times, the foot takes the shape of a spring, twisting, as if wringing out a towel, then launching the body upward and forward in a single step. At other times, the foot spreads and widens to receive the ground's force. The feet need to be both a coiled structure (a more rigid form) and adaptable (a more mobile form) to perform the great variety of tasks required of them in standing, balancing, and moving.

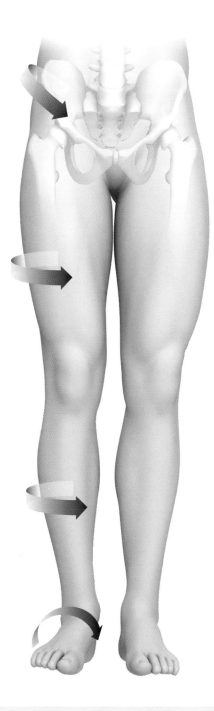

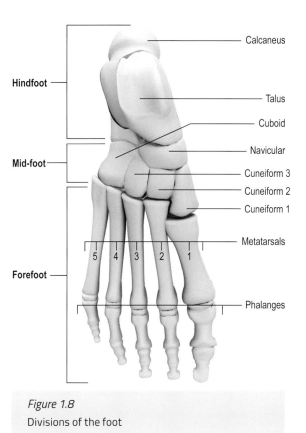

	Calcaneus
Hindfoot	Talus
	Cuboid
	Navicular
Mid-foot	Cuneiform 3
	Cuneiform 2
	Cuneiform 1
	Metatarsals
	5 4 3 2 1
Forefoot	Phalanges

Figure 1.8
Divisions of the foot

Rigid feet with high arches are held perpetually in a pointed position called plantarflexion. This position prevents the body from standing centered over the bones meant to support its weight. The overly flexible foot, on the other hand, has lost its arch support. It maintains a flexed ankle position called dorsiflexion, which inhibits the spring-like action required for healthy hip motion. Some investigation is usually required to identify the source of either type of position. In other words, finding the solution to the local issue – in this case in the foot – requires a global solution by looking to other areas of influence.

We should begin by understanding the foot itself.

The foot includes three areas: the rear foot, the mid-foot, and the forefoot (see Fig. 1.8). The rear foot is made up of the heel bone (calcaneus) and ankle bone (talus). The mid-foot comprises five small bones that together form a transverse arch. On the inner side of the arch is the navicular with three cuneiforms. In the

Figure 1.7
1. Right side of ilium anteromedial 2. Hip joint and femur internally rotated. 3. Tibia internally rotated. 4. Foot pronated

outer side of the arch, one bone is the cuboid. The pad of the foot, or forefoot, contains the five metatarsal bones and the toes (known as phalanges).

The rear foot: ankle

Where exactly is the true ankle joint? The motion of squatting, lunging, or simply pointing and flexing the foot, is happening in the rear foot, the ankle. The layperson may think of the ankle as being the knob visible on the outside of the foot; however, this is actually the end of a slim longer bone (the fibula) of the lower leg, where the lower leg, made up of the larger bone (the tibia) and the bone next to it (the fibula), meets the foot. The tibia hovers over the top of the talus while the sides of the talus are gently held by the lower part of the tibia and fibula. In a squat, the foot is more stable or fixed while the tibia slides over the top of the talus as the ankle bends. At the same time, the lowest part of the fibula (fibula malleolus) moves in a greater distance than the medial malleolus due to the length of the lateral top of the talus. The movement of the tibia and fibula is not purely a rolling on top of the talus but a helical motion, allowing for the talus to move back for a deeper bend at the ankle (Kessler and Hertling, 1983) (Fig. 1.9 A). To rise onto the ball of the foot, as in a heel rise or relevé, the tibia slides over the talus as the talus rolls forward. The medial and lateral malleolus (the lowest part of the tibia and fibula) travel a very small distance, becoming closer to the talus, acting as arms holding the bone in place (Fig. 1.9 B). The helical motions of the talus, along with the tibia and fibula, are also significant for healthy knee movement.

The "true" ankle joint (the subtalar joint) is centered between the calcaneus and talus, underneath the talus. The talus is a rounded bone shaped like a turtle's shell, with a neck and head, called the head of the talus – imagine the turtle looking out of its shell (Fig. 1.10). The talus is unusual in that no muscle is attached to this bone but it is surrounded by muscles that pass from the leg to the foot, making it look like a "caged bone" (Kapandji, 1987). Its movement is initiated by the other structures connected to it, the heel (calcaneus) and the crest of the turtle, the navicular. It is also supported by a strong group of ligaments.

The shape of the calcaneus and its offset position to the talus allow for movement around three axes. Three articulating surfaces of the calcaneus and talus, known

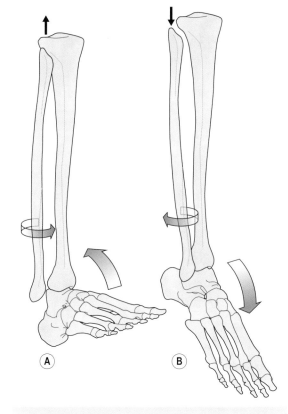

Figure 1.9
A Dorsiflexion
B Plantarflexion

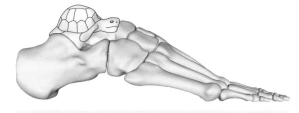

Figure 1.10
Talus turtle

as facets, glide and rotate as the foot moves. As described by Kapandji, the calcaneus is "pitching, turning, and rolling," and that initiates a spiral motion of the foot (Kapandji, 1987). Imagine the calcaneus as a catapult and the talus as the stone being launched. When the foot springs into action, in push-off to step forward or jump into the air, the calcaneus tosses the talus forward into a supinating, spiraling action. The arches roll out, the inner heel bone lifts, and the navicular moves toward the midline of the foot, away from the floor. The cuboid slides toward the toes and to midline. These small rotations of the mid-foot bones create a strong and stable structure, winding up the spring to facilitate movement.

 Spiral of foot
VIDEO LINK V 1.1

Conversely, when landing from a jump, or when placing the body weight onto the foot, the calcaneus rolls out from under the talus in a reverse spiral motion. The cuboid is pulled out, away from the midline and down toward the floor, drawing the navicular with it. The calcaneus moves back into the floor as the talus moves into a neutral position (Gorman, 1981).

Prone heel lowers

An ideal movement to observe this spiral motion is heel lowers and lifts while lying prone on the Reformer with the metatarsals on the bar. An alternative is standing on a ledge or slant board where the heels move below the level of a floor, then lifting up (in Pilates it is called "heel lowers"). To observe the movement clearly, view at the level of the ankle. The Reformer is the best set-up for observation at this level.

Prone heel lowers are an excellent way to observe the motion of the foot through the rear foot motion traveling up the leg to the pelvis. Additionally, it is a whole body exercise requiring trunk stabilization. In balance training, the focus is placed on hip strength, with too little attention being paid to the lower legs and feet. Adding heel lowers and lifts to a regular program is important for whole leg strength.

- Place the box in the long position with two red springs, or add one blue spring for more resistance. Use caution, though – if resistance is too strong, the body's efforts may make a clear reading (seeing) of the spiral difficult to achieve.

- The client lies prone with the metatarsals on the bar (Fig. 1.11).

- The body position is held as if standing in an upright position, with the whole body engaged in maintaining a good form.

- Simply lower the heels (dorsiflexion) and rise onto the balls of the feet (plantarflexion) (Fig. 1.12).

- Observe the inner heel moving toward the inner ankle bone (medial malleolus).

- Observe the line of the metatarsals along the bar:

  - Are all the metatarsals meeting the bar? If not, this is a sign of forefoot varus or valgus.

  - Are the bones centered through the second metatarsal with solid contact of the first and fifth metatarsals with the bar?

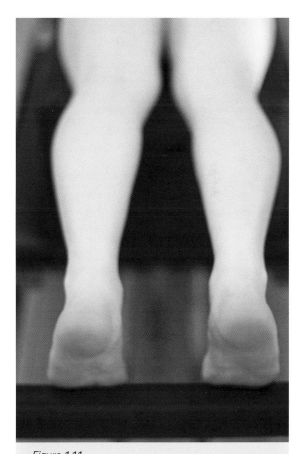

Figure 1.11
Prone heel lowers: start position

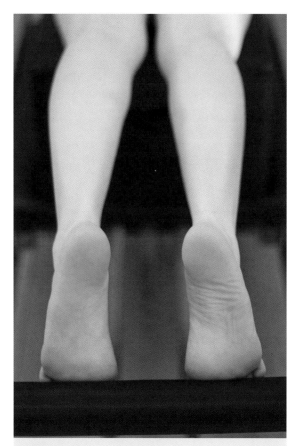

Figure 1.12
Prone heel raise

- Observe the mid-foot bones:

  - If the bones of the mid-foot move beyond the first metatarsal medially, the mid-foot is moving more than the calcaneal spiral.

Practitioner note

Observe the metatarsal placement as the foot spirals into a heel lift. The mid-foot may be hypermobile due to the lack of micromovement of the subtalar joint. Hold the mid-foot bones to draw them closer to one another then observe how the heel spirals (or not). Then perform the calcaneal spiral technique below and repeat the prone heel lowers to observe the change in the contact positioning of the metatarsals. Also, observe the whole leg as the heel rises. The spiral may be happening through an external rotation of the tibia at the knee.

Wash Rag Foot: spiral motion

Although the athletic footwear industry has taught the public to think of pronation as unhealthy, in fact the feet move continually through a twisting (higher arch) and untwisting (lower arch) motion. Even those with apparent flatter feet while standing may move well in the spiral. More important than the foot's appearance is the way in which the foot moves. The potential dysfunction of a flat foot is an arch that is too flexible and fails to twist, continually pulling the whole leg inward (see Fig. 1.7) and over time potentially straining the knee or hip. When the calcaneus and talus do not pitch, turn or roll, this inhibits the ability to spring or not spring. Then the foot compensates by moving too much in the mid-foot, collapsing the inner arch and possibly causing foot pain. Poor ankle positioning and lack of spiral motion may place stress on structures above, including the lower back.

The calcaneus lies in the sagittal plane while the forefoot is in the transverse plane, and this combination produces the spiral motion. It is a perfect example of function following form. The twisting occurs around a central line of the foot at the third toe (to help visualize the movement of the foot's twist, imagine a wash rag as it is wrung out). The rear of the foot will move up toward the inner ankle bone (medial malleolus) while the top of the toes moves down. Both ends move toward one another when viewing the bottom of the foot. In unwinding the spiral, the opposing ends move away from one another.

Try it!
Self-mobilization of the foot

Sit down, then cross one leg over the thigh to be able to hold the foot with both hands. If the right foot is first, cup the heel with the left hand and place the right palm over the base of the toes, primarily near the first toe (Fig. 1.13). Begin wringing the foot. Turn the heel up and in and, at the same time, the toes down and in (Fig. 1.14). Repeat many times until the whole foot feels the suppleness of the twist.

Calcaneal spiral on Cadillac

 Calcaneal spiral on Cadillac
VIDEO LINK V 1.2

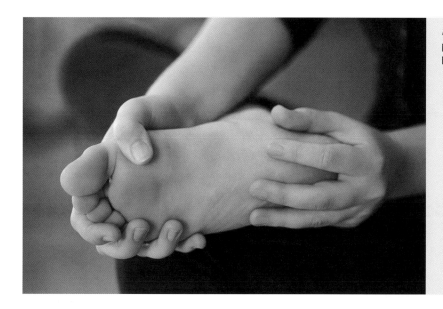

Figure 1.13
Hand placement for Wash
Rag Foot exercise

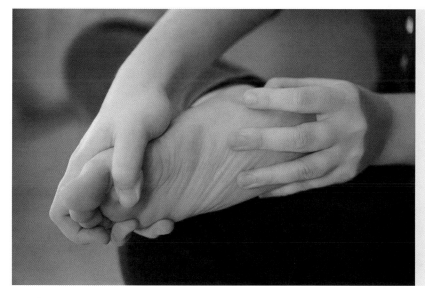

Figure 1.14
Wringing action

A simple movement technique called the "Calca-neal Spiral," assisted by an experienced Pilates or movement/bodywork practitioner, unlocks the heel and spiral of the lower limb. This movement rotates the hip inward and outward, creating a motion that moves down the leg and through the talus, unlock-ing the calcaneus. This technique is performed on the Pilates apparatus called the Cadillac. This specialized movement technique releases the immobility of the true ankle joint (subtalar joint), the articulation of the talus and calcaneus. The release of the subtalar joint will assist in restoring knee and hip function.

Apparatus set-up on the Pilates Cadillac

Set the tower bar with the safety strap and load the bar from the bottom with one blue spring (Fig. 1.15). The bottom-loaded bar is providing a force through all the joints from the foot into the hip. Test the leg position by holding the bar and gently pull down on the bar to move the force through the leg (Fig. 1.16). See and feel the movement of the force vector from the bar as it passes through the leg joints. It is important that the hip respond to the movement and weight of the bar. If the transfer of force is stopping at the knee, then the

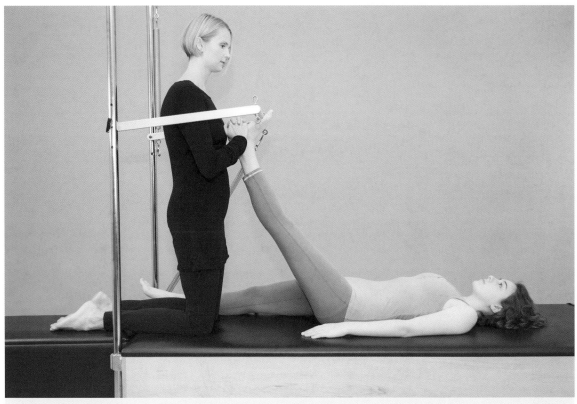

Figure 1.15
Cadillac set-up for calcaneal spiral

client needs to move closer to or further away from the bar. Try a few positions until the force of the bar moves into the posterior hip.

- The client lies supine (on the back) with the feet toward the push-through bar.

- Place the toe balls (the metatarsals) of the ankle to be worked on the bar.

- Observe the alignment of the center of the foot, between the second and third metatarsal, lining up with the center of the knee, and the center of the hip joint (acetabulum).

- The knee is fully extended and there is approximately 60° of hip flexion.

- The other leg is resting on the table fully extended.

- Release at the ankle so that the ball of the foot on the bar is not pressing the bar up.

- The practitioner kneels at the bar end facing the client to hold the heel (see Fig. 1.15).

- The grip is cupping the calcaneus to stabilize the foot by interlacing the fingers and firmly holding with the base of both palms.

- As the client moves the hip in (Fig. 1.17) and out (Fig. 1.18), the pressure in the hand changes to resist any movement of the calcaneus; if the client presses beyond the interbarrier range of the hip, then it is felt in the hands with a hard increased pressure with no movement.

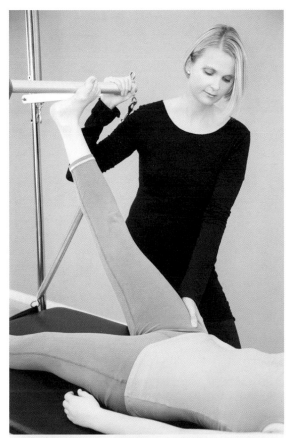

Figure 1.16
Testing the starting position using the bar

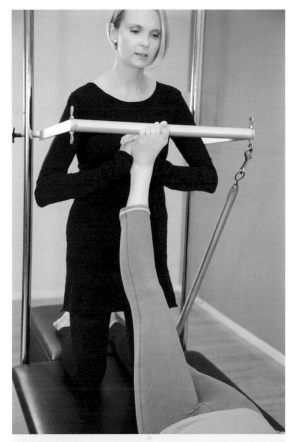

Figure 1.17
Spiraling leg turning inward

Note

The interbarrier zone is prior to the barrier of a person's available movement. The barrier may be an anatomical barrier or a physiological barrier. With your hands, feel how the body moves into a direction; pause before you reach the end of the joint or tissue range (the barrier) and work from this place. Many people push pass the barrier, producing over-movement, which then sends the effort into a different direction of the body than the one needed to achieve the precision of being at the place necessary for effective change in the tissue.

Practitioner note

The emphasis of the internal and external motion is seeing the whole leg moving from the hip through the lower leg. Be attentive to the end range of motion. Coach the person to feel the end of hip joint movement and reverse the direction of the rotation slightly before coming to the end, moving in an interbarrier range. There is no over-movement. The femur is spiraling in and out and that translates through the tibia on the talus and talus with the calcaneus. Repeat several times until ease is present in the motion of the whole leg.

moment of gait, the soleus and gastrocnemius (triceps surae) maximally contract as the back leg extends and this is combined with the all-important adduction and supination of the bottom of the foot, the spiral.

Training the soleus within the timing of the calcaneus spiral is important to increase the capability of pressing off the foot in movements such as walking, jumping or climbing. It is an integral part of the propulsive force of gait.

Soleus release on the Wunda Chair

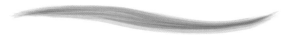

- Set the Wunda Chair with one light to medium spring (the resistance needs to be light enough to allow for the heel to spiral without engaging global muscles such as the quadriceps but strong enough to challenge the soleus) (Fig. 1.19).

- Have Biotone ® or massage cream available for use.

- Sit on the floor behind the client to access the posterior lower leg.

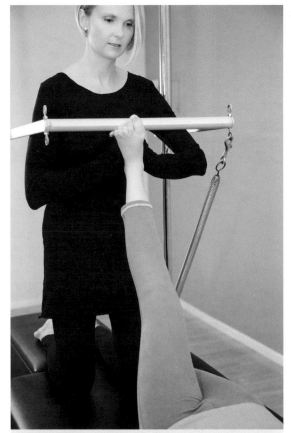

Figure 1.18
Spiraling leg turning outward

Soleus adds to the spiral

The soleus muscle arises from a deep fascial compartment underneath the gastrocnemius on the back (posterior) of the tibia, fibula and the fibrous band between the two bones. The soleus joins the gastrocnemius in a common tendon, the Achilles tendon. The tendon attaches to the posterior aspect of the calcaneus and it continues into the fibrous boundary of the fat pad, called a septa and plantar aponeurosis (Stecco and Stecco, 2012). There is mixed evidence concerning the fibers connecting to the plantar fascia, and it is thought that this is perhaps age-related. The fibers of the soleus are spiral in nature, which produces the elastic quality. The triceps surae (gastrocnemius and soleus) directly acts on the ankle joint through the subtalar joint (Kapandji, 1987). In the push-off

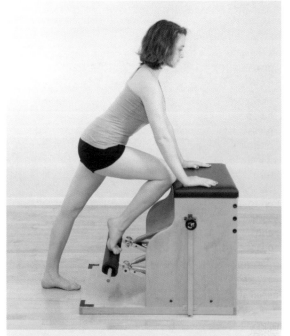

Figure 1.19
Starting position for soleus release on Wunda Chair

- The client stands in front of the chair in good form.

- Place a pad on top of the chair to rest the knee on.

- Rest the knee on the pad and place the ball of the foot on the bar.

- Form is important to align the force in the spiral direction.

- Starting at the metatarsal transverse arch, observe the toe balls in contact without an angle deviation (see forefoot, below); propping of the metatarsal transverse arch may be necessary for optimal contact.

- The front of the ankle is relaxed in the client's available dorsiflexion.

- The femur is aligned on center of hip joint; observe the line of the knee to the hip.

- The pelvis is level.

- The spine is elongated, including the head (clients like to look down to see the movement).

- The client presses the foot bar down with the ball of the foot (plantarflexion).

- The client resists the bar on the return.

- Repeat 15–20 times.

> **Practitioner note**
>
> At the start of the exercise the Achilles tendon should be straight vertically. If it is bowed then change the pressure of the foot on the bar and use a lighter spring; most likely the ankle is not gliding well in dorsiflexion; it will change with the fascial stroke. Observe the spiral of the heel as the ankle plantarflexes, pressing the bar down, and the medial side of the calcaneus moves up toward the medial malleolus; on the dorsiflexion, as the bar returns, the medial side should lengthen and return to a straight Achilles tendon; be sure quadriceps are not assisting movement.

Fascial stroke of soleus on Wunda Chair

Soleus fascial stroke
VIDEO LINK V 1.3

Begin on the concave side of the Achilles tendon. Cue the movement so that the spiral movement is apparent and where the weight is in contact on the metatarsal arch. Use a light coating of massage oil on finger pads and a small amount on the client's skin.

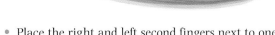

- Place the right and left second fingers next to one another, creating contact of all the finger pads with the fascia of the soleus.

- Starting at the medial/superior aspect of the Achilles tendon (Fig. 1.20), stroke superiorly/laterally as the client slowly dorsiflexes.

- Maintain contact with the tissue and move with the gliding of the movement.

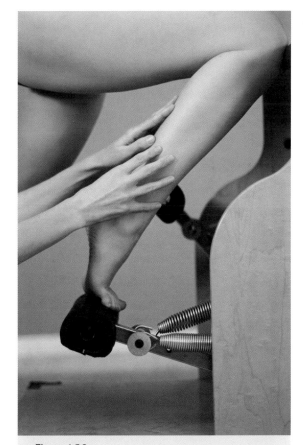
Figure 1.20
Fascial stroke

- Follow the glide to the top of the soleus.

- Repeat, changing the line of stroke slightly laterally.

Seated soleus on tower bar and box

Set the Cadillac push-through bar with a red or medium bottom-loaded spring and safety strap. Place the Reformer box on top of the table in the long position near the bar so that a client sits on the box with the tower bar placed on top of the knee. When seated, be sure the tibia is in a vertical orientation to the table with the ankle in neutral position, and the arches neither in nor out. Using a pad or towel between the bar and the thigh may be more comfortable for some people (Fig. 1.21).

- Press the foot into plantarflexion with the heel spiral, which lifts the bar (Fig. 1.22).

- The weight is on the first metatarsal and phalange of the big toe through the transverse arch with light contact of the fifth metatarsal.

- Slowly lower the heel, unspiraling the heel into dorsiflexion.

- Repeat 15–20 times or until fatigue is apparent.

Soleus bend and stretch

Set the Cadillac push-through bar with a blue or light-to-medium bottom-loaded spring with safety strap (Fig. 1.23).

- Lie under the bar supine (on back) with the head at the end of the table.

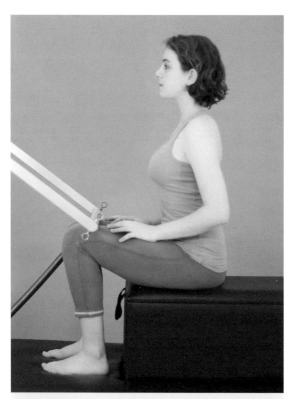

Figure 1.21
Starting position for seated soleus on tower bar and box

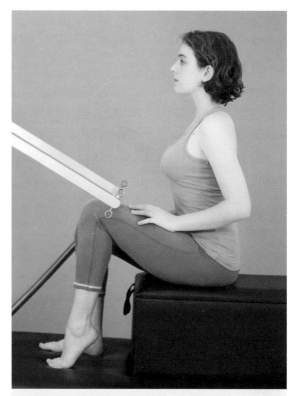

Figure 1.22
Raising the heel

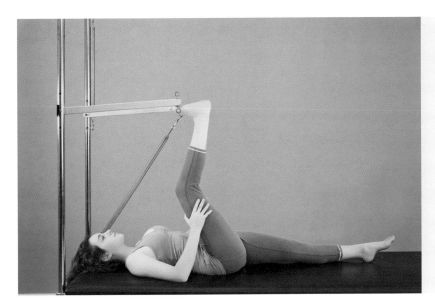

Figure 1.23
Starting position for soleus bend and stretch on Cadillac

- Place the metatarsals on the bar and pressing the bar up, extend the leg to approximately 110° hip flexion.

- The hamstrings should not be overpressured during the stretch; adjust the body position further under the bar, using a headrest if needed, to find a comfortable position.

- The sacrum is anchored along with the lowest posterior ribs.

- The pelvis is level.

- Hold the knee with the hands to stabilize the femur.

- Isolate to plantarflex the ankle and slowly dorsiflex the ankle, resisting the bar, thus creating an eccentric contraction of the soleus (Fig. 1.24).

Practitioner note

This position is not for all bodies and some clients may find that it is at the extreme end of their range. Be mindful and observant of any overpressure of the hip and back. It is very important that the starting position is within the range of the person. When the ankle bends into dorsiflexion the femur and pelvis do not change position. For most people, the seated soleus on the Cadillac is the better choice.

Mid-foot

The mid-foot is the region of the foot that tends to become mobile when the calcaneal spiral is restricted. It comprises a series of small bones that adapt to the movement of the ankle joint and toes. These include: the navicular, three smaller bones (the cuneiforms) articulating with the first three metatarsals, and the cuboid bone articulating with the fourth and fifth metatarsals. All of these bones either lock into place when the foot springs into a higher arch or move freely, lowering the arch closer to the ground. This movement varies while walking, influenced by the motion of the ankle joints (subtalar joints) and how the body weight is transferred. During gait, the weight is transferred from the outer heel point through the foot toward the first toe (Fig. 1.25). This motion through the foot establishes a specific sequencing of whole body dynamic recruitment for movement.

Standing well on our feet supports our body's weight without causing excess stress to the joints above and improves our balance. The foot has an interesting arrangement to support the weight and at the same time provide a template for movement. A line of separation exists between the third and fourth metatarsal bones (Fig. 1.26). Looking up the chain of bones, the inner half of the foot aligns with the tibia clearly through the talus side. The outer side aligns the fibula with the calcaneus and cuboid. The body's weight is

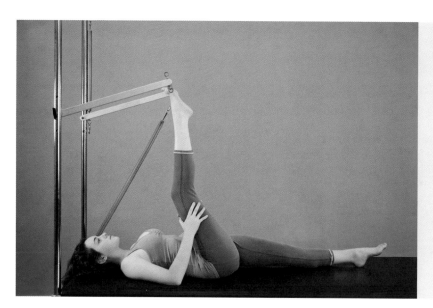

Figure 1.24
Raising the heel

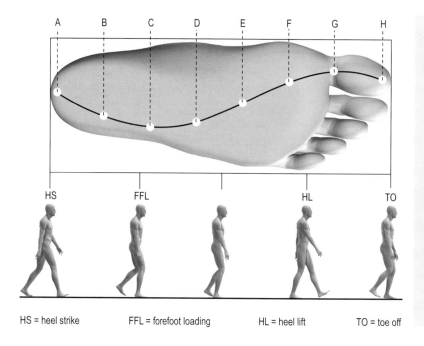

Figure 1.25
Weight points on the bottom of the foot during the gait cycle

HS = heel strike   FFL = forefoot loading   HL = heel lift   TO = toe off

supported through the pelvis onto the femurs, on top of tibias that sit directly on top of the tali (plural of *talus*). This becomes a challenge for the inner arch. The lateral side of the lower leg is the thin fibula, clearly not a weight-bearing bone. The lateral part of the foot meets the ground and plays a role in transferring the weight moving through the foot. In standing, in order to support the weight of the body, weight is distributed between the outer arch where the heel meets the cuboid and the base of the big toe.

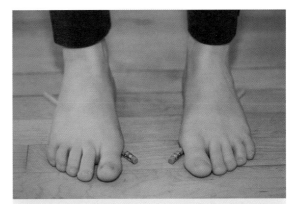

Figure 1.27
"Standing on Pencils" for a felt sense of balanced standing

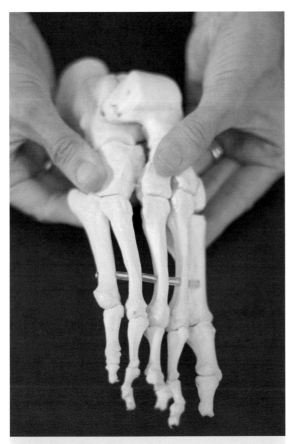

Figure 1.26
Division of the bones of the foot

Practitioner note

To find the cuboid bone, lift all the toes up with the metatarsals on the ground. Look on the outer edge of the foot, where you will see a small muscle pop up (Fig. 1.28). It looks like an oyster. The cuboid bone sits underneath this muscle (called the extensor digitorum brevis and extensor hallucis brevis). Ideally, standing on the bones that meet the ground then distributing the body weight through the foot gives a grounded sense of balance.

Forefoot

The forefoot consists of five long bones that make up the pad of the foot, called the metatarsals, and the phalanges (see Fig. 1.8). The transverse row of metatarsals is important for allowing the talus to be held in a more neutral position while standing. When the talus is in a neutral position, all the bones of the feet are held together in relationship to one another by gravity rather than by tension in the ligaments. The neutral talus can be seen when the first toe ball (metatarsophalangeal, or MP, joint) is planted on the ground with the inner arch lifted. In this position, the tendons at the front of the ankle joint are not tensed. In a healthy foot, this position is stable and can be maintained without fatigue for long periods of time.

Over time, inefficient weight bearing, an ankle out of balance (talus not sitting properly) and little or no

Try it!
Standing on Pencils

"Standing on Pencils" is a felt sense exercise to help feel how to distribute the weight in standing. Place one pencil under each foot. The pencil will run on a diagonal, starting with one end of the pencil under the base of the big toe and the other where the heel meets the cuboid (Fig. 1.27). Stand tall, look straight ahead (not at the feet) and distribute the weight evenly over the pencils. Play with the position: first stand back on the heels more and feel where the body has to work to balance. Then reposition the weight to be evenly distributed over the pencils. Notice now how the core naturally supports. Standing well will increase the body's natural ability to engage the core.

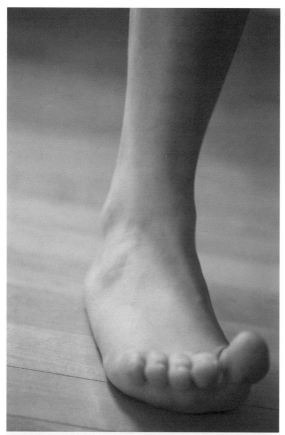

Figure 1.28
Extensor hallucis brevis, extensor digitorum brevis for identification of cuboid bone

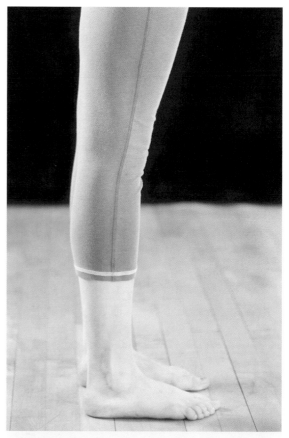

Figure 1.29
Standing in neutral talus

spiraling of the foot cause a compensated foot. The forefoot potentially becomes malformed (for example, a bunion may develop). Feeling the whole lower limb over a balanced foot (dynamic neutral talus position) is important to achieve better feet.

Feeling dynamic neutral subtalar joint (ankle)

A simple exercise taught by Naja Cori, an original teacher of Joseph Pilates, called "Arches In and Arches Out," mobilizes this area and teaches how to feel where the congruent placement of the talus sits on the calcaneus.

Try it!
Arches In and Arches Out

Stand with the ankles in a neutral position and the legs straight (Fig. 1.29). Roll the arches out and in. Feel the rocking and rolling of the ankle. Using the images of the bones or arches, visualize and feel the arches moving up and down. Allow the movement to flow up the body naturally, feeling how the feet create motion up the legs, pelvis, and spine (Figs 1.30 and 1.31). Find the best position, in the middle of arches in or out, and think "Standing on Pencils."

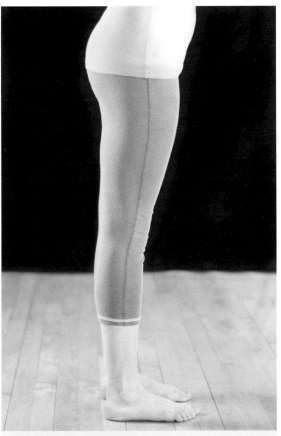

Figure 1.30
Standing in "Arches In"

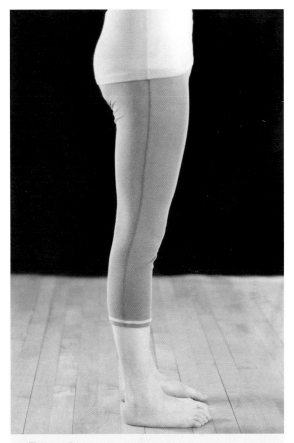

Figure 1.31
Standing in "Arches Out"

> **Note**
>
> Naja Cori, also known as Dolores Cori, was chosen by Mr. Pilates to open the new studio in Bendel's department store in New York City in 1967. She continued teaching the Pilates Method in the city at her own studio until her death in 2009.

In the arches in and out movements, a tensile pull can be felt from the foot upward into the pelvis and spine. During the movement, feel when the arches are rotated inward (Arches In) (see Fig. 1.30). The pelvis is pulled toward the floor in an anterior tilt. In the Arches Out position, the pelvis is pulled back in a posterior tilt, tucking the pelvis (see Fig. 1.31). The pelvis position is vital to the health of the knees, hips, and spine. A part of restoring a functional pelvic motion includes working with the feet. Standing in neither Arches In nor Arches Out creates a better position of the talus.

 Spiral of foot
VIDEO LINK V 1.1

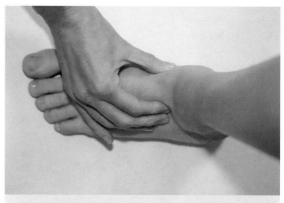

Figure 1.33
Moving talus side to side, inward direction

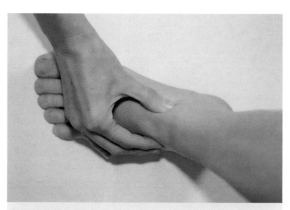

Figure 1.34
Moving talus side to side, outward direction

Fixed forefoot position

In any movement where the forefoot is placed as a fixed point, as in the small "v" or prehensile positions on the Reformer, compensation of the forefoot changes the talus out of neutral. The talus will either drop toward the inner arch (Arches In) or drop outward (Arches Out). In either position, the talus has lost its neutral alignment, creating a dysfunctional movement pattern where the functional recruitment of the legs will not be accessible, minimizing the intended strengthening. Be sure to maintain the dynamic neutral

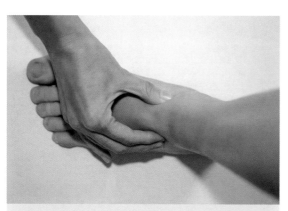

Figure 1.32
Hand placement for hands-on talus

talus when the forefoot is placed on a bar or in a loop (Figs 1.35–1.38).

The forefoot is either at the beginning or at the tail end of the lower limb spiral, depending on your view. In either perspective, as the heel twists and untwists in a fixed forefoot position, the forefoot responds by transferring weight along the transverse arch in an effort to keep the big toe ball and the little toe ball in contact with the floor in a movement. In losing one's balance, the foot usually loses the contact of the big toe with the floor. In lifting and lowering the heels, if the forefoot cannot maintain contact, the mid-foot will take up the slack. This is one cause of exaggerated pronation or supination. To compensate, the talus

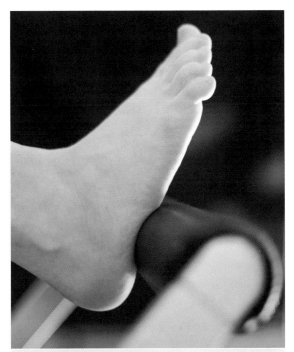

Figure 1.35
Neutral position of feet on Reformer foot bar

is pulled out of its neutral position, either toward or away from the floor (Figs 1.39 and 1.40).

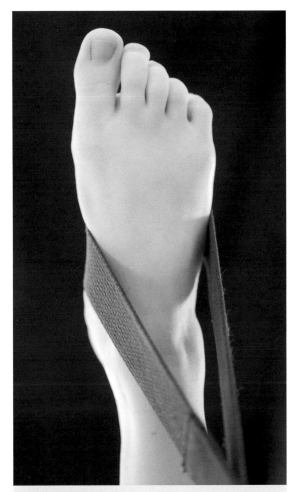

Figure 1.36
Foot in loop neutral position

> **Try it!**
>
> Kneel on the floor, tucking the toes under and with the ankles flexed (Fig. 1.41). Look at the line of the toe balls on the floor, heels straight up, and see if the pelvis can sit on the heels. This is normal positioning of the forefoot and whole leg. (It may hurt!) Slowly introduce this position to the feet. It is used in Pilates kneeling work on the Reformer. Introduce the foot position by sitting in the kneeling squat with the toes tucked under.

Props for forefoot varus and valgus

Any time the forefoot is in contact with a surface, such as the foot bar on the Reformer or even the floor, in a more balanced foot, the talus is in neutral with the transverse arch level (Fig. 1.42). When the forefoot is compensated use a prop to improve the position of the talus and observe how the movement of the ankle is improved. Placing a small soft prop such as a foam cat toy ball or a folded cloth under the big toe ball for the varus forefoot, or little toe ball for valgus forefoot, will assist in maintaining the talus in neutral position (Figs 1.43 and 1.44). Use the props as a temporary measure until the foot has adapted and changed form through the foot practice in this book.

Improving the health of the feet involves a combination of looking at the forefoot balance, the talus and calcaneus motion, and the whole body alignment to identify the possible link to unlocking the recurring

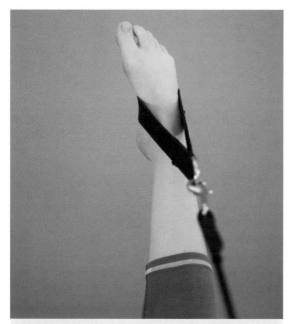

Figure 1.37
Foot in loop supinated/inverted

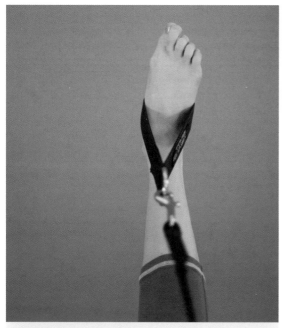

Figure 1.38
Foot in loop everted

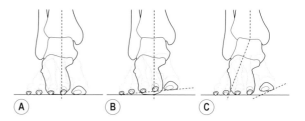

Figure 1.39
A Neutral talus and forefoot meeting ground equally
B Neutral talus with forefoot varus
C Compensation of forefoot, talus and navicular falls medially

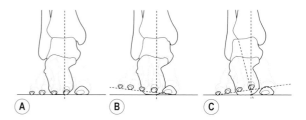

Figure 1.40
A Neutral talus and forefoot meeting ground equally
B Neutral talus with forefoot valgus.
C Compensation of forefoot, talus and navicular falls laterally

faulty movement. Movement patterns are embedded in our brain and it takes consistent movement practices to transform the transverse arch, spiraling of the whole lower limb, and pelvis–leg motion. Practice the following series of foot exercises daily. If the feet are extremely tight and weak, start with the "Doming" and "Inchworm" exercises and gradually add the other movements. If the foot cramps, repeat the "Small Ball Foot" exercises from earlier in this chapter. For overly flexible feet, begin with the foot strengthening work.

Exercises for the feet

Doming

The dome of the foot may become immobile and weak. The dome of the foot is made up of a vaulted

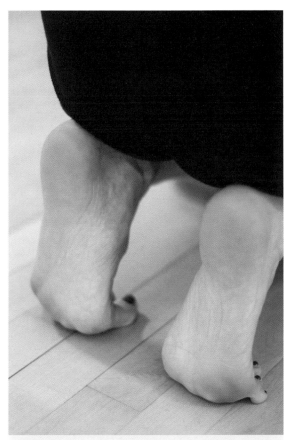

Figure 1.41
Alignment of the balls of the feet in a kneeling
sitting position

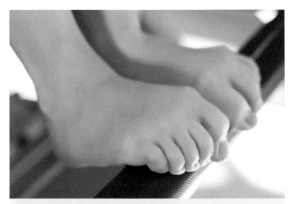

Figure 1.42
Neutral talus in prehensile position

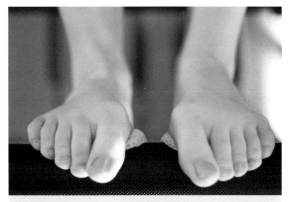

Figure 1.43
Props for forefoot compensation: varus forefoot

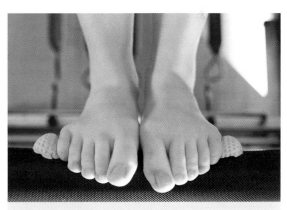

Figure 1.44
Props for forefoot compensation: valgus forefoot

triangular shape that runs underneath the foot with
a tri-bone contact: the center of the heel, the first toe
ball joint and the fifth toe ball. The vault looks like a
backpacking tent in its connections from the points
upward creating a dome shape.

To begin, feel for the doming action, the lifting of the
bottom (the plantar surface) of the foot. A seated position is recommended although it can also be practiced
standing. No shoes and socks are to be worn. Sit with
an elongated spine and good foot contact on the floor.
The lower leg bone (the tibia) is vertical and perpendicular to the floor.

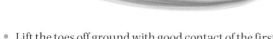

- Lift the toes off ground with good contact of the first toe ball (metatarsophalangeal, or MP, joint) and fifth toe ball on the floor (Fig. 1.45).

- Distribute the weight through the pad of the foot with more weight on the first MP joint and less on the fifth.

- Maintain this position of contact and visualize making a tent or dome underneath the foot.

- Keep a nice high dome and simply lower the tips of the toes to the floor without disturbing the weight distribution of the foot (Fig. 1.46).

- Practice several times.

Inchworm

- Lift the dome like a parachute inflating (Fig. 1.47).

- Toes are in contact with the floor, anchoring the first and fifth toe balls without tensing or curling the toes.

- Slide the heel toward the metatarsals without moving the toes, which shortens the plantar vault and increases the height of the dome – this is a small movement, like "scooching" the heel forward.

- Then allow the toes to move away from the heel and relax the arch (Fig. 1.48).

- Repeat the motion of expanding the arch and inching the heel forward; the foot moves forward as an inchworm moves (Fig. 1.49).

- Reverse the inchworm by anchoring the heel position first and inch the toes toward the heel until the tibia returns to the vertical starting position.

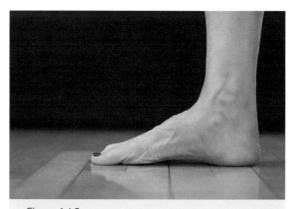

Figure 1.46
Dome of foot with the toes down

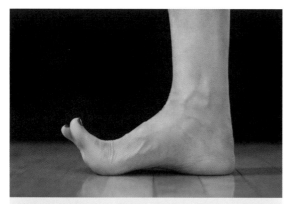

Figure 1.45
Dome of foot with the toes up

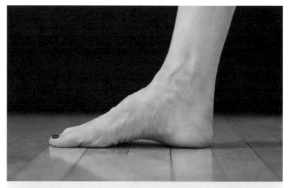

Figure 1.47
Inchworm: starting with doming and moving heel toward toes

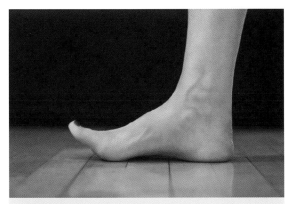

Figure 1.48
Inchworm: releasing toes to move foot forward

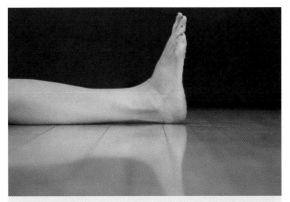

Figure 1.50
Forward Toe Waves: dorsiflexion

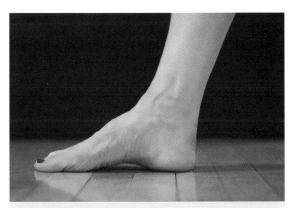

Figure 1.49
Inchworm: moving forward

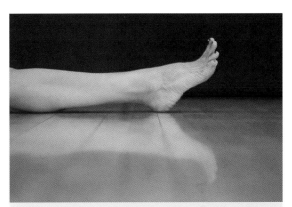

Figure 1.51
Forward Toe Waves: pressing through balls of the feet

Toe Waves

This movement articulates the whole foot, creating a wave motion of plantar/dorsiflexion with toe flexion and extension. It is performed in a forward direction (the forward wave), and a backward direction (the backward wave), and it challenges the brain's coordination and motor control.

Forward Wave

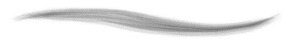

- Sit with the legs straight in front and the ankles flexed (dorsiflexion position) (Fig. 1.50).

- The forward wave starts moving into plantarflexion by pressing into the balls of the foot with the toes pulled back (extended) (Fig. 1.51).

- Complete the movement into a pointed foot, toes pointing toward the floor (Fig. 1.52).

- From the pointed foot, keep the toes pointed downward and dome the transverse arch (top of the toe knuckles rise up) as if picking something up with the toes (Fig. 1.53).

- Uncurl the toes into dorsiflexion position.

- Practice and repeat the forward wave several times to imprint the coordinated movement.

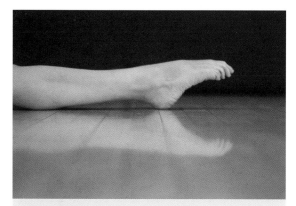

Figure 1.52
Forward Toe Waves: pointed position

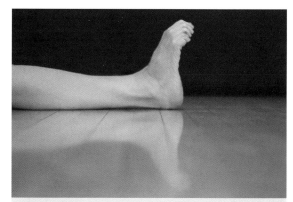

Figure 1.54
Beginning of curling toes down for Reverse Wave

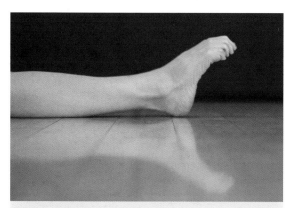

Figure 1.53
Toe Waves: starting with transverse arch curling and reversing toe waves moving curled toes into plantarflexion

Reverse Wave

- Starts in dorsiflexion (see Fig. 1.50).

- From the tips of the toes, curl the toes first into the pointed foot (Fig. 1.54).

- Move the foot into a full pointed foot (see Fig. 1.52).

- Uncurl the toes first in the pointed position (see Fig. 1.51), toes pull back.

- Leading with the tips of the toes, complete the movement into a dorsiflexed position.

- Practice and repeat the reverse wave several times to imprint the coordinated movement.

Foot challenge

- Move the feet, alternating the forward wave followed by the reverse wave.

- Try moving only the right foot in forward wave while the left foot performs the reverse wave.

- Reverse the foot action, left forward, right backward (Figs 1.55 and 1.56).

Exercises for strengthening the arch and lower extremities: toe extensors and flexors

Feet are not that different from hands. The embryological origins of the feet are in the same area of the embryo as the hands, namely the apical ectodermal ridge from the Wolffian ridge (Schoenwolf et al., 2009). It is from this ridge that the upper and lower limbs and the sense organs originated. This highly innervated sensory beginning is present in the feet. Chapters 2 and 6 discuss the growth pattern and origins of the limb buds as they pertain to whole leg movement.

The toes are more web-like than our fingers but move individually, as the fingers do. The possibilities for movement of the foot are similar to those of the hand and great dexterity has been achieved by many people

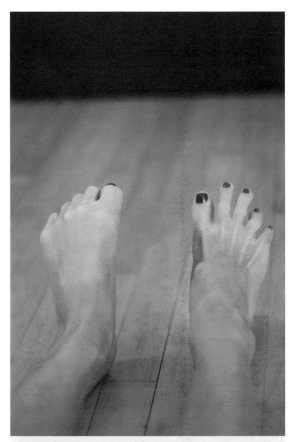

Figure 1.55
Alternating Toe Waves: top view

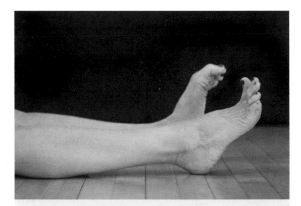

Figure 1.56
Alternating Toe Waves: side view

(see, for example, the movie *My Left Foot* in which Daniel Day-Lewis plays the artist Christy Brown, who despite his cerebral palsy, painted professionally using only his left foot). There are many people in the world with the talent of creating with their feet rather than their hands, and the artistic work thus created can be stunning.

Foot coordination comes from coordinated intrinsic tissues (muscles, fascia, ligaments, nerves) that are highly linked with the motor sensory part of the brain. Moving the individual toes up and down works the flexor and extensor muscles of the toes, which are located on the lower leg and locally within the foot. The muscles that originate on the lower limb have a spiral orientation as the muscles transition into the foot. The synergistic work of these muscles along with the intrinsic muscles of the foot produces the high dexterity potential in the foot.

Synergistic connections of lower leg and foot

The groups of synergistic muscles sharing the same nerve supply are bundled into fascial compartments. The lower leg has four compartments encircling the bone: anterior, lateral, superficial posterior, and deep posterior. Each of the compartments is separated by intermuscular septa fascia. In most places the muscles are free to glide and contract deep into the fascia. Near the joints, such as the ankle, the deep fascia is thickened and called a retinaculum. The intermuscular septa are fascially linked into the musculature of the leg. This continuous relationship of the fascia and muscle spirals from the foot to as far away as the head is movement form expressed in the tissue.

Posterior compartment of lower leg

- The superficial posterior compartment is made up of the gastrocnemius, soleus and plantaris muscles that plantarflex the ankle while acting on the knee and heel of the foot. When pushing off the foot during gait, the posterior compartment initiates the chain of work from the foot through the extension of the hip, activating the posterior hip across the pelvis upward to spinal extensors.

- The deep posterior compartment contains posterior tibialis, flexor hallucis longus, flexor digitorum longus and the popliteus. The flexor hallucis longus, flexor digitorum longus and the posterior tibialis originate from the tibia with tendons attaching on the bottom of the foot. The three tendons spiral around the inner ankle (medial malleolus) to attach to the bottom of the foot; the posterior tibialis attaches to almost all of the small bones except the talus; the flexor muscles reach to the end of all the toes (Fig. 1.57). Posterior tibialis plays a vital role in supporting the transverse arch of the foot along with the peroneus longus and adductor hallucis (Kapandji, 1987).

- The deep posterior compartment continues upward behind the knee, merging with the intermuscular septum between the hamstrings and adductor group (Myers, 2009) (Figs 1.58 A & B).

Anterior and lateral compartments of the lower leg

- The anterior compartment consists of the anterior tibialis, extensor hallucis longus and extensor digitorum longus.

- The anterior tibialis runs along the front of the tibia (coming from its fascial continuum of the iliotibial band – see Ch. 2, Lateral Structures of the Lower Limb) to also attach to the underneath side of the first metatarsal and first cuneiform bone; extensor hallucis longus and extensor digitorum longus work synergistically with anterior tibialis at the ankle to stabilize the toes in dorsiflexion, lifting the toes so that the foot is not dropped and dragged during walking (Fig. 1.59 A).

- The lateral compartment is made up of the peroneus (fibularis) brevis and peroneus (fibularis) longus that travel along the fibula (coming from fascial continuum of the biceps femoris – see Ch. 2, Lateral Structures of the Lower Limb, Fig. 2.11) and spiral around the lateral malleolus to attach to first metatarsal and cuneiform bone (Fig. 1.59 B).

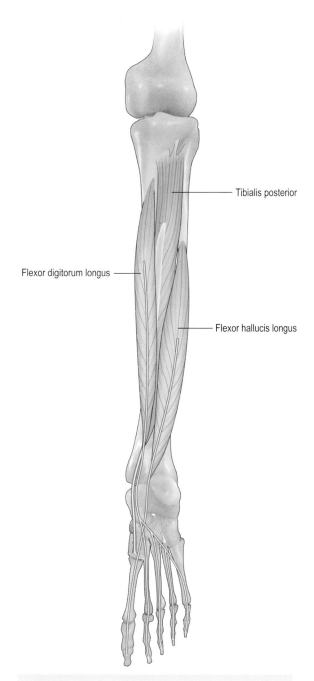

Tibialis posterior

Flexor digitorum longus

Flexor hallucis longus

Figure 1.57
Posterior tibialis; flexor hallucis longus; flexor digitorum longus

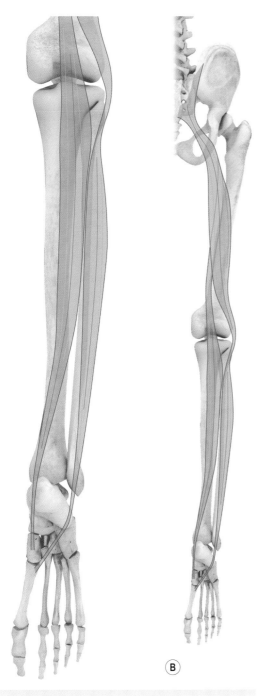

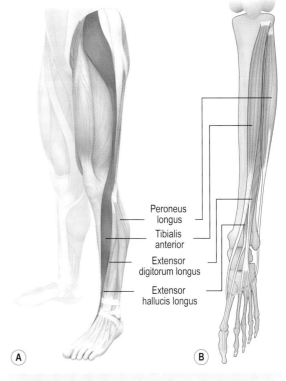

Peroneus
longus

Tibialis
anterior

Extensor
digitorum longus

Extensor
hallucis longus

(A)   (B)

Figure 1.59 A & B
Anterior and lateral compartments

- At the bottom of the foot are the tendons of the peroneus longus (fibularis longus) of the lateral compartment and the tibialis anterior of the anterior compartment which form a stirrup to support the medial arch of the foot (see Fig. 1.59 A) (Myers, 2009).

The intricate relationship of the compartments to one another through the fascial envelopes and the muscle attachments from the sole of the foot up through the leg into the pelvis form a woven system interacting, moving, and stimulating movement. It is important to move the toes and ankles for stimulation and gliding of the tendons, muscles, and fascia for improved movement, circulation, and overall feeling of well-being.

Toe exercises

The toe exercises stimulate the compartments by moving the toes in a variety of directions, facilitating the fascial envelopes of the compartments to glide and

(A)   (B)

Figure 1.58

A Deep posterior compartment connecting behind knee into intermuscular septum between hamstring group and adductors.
B Peroneal longus connection with lateral hamstring and sacrotuberous ligament

hydrate the layers. The action of pressing the first toe down activates the posterior compartment (flexor hallucis longus) and lifting the first toe activates the anterior compartment (extensor hallucis longus). Pressing the second through fifth metatarsals activates the posterior compartment (flexor digitorum longus) and lifting the second through fifth toes activates the anterior compartment (extensor digitorum longus). The lateral compartment is participating to track the movement of the ankle working synergistically with both the flexor and extensor movements. Improve motor skills and strengthen the lower leg and foot by practicing these movements. This corrective work is excellent for lower leg problems such as knee issues, swelling, shin splints, foot pain, and general foot weakness. It also improves brain function through movement by stimulating the coordination and motor learning areas of the brain.

Lifting all the toes

- Sit in an upright position, knees aligned over the ankles so that the tibia is perpendicular to the floor.
- Feel the tri-bone contact points on the bottom of the foot.
- Relax the toes.
- Lift all the toes up, feeling the tri-bone contact points (Fig. 1.60).

- Separate and widen the toes, creating space in between them.
- Place the toes down and relax.
- Repeat and visualize the action for spreading the toes, and feeling the big toe ball and little toe ball into the floor.

One Toe at a Time

- Lift all the toes again.
- Lower one toe at a time, starting from the little toe and ending with the big toe (Fig. 1.61).
- Try lowering big toe to little toe; imagine playing the piano with the toes.

Opposing toes

- Press the big toe down, hold it down, and lift the four toes (Fig. 1.62).
- Repeat several times until it feels coordinated.
- Reverse the action, press the four toes down, and lift the big toe up (Fig. 1.63).
- Try working both feet at the same time.

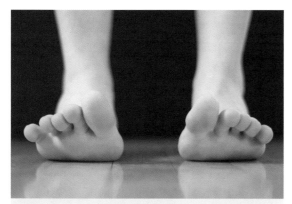

Figure 1.60
Lifting all the toes up

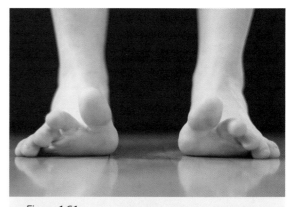

Figure 1.61
One Toe at a Time

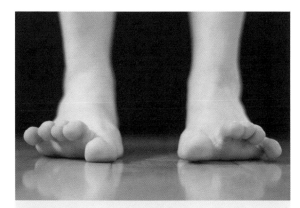

Figure 1.62
Big toe down, little toes up

- Place the foot on the small box (or large book) with the toe balls on the box and the toes over the box.
- Flex the big toe below the box into a larger range of motion.
- Place the loop or rubber band around the first toe, creating resistance as the toe flexes over the box (Fig. 1.64).
- Watch for the big toe curling downward over the box (or book). All the toes may be worked in this way.
- Repeat 10–20 times.

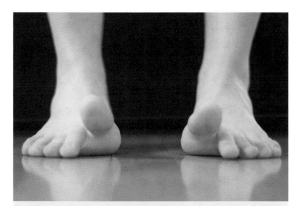

Figure 1.63
Little toes down, big toe up

- Try doing one action with one foot and the opposite action with the other foot; this is challenging the coordination brain!

Pilates Toe Corrector

The strength of the first toe pressing downward is critical for the push-off phase during the walk cycle. Strength also improves the arch of the foot. The ability to flex all the toes increases the strength of the arch.

Props needed for this exercise are a small box or large book, a Toe Gizmo™ or a small, thick rubber band, such as the kind that is wrapped around broccoli.

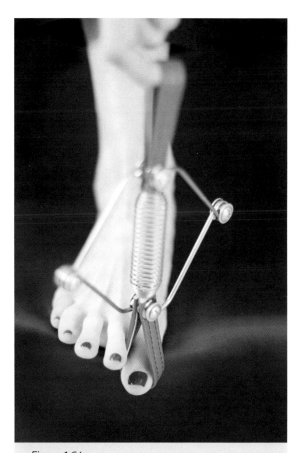

Figure 1.64
Toe Corrector on the box

Specific movements for bunions

Where there are bunions, the first toe joint has developed an excess amount of bone on the side of the toe along with a misalignment of the toe, which bends toward the other toes. This joint also loses mobility. The stiffer the joint becomes, the more painful it may be. Restoring the alignment of the first toe joint and increasing the mobility will help in easing discomfort and restoring function. As part of a whole approach to correcting the bunion, the whole foot needs to be addressed as to its strength and spiral motion ability. Many people with bunions have weak and hypermobile feet but the first MP joint is hypomobile. Performing the corrective exercises will be beneficial.

Self-mobilization of first toe joint

Sit comfortably, preferably on the floor, so that you can hold the foot. Visualize the first toe joint while working (Fig. 1.65).

Working the right toe, place the left thumb on top of the first MP joint (toe knuckle) and the index finger of the same hand on the bottom of the joint to stabilize the joint while the other hand mobilizes. With the right thumb and index finger make a pincer shape. The right thumb is on top and the second finger underneath, covering the big toe as if the toe is in a toe sock (vertical position). The left finger pincer shape holds the first MP joint (toe knuckle) in a horizontal orientation, thumb on top. The two thumbs are close together at the joint line (Fig. 1.66). Hold the joint firmly, in a stabilizing pincer grasp, with the left hand on the right foot. With the mobilizing hand (the right

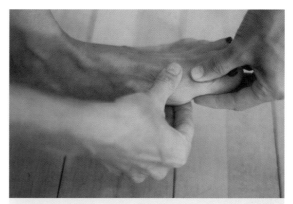

Figure 1.66
Hand position for self-movement of the MP joint

hand), move the toe toward a better alignment without overpressure. Gently compress the joint together by lightly pressing the toe into the joint for 5 seconds. Release the compression while maintaining the placement of the hands. Distract (pull gently) the phalange (toe) away from the metatarsal for 5 seconds with the intention of creating joint space. Repeat 3–4 times. On the last compression–distraction, move the toe away from the second toe.

Repeat the pattern several times: compress, distract and move the toe away from the second toe. Another movement to add is a circle and twist. An experienced practitioner may perform this for the client (Fig. 1.67).

Active toe movement

Follow the mobilizing of the toe with active movement of the toe.

- Place a finger on the side of the first toe and press the toe into the finger (Fig. 1.68).
- Move the first toe away from the second toe without curling up off the floor.
- Practice the movement until the coordination of the movement is clear.
- Add resistance using a Pilates Toe Gizmo™ or a small, thick rubber band.

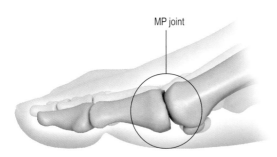

MP joint

Figure 1.65
Metatarsophalangeal (MP) joint

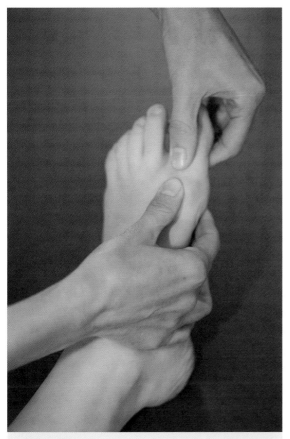

Figure 1.67
Practitioner hands-on

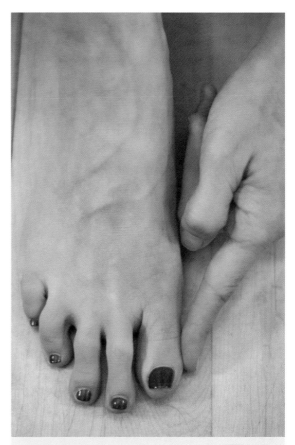

Figure 1.68
Moving first toe outward

- Sit with feet flat on the floor. Place the loop at the end of the Toe Gizmo™ around the first toe horizontally across the remaining toes; the other loop is held by the hand near the little toe.

- Pull the loop on the Toe Gizmo™, stretching the spring, creating resistance.

- Press the toe against the loop moving away from the second toe (Fig. 1.69).

Toe taping

At night, prior to going to sleep, tape the toe into a comfortable position as close as possible to the proper alignment of the toe. To do this, cut three pieces of first aid tape: two short pieces of tape to make rings that will wrap around the first toe and a third long piece of tape that can reach from the side of the toe ball joint along the inner edge of the arch, around the heel to the outside of the heel near the ankle bone.

First, make one ring and attach it around the base of the big toe (Fig. 1.70). Stick the long piece of tape to the side of first ring of tape (Fig. 1.71). Secure the long tape with the second short piece of tape making a ring around the first ring. The long piece of tape is in between the two rings. Pull the long piece of tape laterally to straighten the big toe alignment and firmly attach tape around heel to the other side of ankle (Fig. 1.72). The body will be at rest, passively moving the toe into a better alignment. You should only wear the tape while sleeping, not during the day.

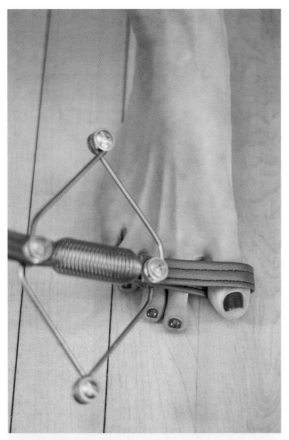

Figure 1.69
Toe Corrector

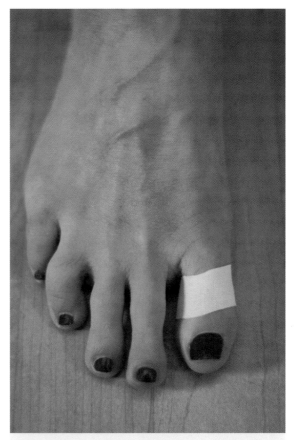

Figure 1.70
Toe taping first step: the small ring

CLIENT STORY

A female client with a significant bunion came to see me to practice Pilates. Her feet were hypermobile with a rigid bunion. When we placed her feet in the Pilates prehensile position (toes wrapped around the bar), it caused her such great discomfort that she refused to work in the prehensile position. She wanted to make changes to her foot but preferred not to resort to surgery. She therefore diligently practiced all the foot exercises to strengthen her feet, especially the "Active Toe Movement" exercise (see Fig. 1.68). We continued to balance her whole body, starting by working on global healthy movement patterns. We then reintroduced the prehensile position. Her foot was now able to dome around the bar, and maintain the position as she straightened and bent her knees performing the footwork series on the Reformer. She no longer has discomfort or pain in her toe joint. Her toe is better aligned and she can bend it in many ways. She still has the bump of bone, which will never go away, but the important point here is she restored her foot function through a whole body approach with specialized focus on the local area.

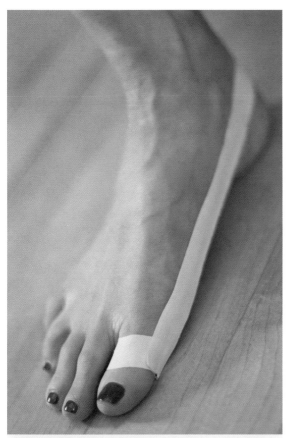

Figure 1.71
Toe taping second step: long tape with second ring

Hammer toes

The condition known as hammer toes is the tightening of the toe flexors that are on the bottom of the toes and the dropping of the metatarsal arch (toe balls). Work to release the tightness of the toes by massaging them from underneath into length (Fig. 1.73). Massaging the toes in a crosswise direction helps with realigning the fibers of the fascia of the toes, stimulating a release of the shortening tissue. Prehensile work in Pilates is the best position to exercise the lower limb. You can work the prehensile position on a small pinky ball.

Prehensile position on pinky ball

In a seated position, place the metatarsal arch over the top of the ball. Using hands-on, stretch the toes into a lengthened position around the ball (Fig. 1.74). Repeat the hands-on stretching of the toes over the ball until the toes become more supple. Then, without the hands-on, actively dome the toe balls over the ball and lengthen the toes over the ball as if trying to grasp the ball without shortening the toes. Practice the "Toe Exercises" and "Foot Exercises" described above daily. While sitting at a desk, you can have the ball under the desk; roll the arch and lengthen the toes over the ball while you work.

Bridging to Chapter 2

Restoring the foot to a flexible, agile and balanced state allows the whole body to be supportive. Practice

Figure 1.72
Toe taping: completed

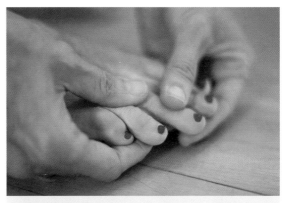

Figure 1.73
Self-massage of toes

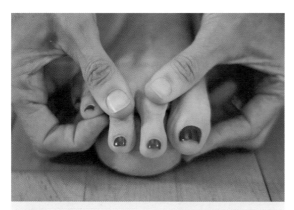

Figure 1.74
Using a pinky ball for the transverse arch and lengthening toes

these foot exercises daily and see the whole body shift into a new and improved stance. Starting at the feet provides a window of opportunity to access the intelligent body system that, given the right stimulus, will follow through in an optimal way. At times, the pathways along the way are blocked so that the signal from the feet may be diverted, or the feet are the derailing factor. Pay attention to following the path of movement through the body, identify the restricted place, and move wisely toward function: this is the art and practice of "centered."

The next step along the path is paying attention to the knee and hip in relation to the feet and lumbo-pelvic area.

Motion of the leg

"The spine is an engine driving the pelvis. Human anatomy is a consequence of function. The knee cannot be tested in isolation. It is part of the overall function and purpose of the musculoskeletal system."

Serge Gracovetsky

Contemplative awareness: successive motion

Movement of the legs may be initiated from the soles of the feet, led from the knee joint, or propelled from the trunk, but wherever initiated, it produces transference of motion throughout the body, changing it both in and through space. The action of locomotion is movement spread throughout the body in a process that is simultaneous, successive, and sequential. The legs give access to moving in space in multiple directions while supporting the weight of the body. The sequence of lower limb movement is spiral in nature with reciprocal motions. As a whole body mover, a distribution of force progresses through the body via a wave of motion occurring in the spaces between the connecting parts. In order for the body to move well and maintain healthy knees and hips, however, some fine-tuning of the foot/ankle, knee, and hip/pelvis acting in concert is necessary.

This spiral orientation and the template for limb movement are first seen during the development of the embryo. The limbs begin as buds that gravitate outward and away from the body (Fig. 2.1). An early limb bud is located in the correct place for movement, as a control point to take the embryo into movement. The initial movement orientation of both the upper and lower limbs is sideways and flat. The lower limb rotates inward (medially), orientating the knee in an upright (caudal) position. It also spirals around its own long axis (Schoenwolf et al., 2009). The soft tissue, myofascia, and bone all have the spiral as their structural form. The direction of growth is spiral and moves in the direction of the knee, developing downward from the hip toward the knee and at the same time upward

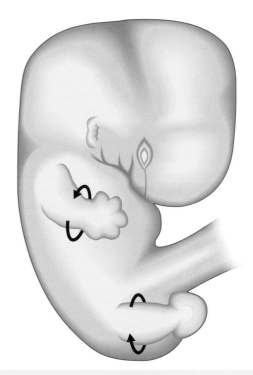

Figure 2.1
Upper limb buds; lower limb buds

from the foot (Phillip Beach, 2013, workshop presentation in Long Beach, CA, USA). This growth pattern compresses the knee, preparing it for its job of weight bearing from above and relaying the ground forces from below. Understanding that the legs are in a spiral pattern and the knee is a joint of compression helps us to direct healthy movement patterns to increase the capacity of normal movement for life.

Ease the knees

The knees can also be understood metaphorically, representing the ability to be flexible in life, to be mobile and move toward a purpose. If we are presented with a threat, our instinct is to run away or move toward a positive desire. Since the nervous system is wired with emotions and initiating movement responses, body motion also influences memory and feelings (Casasanto and Dijkstra, 2010). The emotion of fear represented in the knees will prevent movement in the knees; this is the fear of moving forward in life or of taking the necessary steps toward a goal. Locked knees make it impossible to move forward and mean one can easily be knocked over. Being mentally "locked into" one way of thinking or feeling inhibits movement. Having flexible knees gives the feeling of freedom to choose to move in any direction and to be poised for any possibility, while adapting to change. Having an awareness of the connection between personal life resistances, stuck patterns, and stress manifesting in restrictive body motion gives one an opportunity to look deeper into oneself. The integration of self-study with physical training that focuses on balancing the body's form and function enhances healing potential. Reciprocally, the body's capacity for better movement will help support healthier emotions.

Knee as a pulley wheel

The usual movements of daily living require the body to bend toward the floor and move from sitting to standing many times a day. The knee is the intermediary of the foot, ankle, and hip. In gait, it is the "shortener" and "lengthener" of the lower leg, and it allows the distance between the trunk and the ground to be varied. Being the joint of compression, the knee receives and absorbs very strong forces as the foot strikes the ground and pushes off. The spiraling movement in gait is present at the knee, and thus the knee is not only a hinge joint, to flex and extend the leg, but also moves on the rotational axis. Other motions of the knee include a specific timing of sliding and rolling.

If we look at the bones of the femur and tibia that make up the knee joint, we can see that the shape is asymmetrical. The distal femur (the lower end of the femur) has two convex parts similar to a grooved pulley wheel.

The inner wheel is called the medial condyle and the outer the lateral condyle. The medial condyle is longer by about half an inch (1.27 cm) (Hoppenfeld, 1976). The inner side of the femur bone is lower than the outer side; however, with the femur's natural oblique position the two condyles lie practically in the same horizontal plane. The tibia part of the knee (called the tibial plateau) has surfaces that are reciprocally curved, forming a gutter shape where the menisci and ligaments live. The femur wheels are not level and do not sit in the gutter equally. The wheels not only roll but slide across the surface due to the shape differences, thus creating the very small (micro-) movements – rolling, sliding, and rotation – that are essential to knee health. If the knee lacks these micromovements, then the probability of damage to the structures of the knee, such as the meniscus, increases. Improving the micromovements of the knee is part of the fine-tuning of leg motion.

Path of straightening and bending

The knees bend and straighten with the feet on the ground, as in a squat or sitting down action (closed chain) (Fig. 2.2), or by freely kicking the legs, as when kicking a ball (open chain) (Fig. 2.3). In closed chain, the lower leg is fixed, meaning it remains in constant contact with an immobile surface, such as the floor. Movement takes place at the hip, knee, and ankle with the femur moving on the tibia. When moving the lower leg freely (open chain), think of the movement of a dancer doing the Can Can – here the tibia is moving primarily on the femur.

Rolling, sliding, and rotating

Imagine a set of wheels and the motion that is conjured up is rolling. If a runaway shopping cart's journey ends and the wheels continue to move, a reverse motion of the wheels, sliding back, will stop the forward motion of the cart. If the femoral condyle only rolled, it would fall off the back of the tibial condyle when in a greater range of flexion. The ratio of rolling to sliding varies during flexion and extension and also varies between the medial and lateral condyles. Beginning in standing with legs straight, as the knees bend, the femoral condyle (wheels) rolls without sliding. Then, as the knee movement progresses into deeper bend, the sliding becomes more important than the rolling (Fig. 2.4).

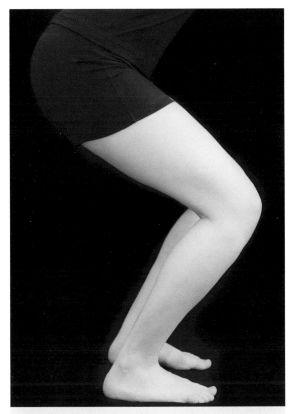

Figure 2.2
Closed chain knee movement

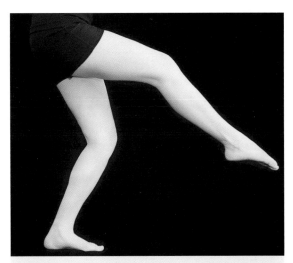

Figure 2.3
Open chain knee movement

(Kapandji, 1987). The lateral condyle rolls further and covers more distance than the medial side. The difference in motion is necessary for the motion of automatic rotation of the knee, and is significant for the function of the knee joint where stability and mobility are a requisite for healthy knees. The degree of rolling matches the degree of knee flexion necessary for walking without scraping the foot along the ground.

The cruciate ligaments are a central link in femoral and tibial movement. The role of the cruciate ligaments is to pull back the bones and cause them to slide on the tibial plateau in the opposite direction of their

There is more rolling on the lateral condyle, from 0° to 20° of flexion, compared to the medial condyle, where pure rolling occurs during the first 10–15° of flexion

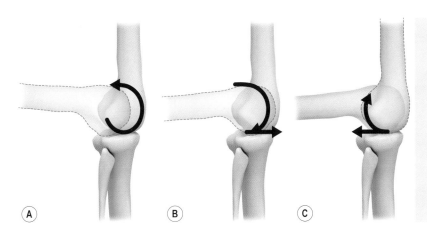

Figure 2.4

A Rolling without sliding
B Rolling and sliding anterior during flexion
C Rolling and sliding posterior during knee extension

A   B   C

rolling movement. In active knee flexion, the flexors of the knee pull the shin backward (posteriorly) and the anterior cruciate ligament slides the femoral condyles forward (anteriorly) or the tibia backward (posteriorly), to change the rolling motion to sliding. While straightening the knee, extension is produced by the extensors of the knee, which pull the tibia forward (anteriorly) under the femur during extension (Kapandji, 1987). Cruciate ligaments also prevent medial rotation of an extended knee. Medial rotation of the tibia stretches or elongates the anterior cruciate and relaxes the posterior cruciate. In lateral rotation of the tibia the opposite occurs, as the anterior relaxes and the posterior elongates. The cruciate ligaments are, in effect, the brakes for the knee joints.

Screw home mechanism

As the knee moves into full extension (straightening of the knee), external rotation occurs at the tibia on the femur. This happens because of the configuration of the tibia and the collateral ligaments but also the differences in the bone shape. Therefore, as the tibia moves on the femoral condyles into full extension, it uses all available articulating surfaces on the lateral side (outer), while leaving about a half inch (about 1.25 cm) on the medial (inner) side (Fig. 2.5). To use the remaining articular surface on the medial side and reach full extension, the medial side must rotate laterally around the lateral femoral condyle. This allows the knee to reach full extension – "home." This motion is commonly called a "screw home mechanism." The screw home mechanism allows a person to stand with the knee extended for long periods of time without activating many muscles.

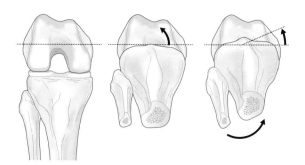

Figure 2.5
Screw home mechanism

Practitioner note
Test for screw home mechanism

Have a person sit on a table or high chair with the feet dangling above the ground. Place a dot at the center of the kneecap (patella) and a second dot at the tibial tubercle (Fig. 2.6 A). Notice first if the dots line up. If the tibia dot is on the outside of the patella dot, then the person's tibia hangs in external rotation. This is an indication of an imbalance of the hip and knee arising from the pelvis spiraling inward and the tibia outward. This position of the tibia is being laterally suspended by the gluteus maximus, the tensor fasciae latae (TFL) as it spans downward into the iliotibial band, and the biceps femoris. The attachment of the biceps femoris is continuous at the fibula head with a direct fascial attachment with the peroneus longus, also known as fibularis longus (Myers, 2001).

Ask the person to extend the knee (Fig. 2.6 B). The lower dot on the tibial tubercle will move to the outside of the patella dot, demonstrating the tibial external rotation on the femur.

Restoring the internal rotation of the tibia using functional foot plate

 Restoring internal rotation of tibia using the foot plate
VIDEO LINK V 2.1

- The client is seated with the foot of the side to be worked on a functional foot plate.

- Align the client's leg from the hip through the foot.

- Hold (or have the client hold) the thigh to stabilize it; do not allow it to move.

- Cue the client to move the tibia inward (Fig. 2.7 A).

- Only move to within the range of internal rotation where the foot remains normal; do not allow supination of the foot.

- Move into the range prior to supination; place the hand on the outer edge of the plate to maintain that position of the plate.

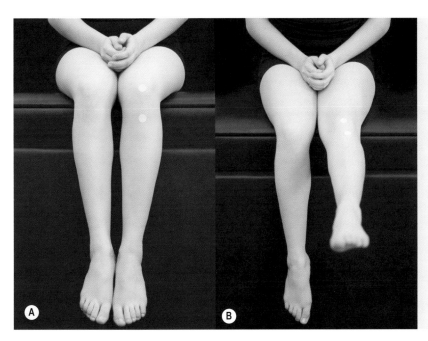

Figure 2.6
A Observing motion of knee
B Extension of the knee
with tibial tubercle
moving laterally

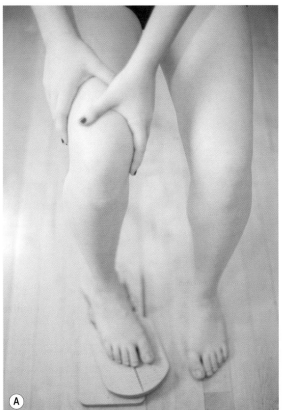

- Cue the client: "I am going to move the plate further into internal rotation – don't allow it to move" (the client moves outward, and you block the motion) (Fig. 2.7 B).

- Hold the isometric contraction for 5 seconds.

- Stop resistance but stay at that range.

- Move the tibia into more internal rotation without supination to a new range.

- Repeat the resistance and movement 3–4 times.

- Add a reciprocal resistance by staying at the new increased range, place the hand on the inner edge, and reverse the isometric contraction to set the new length.

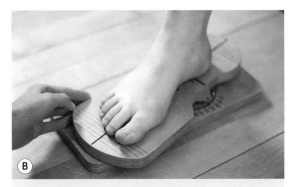

Figure 2.7 A
Foot plate work for internal rotation of tibia

Figure 2.7 B
Hands-on

Lateral structures of lower limbs

The outer line of the whole leg is made up of powerful continuous layers and expansions of fascia (connective tissue). The density varies depending on the location of the fascia. On the whole side of the thigh, a strong fibrous band called the iliotibial band supports and reinforces the lower limb. The iliotibial band is part of a whole fascial system, completely encircling the thigh but diving deep, attaching to bone, encapsulating layers of muscles, nerves, and vessels. The band may be considered the long tendon of the gluteus maximus and TFL (Stecco and Stecco, 2012), running from the pelvis to the outer knee. As the band runs from the pelvis to the knee, it provides extensive attachments and origins of several muscles through its intermuscular septum. On the anterior lateral side lies the lateral quadriceps, vastus lateralis, attaching to the fascia lata deep intermuscular septum. On the posterior lateral side, the band separates the lateral hamstring, biceps femoris, from the lateral quadriceps. The gluteus maximus and TFL pull the band upward while the vastus lateralis and biceps femoris pull it down (Willem Fourie, 2014, Fascia Research Summer School, Ulm, Germany).

> **Try it!**
>
> Stand with the legs straight. Place an index finger vertically along the front edge of the band and the middle fingers at the back edge of the band. Bend the knee to 40°. Feel for the tension changes. Notice that when the knee is straight the front edge of the band is prominent, while in knee flexion the back edge is more prominent (Figs 2.9 A and 2.9 B).

The merging of iliotibial band and myofascia at the lateral knee, blending into the retinaculum of the knee, has a strong influence on the lateral tibial condyle and fibula head (Fig. 2.8). This confluence of tissue is important in inhibiting or assisting healthy knee motions. When the knee and hip bend and straighten, the band appears to move forward and back. According to Fairclough et al. (2006), the iliotibial band movement is an illusion. What is seen is the tension shifting between its anterior and posterior fibers as the knee bends. When the knee is slightly flexed, the TFL muscle force is greater than that from the gluteus maximus. The anterior side of the band becomes more apparent. As the knee bend deepens, the tension is greater from the gluteus maximus, making the

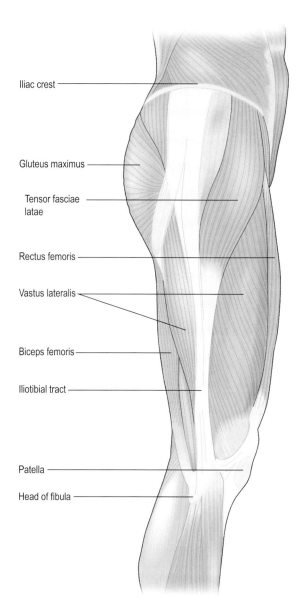

Iliac crest

Gluteus maximus

Tensor fasciae latae

Rectus femoris

Vastus lateralis

Biceps femoris

Iliotibial tract

Patella

Head of fibula

Figure 2.8
Lateral hip to knee connections

posterior fibers more prominent. Athletes and dancers who jump high (think of basketball pros) bend very deeply to use the power of the gluteus maximus to explode up into the air.

The iliotibial band, with its attachments, needs to be able to glide, lengthen, and slide with the increase of distance between the knee and the pelvis as the knee bends deeply. For many people, the

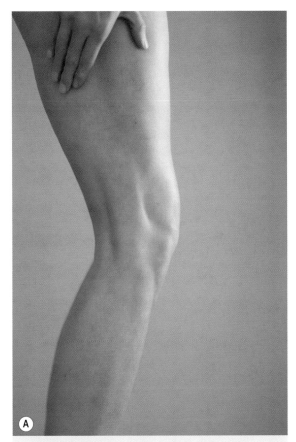

A

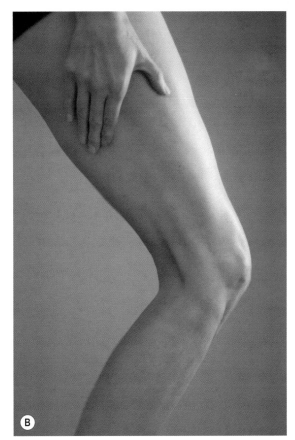

B

Figure 2.9 A & B
Iliotibial band tension changes

tissue becomes stiff and dry, losing its elastic quality. Movement of the hip and knee in all directions of the leg will enhance the gliding and length of the lateral leg.

Tensor fasciae latae releases

Muscle energy technique (MET) for the tensor fasciae latae

The client lies supine on the edge of the table closest to the practitioner (Fig. 2.10 A).

- The practitioner stands to the side of the client, holding the leg in neutral with the inferior hand and with the superior hand placed on top of the anterior superior iliac spine (ASIS).

- Move the leg into slight flexion, abduction, and internal rotation to the interbarrier zone (the place prior to muscular contraction) (Fig. 2.10 A).

- Cue the client to resist the movement of the leg as it is moved toward the midline; TFL contracts. Palpate the TFL or see it contract; hold 5–10 seconds.

- Release the contraction and lengthen the lateral leg by moving the leg toward the midline (Fig 2.10 B).

- Repeat 3–4 times.

- On the last set, ask the client to resist lightly but allow a slow movement of the leg toward the midline (eccentric contraction); cue "meet my resistance and move slowly." If very tight, repeat this 2–3 times.

- Finish with a reciprocal MET; hold the leg in the new length (adducted) and ask the client to resist the movement of the leg outward; try to move it outward and the client moves the leg inward (activating the adductors).

Tensor fasciae latae and iliotibial band on Small Barrel

 TFL and iliotibial band on Small Barrel
VIDEO LINK V 2.2

The Small Barrel is placed on top of the Cadillac or a massage table with the arc side at the edge of the table. (The same release can be performed on the Large Barrel for a greater range of stretch or on a bolster for a smaller range of stretch.)

- The client lies on the side on top of the arc of the barrel, with the leg to be worked on top and the greater trochanter over the apex of the arc (ensure there is adequate padding under the hip) (Fig. 2.11 A).

- The top leg is straight; the underneath leg is bent with the ankle hooked onto the ankle of the top leg.

- The whole body is aligned and the head is resting on the elbow of the supportive arm.

- The practitioner stands behind the client.

- Place the superior hand or forearm on top of the pelvis for stability and the inferior hand above the knee joint or below the knee joint on the shin for resistance and stretch (Fig. 2.11 B).

- Cue the client, "I am going to press your leg down – do not let me do it." The client will resist the downward motion of the leg by pressing up, creating an isometric contraction.

- Hold for 5 seconds.

- Release and move the thigh downward into a new length (Fig. 2.11 C).

- Be sure the thigh does not fall inward off the line established at the starting position.

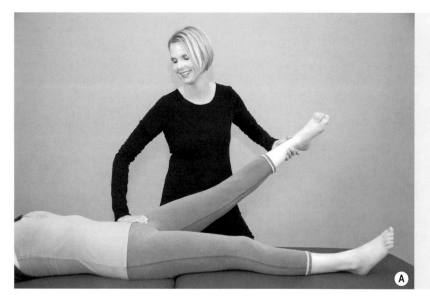

Figure 2.10 A
MET iliotibial band: start position

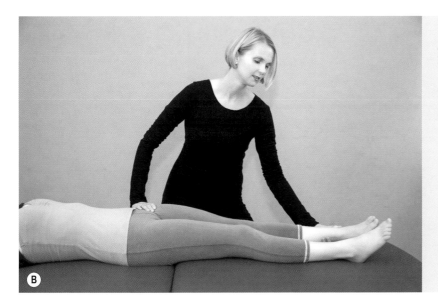

Figure 2.10 B
Adduction of the leg after
the isometric contraction

- Repeat; feel a fascial release by length increasing between the hands or elbow and hand. Repeat 3–4 times.

(Move the femur into different angles to have better effect on the anterior/lateral edge of the band to quadriceps attachment and the more posterior edge at the hamstring.)

Practitioner note

To find the position of the leg, hold the client's femur with both hands just above the knee, and move the femur in internal and external rotation, moving and gliding the lateral tissues of the leg without moving the pelvis. Observe the tension changes or movements. Choose a position that best addresses the line of length; generally it is either more centered or slightly outward; shortened bands roll the leg inward.

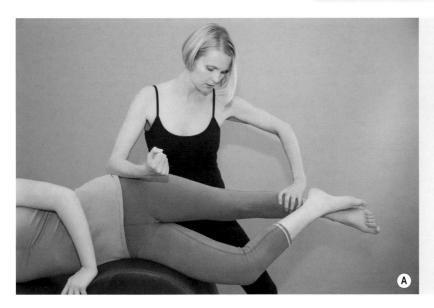

Figure 2.11 A
Small Barrel iliotibial band:
start position

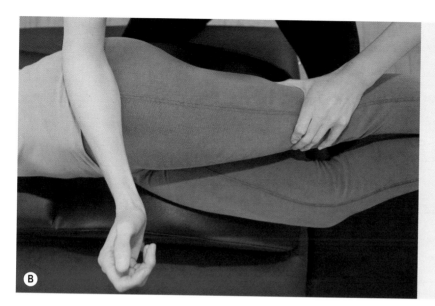

Figure 2.11 B
Hands-on

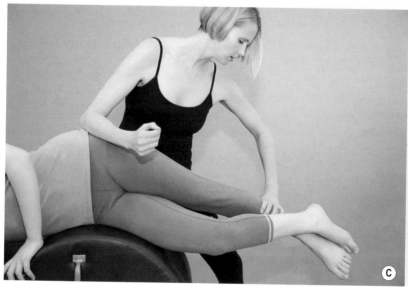

Figure 2.11 C
Lengthening movement

Medial structures of the lower limbs

Similarly, the inner side of the knee has its divisions: the medial intermuscular septum of the vastus medialis and adductors, a convergence of muscles called the pes anserinus, the sartorius, one of the inner hamstrings called the semitendinosus, and the gracilis, an adductor muscle, attaching at the medial side of the knee. It also extends fascially into the inner knee fascia, the retinaculum. Both the lateralis and medialis have fascial connections anteriorly to the patella, blending with the fascia lata contributing to the retinacula of the knee (Fig. 2.12) (Stecco and Stecco, 2012). The spiral of the knee fascia wraps around, connecting the outer and inner sides of the knee.

Back structures of the lower limbs

Completing the continuity of the knee picture is the back of the knee (the popliteal region). The convergence of the other medial hamstring, the semimembranosus, has two expansions into the knee joint capsule forming the popliteal ligament and another into the popliteal fascia. The arrangement of fibers in the back of the knee is a criss-cross webbing of tissues from the inner and outer hamstrings, the smaller popliteal muscle and fascia, and from below, two heads of the gastrocnemius muscle (Fig. 2.13). The lines of force from the hamstrings, both outer and inner, pulling upward, plus the two heads of the calves pulling downward creates a traction of the knee, allowing it to bend. The lines of traction need to be balanced. The function of the criss-crossing is to allow for ease in the bending and straightening of the knee without damaging the ligaments and menisci. Some branches of fibers from the semimembranosus feed into the posterior horn of the medial meniscus. Cadaver studies have shown that some people have attachments to the lateral meniscus as well. The popliteus is also intimate with the

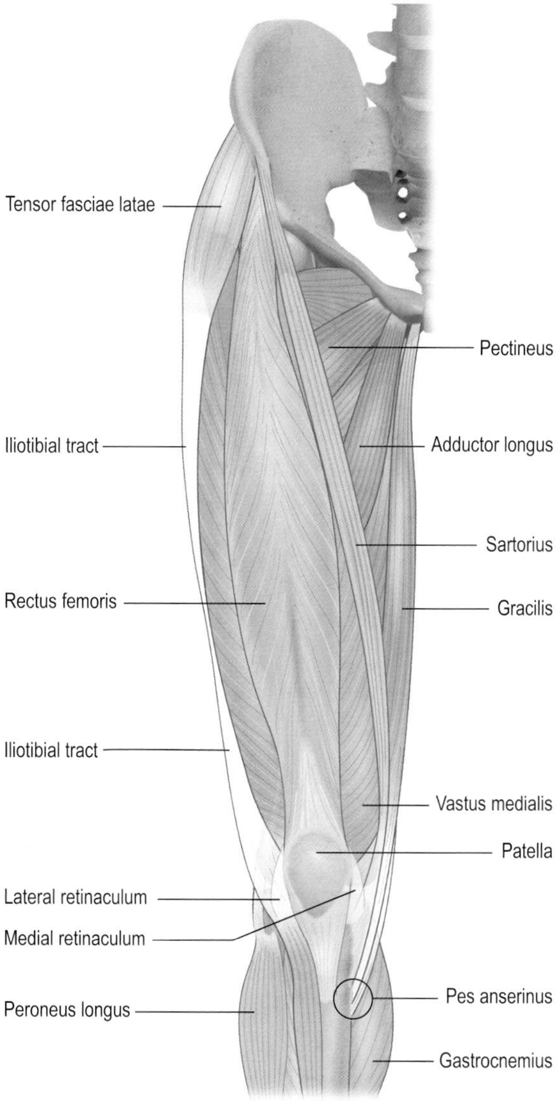

Tensor fasciae latae

Iliotibial tract

Rectus femoris

Iliotibial tract

Lateral retinaculum

Medial retinaculum

Peroneus longus

Pectineus

Adductor longus

Sartorius

Gracilis

Vastus medialis

Patella

Pes anserinus

Gastrocnemius

Figure 2.12

Retinaculum, lateral and medial sides of fascial continuum

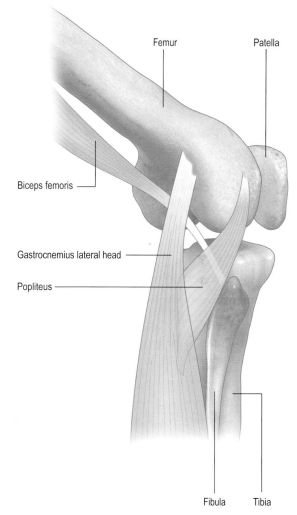

Femur

Patella

Biceps femoris

Gastrocnemius lateral head

Popliteus

Fibula   Tibia

Figure 2.13

Hamstring, gastrocnemius, popliteal muscle criss-cross

meniscus as it runs on a diagonal from the outer (lateral) side of the knee, on the femoral condyle, to the tibia's inner side along the upper line of the soleus. Its attachment to the popliteal ligament, formed by the semimembranosus, is part of the continuum of fascial connections of the lower limb from pelvis to foot.

The first motion of bending the knee is an unlocking of the knee. When the knee is straight, the bones are rotated (femur internally and tibia externally), locking the shape of the joint as if it were a puzzle piece coming together. Bending the knee means an unlocking of the shape that starts with a micromovement of reversing the rotation (internal rotation of the tibia at the femur). The popliteus muscle plays the major role in the unlocking of the knee prior to the hip moving into flexion. Guiding people to bend the knees with the initial awareness of unlocking prior to hip motion is crucial for signaling the pathway of a healthy movement pattern of the whole limb.

Front structures of the lower limbs

Observing the patella tracking shows the direction and timing of the extensor group recruitment and the level of tension in the fascia. The patella sits in a groove, a deep vertical gutter, on the lowest end of the femur. It is

embedded in the capsule of the knee joint and myofascia of the extensor group from above. The fascia continues from the extensor group (quadriceps) to form the patellar ligament. The fascial fibers cross over each other at the knee joint and insert at the tibial tuberosity. The patella is a sesamoid bone (a bone embedded within a tendon), with the bone sitting free within the fascia. Its movement and position rely on the tension of the tissue it sits in. How it moves is indicative of the condition of the contractile ability of the thigh and the folding and unfolding of the capsule (Fig. 2.14).

> **Try it!**
>
> Sit with the legs straight in front and relax them completely. Place one thumb on one side of the patella and the index finger on the other side (Fig. 2.15). Gently wiggle the patella from side to side, up and down, on the diagonals. Notice the directions that are more difficult to move into. Typically the patella is restricted going medial, down and on the oblique angle from upper lateral to lower medial. Patellae tend to be stuck up and lateral. This restriction is tension held from the lateral side of the leg and extensor group tightness. See below for re-education technique.

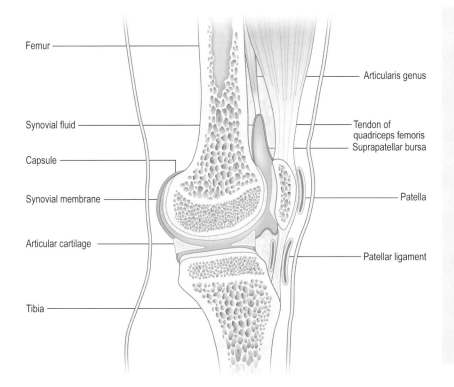

Femur

Synovial fluid

Capsule

Synovial membrane

Articular cartilage

Tibia

Articularis genus

Tendon of quadriceps femoris
Suprapatellar bursa

Patella

Patellar ligament

Figure 2.14
Patella, knee capsule and articularis genu

The joint capsule is a fibrous sleeve, like a cylinder around the knee, filled with synovial fluid to feed the knee joint. It creates a non-bony wall of articular space between the femur and the tibia. Above the patella, the capsule forms the suprapatellar bursa. The patella moves with a vertical force from the extensor group. In knee flexion, the patella moves downward in the groove; the capsule becomes unpleated, allowing the patella to move a distance twice its length. In knee extension, the patella moves upward while the suprapatellar bursa is pulled upward, pleating the capsule so that the bursa avoids being impinged by the femur. The bursa is drawn upward by the articularis genu muscle, which arises from the deep fibers of the vastus intermedalis (Kapandji, 1987) (see Fig. 2.14).

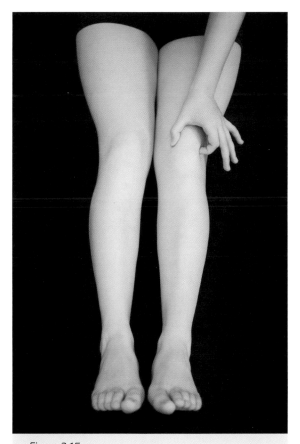

Figure 2.15
Patella passive movement

If the fascia is limited in its elasticity, then the patella is held tightly against the femur, restricting the distance it travels and changing its vertical pull off its centered line. Over time, the underside of the patella becomes worn. There may be a scraping, grinding noise when the knee bends and straightens plus uncoordinated tracking that alters the normal mechanics of the knee.

Seeing the mechanics of the patella movement provides a visual representation for awareness of a normal patella action. To study what is normal and feels right is a powerful way to use the information as a metaphor for movement. Imagine blinds in the window. If one string is shorter than the other, when the cord is pulled the blinds become uneven. So in the body, when one side is tighter than the other the tracking of the knee is compromised. Over time the risk of damage to the knee structures increases. All the tissues are intimately organized as a whole structure for movement and thus a structure with uneven stresses on it will be off center. The whole dynamic function and alignment from the hip to the knee is responsible for the knee joint movement. The tension of the myofascia provides the tensile work to produce the right amount of space in the joint to allow for the bones to roll, slide, and rotate. The lines of traction need to be balanced.

Re-education of patella tracking

The iliotibial band and fascia on the lateral side of the knee may need to be released prior to activating the patella movement.

- The client sits with the leg to be worked extended, the other leg in parallel position; the patella is aligned with the center of the hip joint.

- The practitioner asks the client to pull the patella up and observes how the client glides the patella superiorly.

- If the patella moves lateral first, it is a dysfunction pull of the patella. (The patella should first move at an oblique angle medial/superior to superior to lateral/superior.)

Practitioner note
Hands-on

- Wiggle the patella from medial to lateral and lateral to medial to see ease of the patella motion and to release any holding (see Fig. 2.15).

- Vigorously tap the vastus medialis oblique (VMO) muscle. Place the index and third finger pads on the superior/medial corner of the patella as a tactile cue (Fig. 2.16). Ask the client to first press the finger out of the way as the patella initiates its superior/medial movement. Repeat this until the patella easily glides in the correct direction.

- This is a good home program exercise for re-education of the firing pattern of the quadriceps group.

Strengthen this oblique line of the patella

- Ask the client to lie on the side of leg to be worked.

- The top leg is supported in alignment; use a Reformer box to rest the bent knee on.

- Line up the underneath working leg so that the heel is in alignment with the ischial tuberosity (sits bone) with a soft, slightly bent knee.

- The outer edge of the foot is resting on the mat or table (Fig. 2.17 A).

- Make a pincer shape with one thumb and the knuckle of the index finger; the thumb is touching the side of the knuckle; place it at the bottom (plantar side) of the calcaneus where it meets the talus.

- Cue the client to press the foot into the hand and think of pushing the hand away (slide the heel) (Fig. 2.17 B).

- The heel moves in the line of the sits bone, NOT FORWARD as it would in kicking a ball.

- Introduce enough pressure for the client to press against, creating resistance; work along the inner line of the knee to the hip.

- Repeat this 15–20 times.

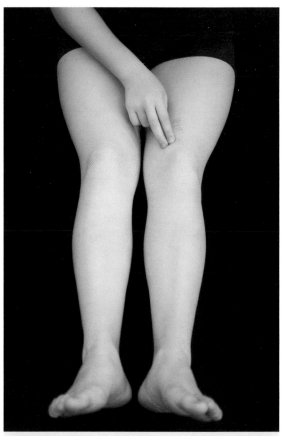

Figure 2.16
Patella tracking medial side

- Follow this work with the Wunda Chair VMO exercise (p. 68) and squats.

Role of the fibula in knee and ankle function

As described in Chapter 1, the lower end of the tibia and talus move in a helical motion to allow for good talus gliding with the subtle motion of the inferior tibiofibular joint for both ankle stability and mobility (see Figs 1.9 A and 1.9 B). At the knee, the superior tibiofibular joint is mechanically linked to the ankle. The lateral side of the knee blends the attachments of the biceps femoris, lateral collateral ligament, thick expansion of fascia from the iliotibial band onto the tibia and a relation to the popliteus muscle on the posterior side. Movement of the fibula is primarily apparent at the

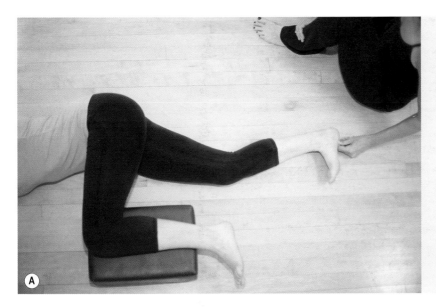

Figure 2.17 A
Side lying knee extension
with hands-on

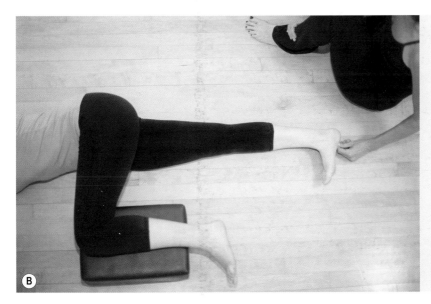

Figure 2.17 B
Movement complete with leg
extended

ankle, with micromovements reflected at the knee
while bending and straightening.

The micromovements are in three directions. The
fibula moves toward (forward) and away (backward), up and down like a piston, and rotates. During flexion of the ankle, the inferior tibiofibular joint
moves away from the medial malleolus, is pulled
upward, and medially rotates. In plantarflexion,

the movement is reversed (Kapandji, 1987). The fibula motion at the knee is influenced by the myofascial tension at the lateral knee. It is common to find
the tibiofibular joint restricted in the up and down
movement, being held up by the lack of fascial gliding of the lateral knee.

In performing a squat, the bending of the knee
includes dorsiflexion of the ankle. The fibula will

move up (superior) and rotate inward (medial), and the top moves forward (anterior) while the bottom moves back (posterior). Standing up out of a squat, the fibula motion returns to its starting position. If one moves into a heel lift (plantarflexion) or relevé, the fibula, at the ankle, will move inferior, externally rotate and move forward. It approximates the bones to wedge the ankle into a more rigid, stable position for balance. This movement of the fibula is especially important in walking at the point of pushing off from the back foot preparing to take the next step. Fine-tuning the fibula micromovement is vital to restoring the movement of the lower limb and easing restrictions of bending down and standing up.

> **Practitioner note**
> **Test the fibula motion**
>
> Sit behind the standing client. Place the index finger of one hand on the proximal end of the fibula head, and the other hand index finger underneath the lateral malleolus (Fig. 2.18 A). Ask the client to bend the knees slowly and feel at the knee for the superior/medial rotation of the fibula head; it will move up into the hand. At the ankle, it will move away from the hand (Fig. 2.18 B). While holding onto a support, ask the client to lift the heels up with straight legs (a relevé). Feel how the proximal (top) end moves away from the hand and the distal (bottom) end into the hand (Fig. 2.18 C). Notice if one leg lacks healthy movement. Is the fibula stuck up? When the ankle moves into plantarflexion, the fibula does not move into the lower hand.

Movement techniques specifically for fibula

First the normal screw home mechanism should be restored prior to the fibular motion.

Movement releases for fibular motion

 Movement releases for the fibula, heel and toe tapping: hands-on
VIDEO LINK V 2.3

- Have the client sit with feet on the floor and knees bent.

- Sit in front of the client.

- Instruct the client to either toe tap or heel tap:
  - toe-tapping will emphasize the posterior–lateral movement of the fibula, thereby moving the fibula up (Fig. 2.19 A)
  - heel-tapping emphasizes the anterolateral motion, moving the fibula down (Fig. 2.19 B).

- Gently grasp the fibula just below the head at the knee and gently rock the fibula in the direction needed.

- The rhythm of the rocking matches the downward movement as the heel or ball of the foot hits the ground.

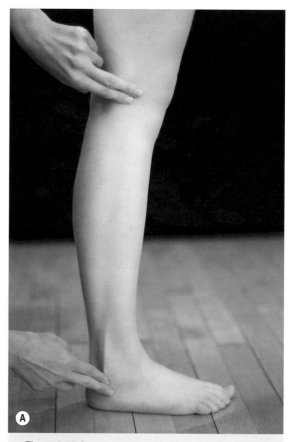

Ⓐ

Figure 2.18 A
Hand placement on fibula

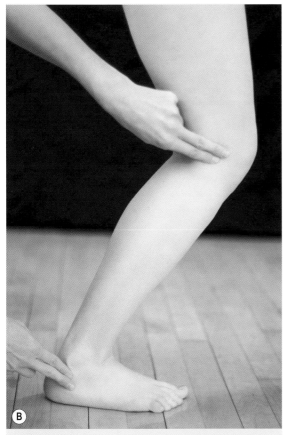

Figure 2.18 B
Bending knee

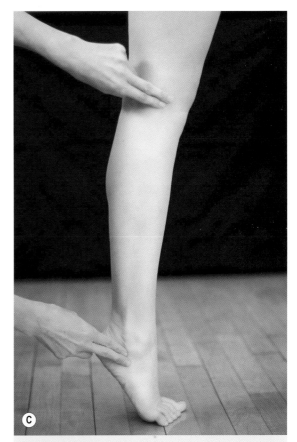

Figure 2.18 C
Heel lifting

- Continue the movement and rocking until the rocking feels easier to do manually.

Mobilization of fibula using a functional foot plate

Release the fascial tightness of the posterior-lateral side of the fibula head and lateral hamstrings.

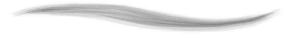

- The client is seated with knees flexed, with the side to be worked placed on a rotational disc (functional foot plate).

- Sit in front of the client's foot.

- Place the palmar side of the fingers along the posterior surface of the fibula; the thumb may rest on the front side of the fibula head (Fig. 2.20 A). BE GENTLE on hand hold – behind the fibula head lies the common fibular nerve.

- The other hand is placed on the client's forefoot or on top of the femur for stability.

- Have the client turn the foot plate inward to internally rotate the tibia (Fig. 2.20 B).

- As the tibia is moving inward, gently stroke from a medial to lateral direction to separate the lateral hamstrings from the midline; also, the movement will enhance the forward motion of the fibula.

- As the tibia moves toward external rotation, using the thumb contact, press into the front of the fibula head, encouraging a posterior position of the fibula.

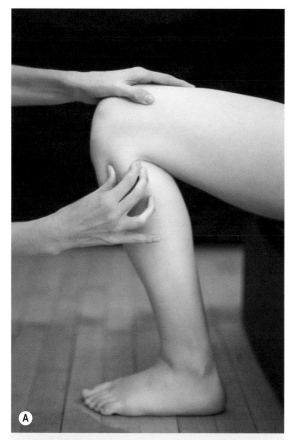

Figure 2.19 A
Fibula release: toe-tapping

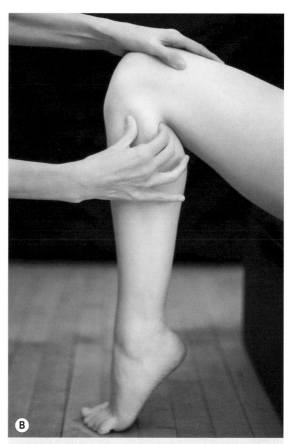

Figure 2.19 B
Fibula release: heel-tapping

- If the fibula head is stuck forward (anterior) using the thumb contact, hold the fibula head back as the foot rotates inward on the disc.

- If it is necessary to move the medial hamstrings from the midline, change the hand position to the medial side to stroke as the tibia externally rotates.

Exercises for tuning the legs

Remember to always include the foot exercises from Chapter 1.

Standing Knee Circles (1)

- Standing with the feet together, lean forward to place the palms of the hands on top of the kneecaps (Fig. 2.21 A).

- Bend the knees into a pain-free range. At first, keep the heels on the floor. Over time, the movement range and strength improve. Progress into deepening the bend of the knees, allowing the heels to lift off the floor.

- Circle the knees to the side (Fig. 2.21 B).

- Straighten the knees as they move back (Fig. 2.21 C).

- Bend again to the other side (Fig. 2.21 D).

- Return to center knee bending.

- Repeat this 5 times in one direction, reverse 5 times in the other direction.

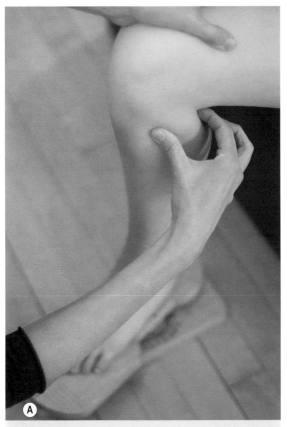

Figure 2.20 A
Functional foot plate fibula release

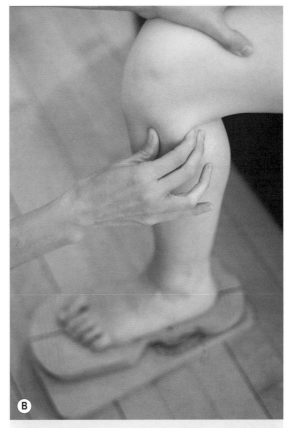

Figure 2.20 B
Internal rotation

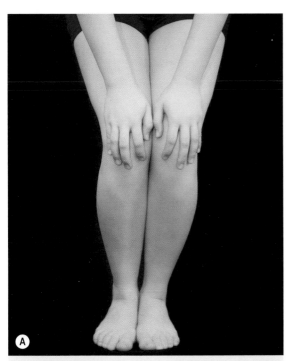

Figure 2.21 A
Knee Circles: start position

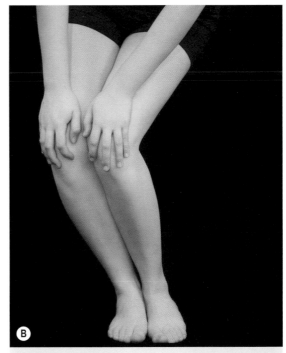

Figure 2.21 B
Circling to one side

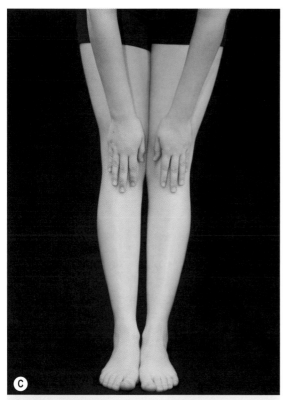

Figure 2.21 C
Knees straight back part of circle

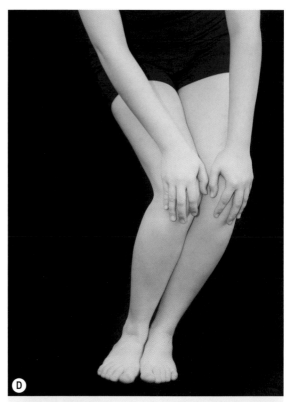

Figure 2.21 D
Other side of circle

CLIENT STORY

Personal story

My knees have served me very well. I danced profes-sionally for 10 years and became an extreme athlete before that term was conceived. I always considered my knees as sound and unimpaired and as benefit-ing from my good mechanics. I could run a marathon one weekend and the next weekend be in a dance performance. Life changes, however, and my level of training became more normal so I could fit in time for my family and work activities. In addition, I was deal-ing with Lyme disease that affected my joints. I was healing, feeling well, and so I began running again in a gentle way to ease back into a regular running routine. One day, my husband and I (both avid hikers)

were hiking a 5-mile trail and I felt a sudden "glitch" in my left knee. I stopped and tried moving it around to figure out what was happening. We had to return to where we started so I continued hiking, but very slowly and mindfully. Later, I had swelling and some pain, primarily on the inner side of my knee but also in the back. I iced it and had to walk very carefully. I knew the inflammation was either a tear or strain of the inner ligaments. I was not considering surgery so there was no need to have an MRI or see an ortho-pedic specialist. I opted for acupuncture to relieve the swelling and movement to restore the mechan-ics of my foot, knee, and hip. I noticed that my hip

(Continued)

felt out of sorts and suddenly weaker. The swelling was resolved after two sessions of acupuncture. This was great because the inflammation was way down, if any was still present, which gave me the opportunity to restore my knee through movement. Nevertheless, I ended up seeking an MRI because the doctor treating me for Lyme disease wanted to know if my knee issue was Lyme-related or an actual biomechanical tear. The examination revealed that I had torn the posterior horn of my medial meniscus. I was relieved, in a way, that it was not related to Lyme disease but to an injury. The orthopedic doctor told me that 52% of people over the age of 45 have a torn meniscus but have no symptoms and that it is no longer recommended to perform arthroscopic surgery for meniscus tears on people over the age of 50 since it may lead to future inflammation in the knee, causing degeneration. He gave me three choices: one shot of cortisone, one shot of another drug, or surgery. The surgery gave me only a 50% chance of being better. The odds were not high enough for me.

I focused all my training around improving my knee. It took me about 2 years to be completely back to full knee bending in a variety of hip positions. I followed my own protocol religiously. Working my foot, ankle, and hip was the key to easing the movement into my knee. What gave me the 100% return to function was restoring the micromovements of the knee, specifically the movement of the femur on the tibia. I was able to bring my knee back to full function, I had no pain and was able to hike, with an occasional run. I also looked deeply into myself and asked what I was not being present to in my life. I saw my purpose evolving into leading other teachers into manifesting their paths in this world of bodywork and Pilates. My passion turned toward writing this book and developing a way to assist Pilates teachers to continue evolving in their own path. And I am staying flexible for the twists and turns in life! Today, I continue to fine-tune my movements of the lower limbs and be mindful to keep my forward movement in life, ensuring that I maintain my healthy knees.

Standing Knee Circles (2)

- Stand with the feet hip-width apart, knees bent, and lean forward to place the palms of the hands on top of the kneecaps.
- The knees circle in opposite directions.
- Bend the knees and allow the knees to move in toward the midline (Fig. 2.22 A).
- Circle them away from each other (Fig. 2.22 B).
- Straighten as the knees circle back (Fig. 2.22 C).
- Roll the thighs inward and bend again in center.
- Repeat 5 times in this direction, circling from in to out.
- Reverse the direction by moving inward and back to straight legs.
- When the knees are extending during the circle, it is important to straighten the knees as the femur moves inward or outward for hip rotation motion.

- The legs roll outward; allow the feet to roll "Arches Out."
- The legs roll inward; allow the feet to roll "Arches In."
- Always be mindful to the feeling of all of the joints of the legs, and the depth of the range of movement possible without strain.

Seated postures

Simply sitting in these postures will allow for the tissue around the knee and hip to change the way the tissues pull from the pelvis through the leg.

Seated kneeling

- Sit back on the heels with a support (yoga block) underneath the pelvis.

- The knees are parallel, the thighs close together, aligned with the center of the hip joint in the front; the tops of the feet are in contact with the floor, especially the tops of the fifth toes.

- Gently press the outer edge of the fifth toe line into the floor using one thumb (Fig. 2.23).

- Breathe and sit for a few minutes if possible; gradually work up to 5 minutes.

- After resting, move into a seated straight leg position and pull the kneecaps up; work on the tracking.

- Repeat the seated posture 3 times and follow with the tracking of the patella.

Kneeling pelvic press

- Sit in a kneeling posture with the hands behind on the floor, or modify by placing a chair behind the body and leaning on it.

- Press the pelvis forward, lifting the buttocks off the heels, making a hinge shape from the knees through the body (Fig. 2.24 A).

- Maintain a long spine, minimizing the curve of the lower back.

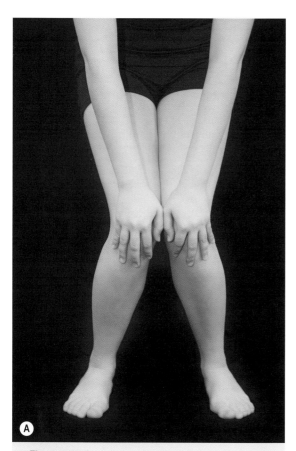

A

Figure 2.22 A
Knee Circles in opposition: inward

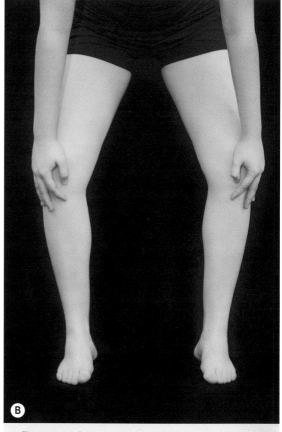

B

Figure 2.22 B
Outward

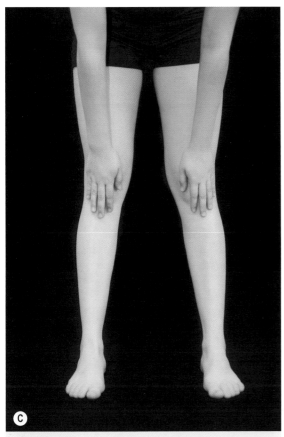

Figure 2.22 C
Straight legs during back part of circle

- Repeat sitting down and pressing the pelvis up.
- After 3 repetitions, stay in the pelvic press position.
- Turn the pelvis to face to the right, feeling the weight on the front edge of the knees; the pelvis stays pressing forward as the pelvis turns (Fig. 2.24 B).
- Turn the pelvis to face left.
- The micromovement is the rotation at the knee, and the hip macromovement of internal and external rotation in hip extension.
- The spine is moving slightly at the lower regions but the ribcage may not shift from side to side; it is an indication that the movement is not occurring at the knee and hip joint.
- Repeat several times in each direction; finish in the center.

In addition to working the knee rotation at the hip, it becomes an excellent anterior hip opener necessary to improve hip spin motion (described in Ch. 3).

Seated Butterfly, single and double

Single Butterfly (Janu Shirshasana A)

- Sit with one leg straight in front and the other in a single butterfly position.

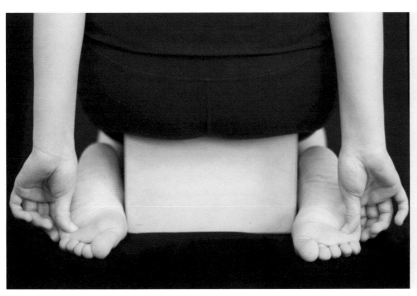

Figure 2.23
Sitting on block pressing fifth toe

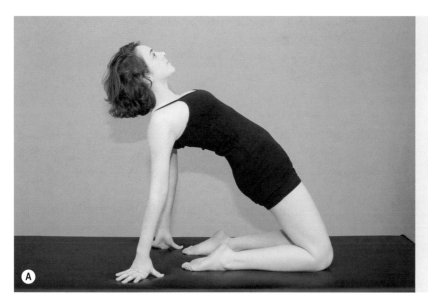

Figure 2.24 A
Kneeling Pelvic Press

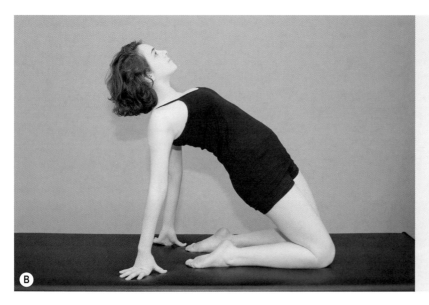

Figure 2.24 B
Kneeling Pelvic Press with rotation

- The sole of the foot on the bent leg is placed against the inner side of the straight leg at a range without any discomfort (I started at the level of the calf).

- The knee is open, the thigh turned outward (Fig. 2.25).

- It is common for the knee to be off the floor; if this is the case, place a prop (a block or pillow) underneath the knee to support the position.

- Elongate the spine and with a long spine lean forward, flexing at the hip.

- Actively lift the patella to contract the quadriceps.

- Sit without discomfort, starting with 5 slow breaths, building to 1–2 minutes.

- Repeat on the other side.

Double Butterfly (Baddha Konasana)

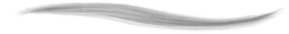

- Sit upright with the sits bones on the edge of a folded towel or blanket.

- Bring the feet together, knees apart; the legs are in a butterfly or diamond shape (Fig. 2.26 A).

- If the knees are higher than the pelvis, increase the height of the prop.

- Start with the feet in a range without any discomfort (the diamond shape of the legs maybe a longer or shorter diamond).

- Place the hands on the inner edge of one of the shins at the lower calf level, both thumbs against the edge of the tibia bone.

- Gently press into the area between the tissue and the bone to roll the tissue and bone away (Fig. 2.26 B).

- Work along the length of the shin toward the ankle (Fig. 2.26 C).

- Repeat on both sides.

- After the repetitions, straighten the legs again, track the kneecaps, contract the top of the thigh firmly.

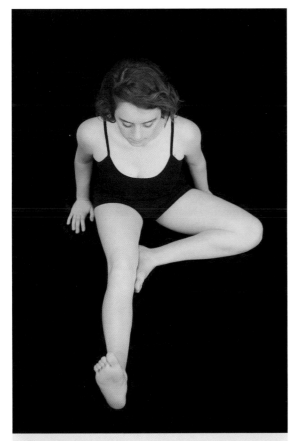

Figure 2.25
Half Butterfly

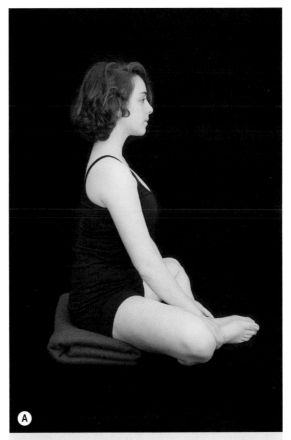

Figure 2.26 A
Seated Double Butterfly

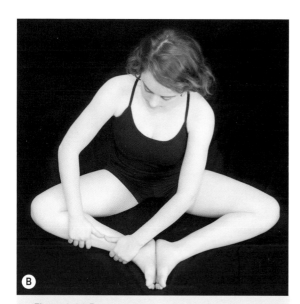

Figure 2.26 B
Hands-on rolling tibia

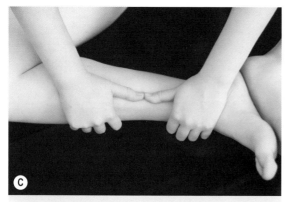

Figure 2.26 C
Hands-on rolling tibia along the shin

Inner/outer leg line activation

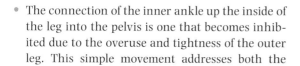

- The connection of the inner ankle up the inside of the leg into the pelvis is one that becomes inhibited due to the overuse and tightness of the outer leg. This simple movement addresses both the

lengthening of the outer leg and contracting the inner.

- Sit on the floor with straight legs wide; feel a light inner leg stretch; place the hands behind the body on the floor; allow the pelvis to be back (do not worry about being vertical).

- Bend one knee so that the foot is standing on the floor in the wide position (Fig. 2.27 A).

- Moving the straight leg, slide the leg toward the bent knee; move as far as possible to touch the bent knee (Fig. 2.27 B).

- Alignment is key here; the knee remains facing the ceiling throughout the range.

- When the knee moves across the midline, the thigh tends to roll inward; turn it slightly outward to maintain the knee facing up.

- When the knee moves outward the thigh rolls outward; spin it in slightly to keep the knee facing up.

- Repeat this 10–20 times on both sides.

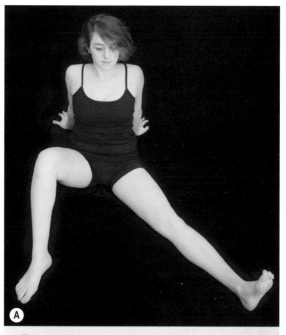

Figure 2.27 A
Inner/outer leg line activation: start position

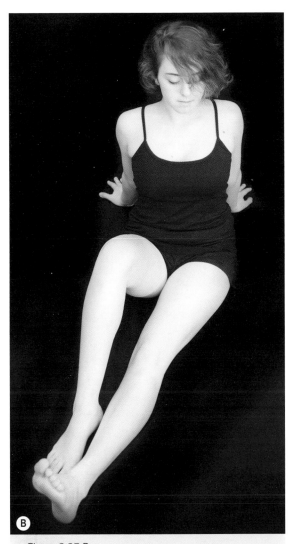

Figure 2.27 B
Movement

Bridging

There are many variations of bridging. All bridging is excellent work when the alignment of the spine, pelvis, and legs to feet is normal. Always concentrate on the places that are the stable points: the feet with the weight distributed across the toe balls, importantly the first toe, and center of the heel; the shoulder blades feeling weighted; and the back of the head. Move through the hips to find a long line from the head through the knees.

- Lie supine (on back), knees bent and feet standing on the floor.
- Either curl from the tail or press through the hips into a straight line bridge (Fig. 2.28 A).
- Reach the knees over the toes while the shoulder blades are anchored.
- Lengthen the spine, avoiding an excessive arch in the lower spine.
- Inhale on the lengthening into the bridge pose.
- In exhaling, either articulate through the spine until the sacrum and tail meet the mat or hinge at the hip to lower the spine long.
- Perform 5–10 times.
- Challenges are to perform the bridge, hold the bridge and unweight one leg, and hold a one-legged bridge (Fig. 2.28 B).

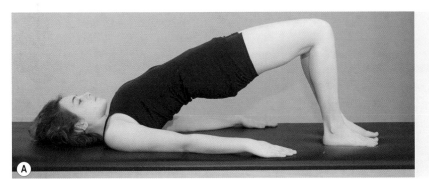

Figure 2.28 A
Bridging

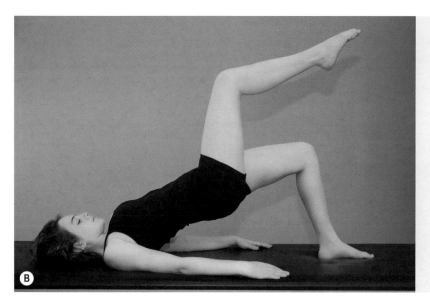

Figure 2.28 B
One-legged bridge

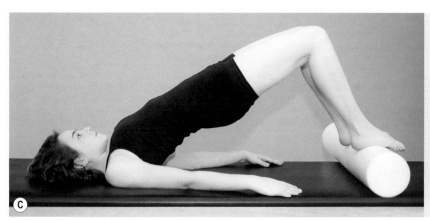

Figure 2.28 C
Using a roller

- Place the feet on a roller and, without moving the roller, move into the bridge (Fig. 2.28 C).

- Advanced bridges are also performed on the Reformer, the Wunda Chair, and the push-through bar on the Cadillac.

Wunda Chair VMO (vastus medialis oblique) exercise

Incorporating the tibia internal rotation to strengthen the internal rotators of the knee.

- Place a pad underneath the bar of the chair (the thickness will vary depending on the person's leg length).

- Sit on top of the chair facing the diagonal.

- Place the heel of the working leg, at the point where the calcaneus meets the talus, on the bar.

- The non-working leg is supported on a small box next to the chair (Fig. 2.29 A).

- Both hips are equally abducted and externally rotated only to the width necessary to achieve lower extremity alignment.

- The practitioner sits at the foot of the chair facing the client; be sure the hip abductors stabilize the femur and slightly internally rotate the tibia without supination of the foot (Fig. 2.29 B).

- Press the bar down, maintaining leg alignment; press into pads underneath the bar to activate full inner line of VMO; cue to press firmly and "squish" the pad.

- With resisting the bar lifting up, return the bar half way up and repeat pressing down.

- Continually monitor the alignment and muscle activation.

- Repeat 8–10 times.

Squats

Squatting is a natural movement necessary for all normal everyday activities. With knee issues, it can be tricky to do well and without stressing the knee. Awareness of how the bones are moving and of the rhythm of the bone movements combine to make up

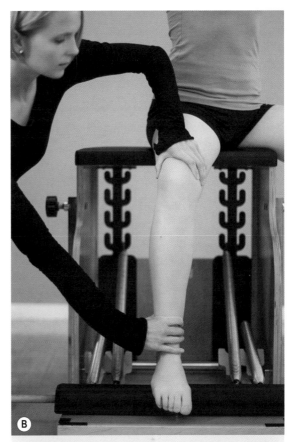

B

Figure 2.29 B
Hands-on and position

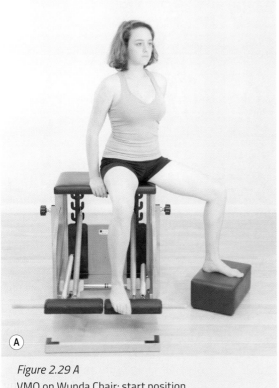

A

Figure 2.29 A
VMO on Wunda Chair: start position

the skill of moving in a healthy range. Always maintain a vertical tibia with the weight over the foot as if "standing on pencils." Move from the pelvis and hip joints. Practice every day to see an improvement.

- Starting stance depends on the flexibility and level of pain in knee bending and straightening; standing with the feet shoulder-width apart or wider if the hips are tighter with slightly turned out feet.

- Hold onto a door jamb or the bars on the Pilates Cadillac to allow bending well in the ankle, knee, and hip (Fig. 2.30 A).

- Begin by moving the tailbone back and widening the sits bones as the pelvis moves back; think of pulling the hips back.

- The trunk may lean forward in an elongated position; if holding onto a support, then work to maintain a more upright torso (Fig. 2.30 B).

- Maintain good body form and weight over the foot; stop the lowering if the weight on the feet shifts toward the heels.

- Press down into the feet as the pelvis rises up to standing.

- Repeat 5–7 times; gradually increase the repetitions.

- Perform additional sets, 1–2 with rest in between.

Russian Squat on the Cadillac

- Stand on the table of the Cadillac, holding the push-through bar without a spring.

- Begin to squat down, maintaining a vertical tibia (Fig. 2.31).

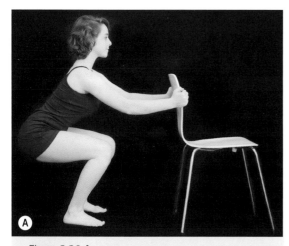

Figure 2.30 A
Squat holding a chair

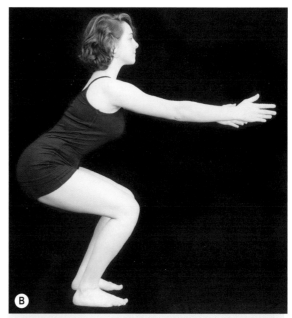

Figure 2.30 B
Squat

- Bend the knees as deeply as possible without discomfort in the knee; heels remain in contact with the table throughout the movement.

- Arms remain straight and the spine long, but may be forward.

- Stand up, moving through the posterior hip; tibias remain vertical.

- Repeat 10 times.

Notes on movement patterning for foot and leg work on Reformer

> Movement patterning on the Reformer
> **VIDEO LINK V 2.4**

Foot and leg work on the Reformer is vital work not only for strengthening the whole leg but also for re-educating muscle and timing the movement sequence of the limbs. The Reformer on its own will not provide the correct patterning. The body

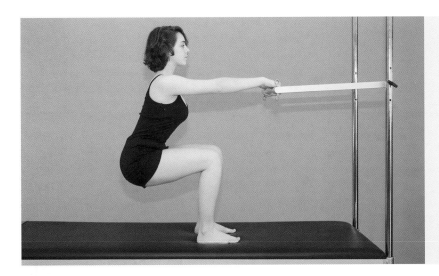

Figure 2.31
Russian Squat on the Cadillac

on the Reformer must be concentrating and feeling the pattern of pressing the carriage out and pulling it back in. The bones move differently on the way out than they do on the way in. Here is where the screw home mechanism comes into play. Review the "Screw Home Mechanism" section above (p. 44) if necessary to fully understand the importance of this function.

As the Reformer is sliding away from the home starting position (Fig. 2.32 A), the springs are increasing in tension, and the body is moving from a squat position to standing. The feet, in this example, are on the bar in parallel, contacting the heel where it meets the cuboid. The feet are stable and therefore the tibia is gliding on the talus and the femur is rotating as the hip extends. At the knee itself, the femur is primarily rotating on the tibia. To straighten the knee, the femur is spinning inwardly to create the external, screw home position at the knee (Fig. 2.32 B). The spiral of the thigh is inward with a balance of an outward spiral of the lower leg, not the foot.

Returning the carriage home, the springs are recoiling, pulling the carriage back home and changing the rhythm of the bones. First, the knee "cracks open," the rotation of the knee unlocks the puzzle pieces, then the head of the femur sinks into the hip socket as it flexes (a posterior inferior spin of femoral head, Ch. 3). The engagement of deceleration begins with the popliteus, stimulating the hamstrings into the gluteus and deep hip muscles through the spine. Now the

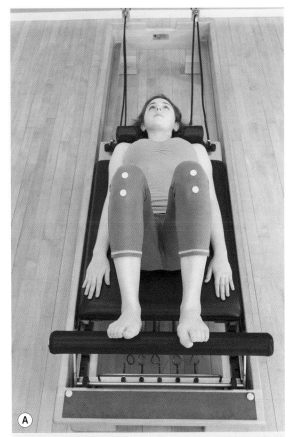

Ⓐ

Figure 2.32 A
On Reformer with the carriage home, observing knee movement

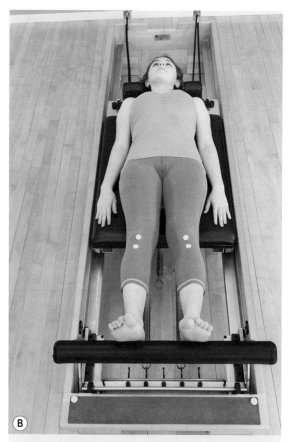

B

Figure 2.32 B
Knees extended

femurs are externally rotating on the tibia to create the internal rotation of the tibia, allowing it to bend.

When you are teaching this recruitment pattern, notice how the pattern allows for the knee to stay in its alignment. It completely eliminates the faulty movement of the knees falling into the midline when bending and rotating too far outward when straightening the legs. There is absolutely no need to place a prop, such as a small ball, between the thighs. In fact, this type of prop placement inhibits the healthy movement patterns of squatting to standing and standing to squatting and places undue stress on the knee.

Simply cueing with the use of a Theraband stimulates the proper timing of the whole leg during foot and

leg work. Using movement-directed cues is the most effective way to cue and recruit the desired muscle patterns, for example, "I am going to move your leg in this direction [hip flexion; demonstrate on them], and now do not let me move you." The client then moves into the opposite direction, stimulating the hip extensors. The initial pressing out is executed by the hip extensors.

Pressing out cues

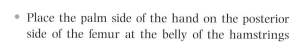

- Place the palm side of the hand on the posterior side of the femur at the belly of the hamstrings (Fig. 2.33).
- Using a movement direction to "do not let me move you" creates a resistance pressure into the hand to initiate the hip extension; allow the carriage to move away from the bar.

Carriage return cues

- Rest the palms of the hands on top of the tibia before the knee bends (Fig. 2.34).
- Cue the client to pull the tibias away from the hands, "soften the knees" or "crack open the knees," and pull the shins away.

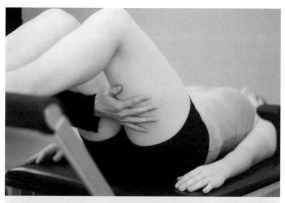

Figure 2.33
Hands-on posterior thigh for cueing

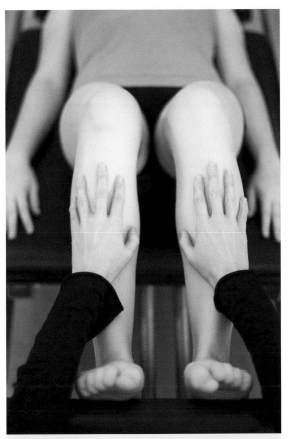

Figure 2.34
Hands-on shins cueing

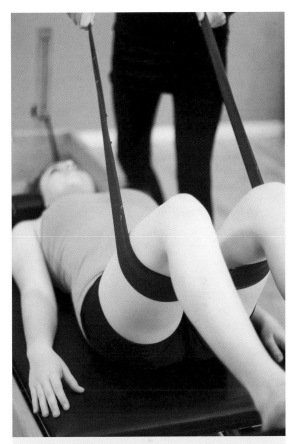

Figure 2.35
Theraband cue

- The action of the intention of moving the shins away recruits the knee flexors.

Using a long Theraband™ for patterning

- Place a long Theraband behind the mid-thigh at the belly of the hamstrings.
- Stand at the head of the client facing the client's feet.
- Holding both ends of the band, give it some tension (Fig. 2.35).
- Prior to moving the carriage, the client presses the thighs into the band and continues the pressing downward as the legs straighten.

- To return, "crack the knees," resisting the band as the carriage slides in.

Cue for internal rotation of the tibia

When the carriage returns and the knees are bending, notice if one or both heels begin to pivot inward, toward the mid-line. This is a dysfunctional tibial movement from the hip and knee.

- Place one fingertip at each outer point on the calcaneus (Fig. 2.36).
- As the knees begin to bend, cue to pivot slightly in the heel as if the foot were on a disc and press into the fingers.

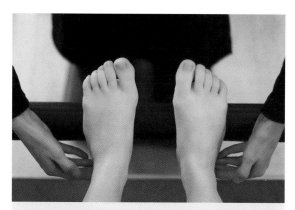

Figure 2.36
Hands-on lateral heel to cue inner spin of tibia

- Be sure the client is doing a pivoting action, not a sideways pressing on the finger.

Bridging to Chapter 3

The power to imprint into body memory a new foot to hip movement pattern is made attainable through practice of this timing of the bone rhythms. In any form of bending and straightening, moving forward, backward, sideways, or in spirals, the good form of motion in the lower leg chain in relation to the whole body will affect strength, flexibility, and tissue health. The body has an original design to move. When we are off center, the lines pull and torque the body, which changes the normal way we move. In Chapter 3, the sole to spine connections are brought together into the trunk.

Whole lower chain

> "With each step you fall forward slightly. And then catch yourself from falling. Over and over, you're falling. And then catching yourself from falling. And this is how you can be walking and falling at the same time."
>
> Laurie Anderson, "Walking and Falling"

MERGING INTO THE CENTER: PART 1

Contemplative awareness: winding and unwinding

Walking is the merging of the legs and the spine. What drives our ability to walk? Rotational or spiral motion is the basis of our human capacity to walk upright and be bipedal. In walking, the pelvis is moved by the spinal torque and compression brought about by the motion of the legs (Gracovetsky, 1988). The spine spirals as it torques and unwinds in a synchronized way, responding to the ground forces in a wave-like pulse that moves and dissipates from the foot through the knee, hip, and pelvis, then ascends the spine sequentially. This allows for a lessening of the impact from the ground forces on any one structure, where a constant load could potentially cause damage. In a balanced body, the torque is spread out during the cycle of each step, minimizing stress.

Movement travels, crosses, and torques throughout the body in any movement form we practice. The center of the spiral changes as we move in different ways. In an anatomical position, the center of gravity is at about the second sacral bone (S2), that is, the center of the pelvis. The center of gravity in the body is ever changing, however, depending on bodily proportions, the body's position, and the pathway of the movement. The lumbopelvic, sacral, and hip joints together form an integral system for the spine to generate the spiral of walking.

Legs connecting to trunk

Our legs provide contact with the ground, support the weight of the body, and swing freely. The legs play a role in modulating the ground pulses, rhythm, and speed, moving the body along a wide range of surfaces. The righting reflexes of the nervous system, the inner ear and the eyes, help guide the proprioception of our step, aided by the flow of information on how best to adjust the body in response to our changing environment, communicated through the fascia (van der Wal, 2012). A web of connective tissues (the fascia, the muscles, and the ligaments, all in relationship) travels from the trunk to the thigh and affects movement of the leg. Oblique lines can be seen in connective tissue, for example in the fibers running from one side of the chest to the opposite side of the pelvis (Schultz and Feitis, 1996). These connective tissues stimulate a continuous and connected motion of the legs into the trunk via the hip joint.

Hip joint

Joints have sensory receptors and mechanoreceptors that send information to our central nervous system to elicit subconscious responses in the body. Restrictions in the joints limit the range of motion, and can inhibit the healthy recruiting patterns that support movement. If this happens, the body's movement pattern becomes compromised and the spiral through the body is no longer continuous. A balance of hip joint mobility and strength is the key for transmission of forces between the foot and the trunk.

Practitioner note

Mobility is simply the active motion that is possible through design of the joint. Hip joint design is for greater mobility than the sacroiliac joint. Mobility is not the same as flexibility. Mobility improves the position of the body and facilitates optimal engagement for better performance.

The hip joints, also known as femoral joints, are ball and socket joints in shape, the ball being the top of the femur and the socket the concave surface of the pelvis (called the acetabulum). The pelvis sits on top of the rounded bones ("head") of the femur. In normal standing, the pelvis is balanced evenly, from front to back and from side to side (Fig. 3.1). The legs move freely in all directions in relation to the stable pelvis. Due to its interlocking position, the hip is quite stable, supporting our body weight, and it is the most difficult joint to dislocate. The hip joint gives us ambulatory action, which is a combination of mobility and stability.

There are three axes and degrees of freedom of movement in the hip joint:

- flexion and extension (forward and back) (Fig. 3.2 A)

- abduction and adduction (side to side) (Fig. 3.2 B)

- lateral and medial rotation (rotating outward and inward) (Fig. 3.2 C).

The freedom of movement in the hip joint is the ability of the head of the femur to have contact with the joint capsule in a way that elongates it and stimulates the fluids of the joint. The micromotion of the hip joint feeds the capsule through blood flow and synovial fluids that lubricate the joint. It is vital for hip joint health to have all degrees of movement available. Moving in all ranges of motion to challenge the hip promotes healthy hips and balance in the body.

Hip congruency and accessory movements

A full range leg movement such as a leg circle involves a large range of motion for the hip (known

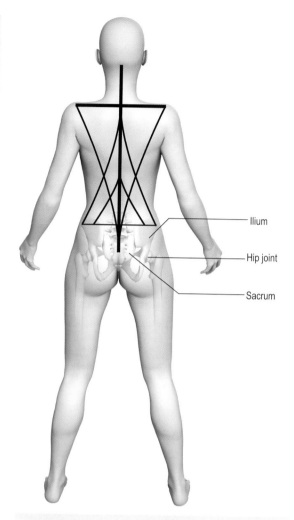

Figure 3.1
Balanced standing

as a macromovement). With all large (macro-) movements, there are small (micro-) movements coupled for transmitting the motion through the body. An accessory movement is the small joint movement necessary for full range of motion. For most people, these movements are involuntary or unconscious. Accessory movements are present in movements such as glide, spin, and rotation. For example, the calcaneal spiral described in Chapter 1 is an important accessory movement of the ankle (subtalar joint) that begins a sequence of motion. A restriction or loss of an accessory movement will inhibit the joint's ability

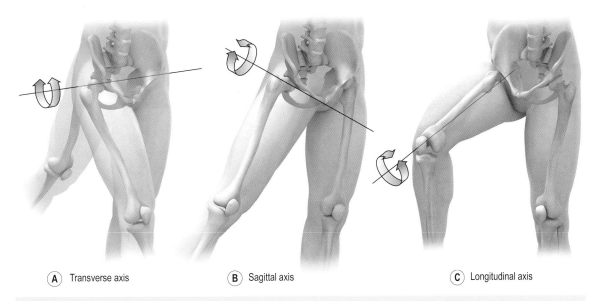

A Transverse axis　　　　B Sagittal axis　　　　C Longitudinal axis

Figure 3.2
A Leg flexion and extension axis
B Hip abduction and adduction
C Lateral and medial rotation

to be congruent and contribute to movement dysfunction. Restoring accessory movements influences the joint position, allowing for improved motion and accessible strength recruitment patterns of the myofascial components. There are many places in the body with accessory motions.

Look how the body alternates its macro- and micro-movements:

- micro: subtalar joint (calcaneal spiral)
- macro: ankle joint, flexing and pointing of the foot
- micro: knee (screw home mechanism and fibula movement)
- macro: hip joint
- micro: sacroiliac joint
- macro: spine
- micro: occipital and first cervical vertebrae.

Hip spin

In normal whole leg movements, the hip joint's component motion is described as gliding or, more accurately, seeing it three-dimensionally, as a spin motion. If the spin does not take place and the person continues to put effort into a movement, the joint stops moving, becomes compressed, and the muscles lose synergistic activation. In some cases, muscle cramping may occur and compensatory movement patterns develop; for example, during hip flexion, if the posterior capsule is shortened (see "Windshield Wiper Legs," below, for release technique), the motion of the posterior inferior spin is inhibited, jamming the femoral head into the anterior hip capsule. If the head of the femur is being held forward and not moving back into the socket, the psoas and gluteus maximus lose the ability to pull the femur into the posterior part of the joint. Then the hamstrings work too hard in order to compensate for the underworking gluteus maximus, which pushes the head of the femur forward. The lateral rotators, specifically the obturators internus and externus, are short and stiff, contributing to the restriction (Sahrmann, 2002).

Femoral head movements:

- Flexion: the femoral head moves posterior, inferior with small medial rotation.

- Hip extension: the femoral heads move anteriorly, superiorly with lateral rotation.

- Leg abduction is a lateral movement of the lower limb with inferior and medial spin of the hip.

- Leg adduction is the medial movement of the lower limb with superior lateral spin of the hip (Sahrmann, 2002).

Quadruped hip movements: pelvis on femur

Performing multidirectional movements that promote hip congruency, mobility, and stability of the hip joint will improve strengthening exercises for the hip. Moving the leg with a fixed pelvis, as in leg circles or side lying leg work, is commonly used to tone the hip muscles. There is an abundance of connective tissue connections running in many directions around the leg, pelvis, sacrum and spine; you can introduce a challenge to the hip by, instead of moving the leg, fixing the leg and moving the pelvis around the head of the femur. (Imagine a mortar and pestle – one can hold the bowl still and turn the pestle or hold the pestle still then turn the bowl around the pestle.) Notice how interrelated hip joint movement is with lumbopelvic motion.

To feel and enhance the femoral head motions, kneel in a quadruped position, with the hands placed under the shoulders and the knees in alignment with the hip joints. The spine and pelvis are in a neutral position, neither rounded nor bowed (see Neutral Pelvis, p. 114) (Fig. 3.3 A).

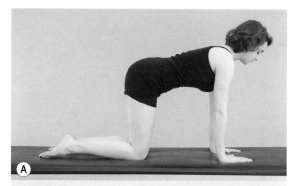

Figure 3.3 A
Quadruped hip movements: starting position neutral spine

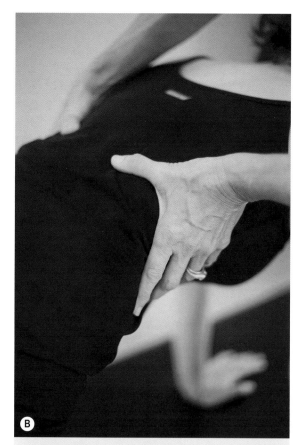

Figure 3.3 B
Hands-on

> **Practitioner note**
>
> For all the movements below, place your hands on the sides of the ribcage at the thoracolumbar junction point and hold it stable as the client moves the pelvis on the femurs (Fig. 3.3 B). Observe how the client moves.

Anterior hip joint movement sequence

- Begin at the tail. Curl the tail downward and under, moving the pelvis into a curl (posterior tilt), which also creates lumbar flexion (Fig. 3.4).
- Feel how the pelvis (acetabulum) is moving over the femoral heads.
- Try to be precise and only move the pelvis and lower spine. Do not move the lowest ribs.
- Return the pelvis to the neutral position by moving from the pelvis first, followed by the tail.
- Using the breath is helpful to enhance and deepen the movement. Inhale at the start; slowly exhale throughout the movement into flexion; inhale as you move into the neutral beginning position.
- Repeat several times until the movement is smooth and clear.

Posterior hip joint movement sequence

- Inhale in the neutral position (see Fig. 3.3 A).
- Start a slow exhale to tip the front and top of the pelvis toward the floor.
- Follow the pelvis motion by the movement of the tail upward or think of the sits bones moving up the wall behind you (Fig. 3.5).

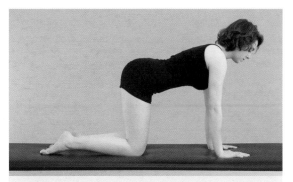

Figure 3.5
Posterior hip movement: extended spine

- The lower spine will bow slightly, but do not allow the lower ribs to move downward.
- Try to be precise; visualize the pelvis bowl tipping down toward the floor as the sits bones move up the wall, with the acetabulum moving anterior over the femoral heads.
- Inhale at the end of the movement.
- On the exhale, begin the return to neutral by curling the tail first, followed by the pelvis as in the anterior hip movement cues above; however, stop in neutral and do not continue into the full anterior movement of the hip.

Lateral and medial joint movement sequence

- From the starting neutral position, the pelvis will now stay level (see Fig. 3.3 A).
- Visualize the movement initiating from the top of the pelvis, not the tail.
- On an exhale, sway the pelvis to the right; the weight is more on the outer edge of the right knee and inner edge of the left knee (Fig. 3.6).
- Check how level the pelvis is (the tendency is to hike one hip up toward the lower ribs).
- Maintain the length of the waist on both sides.
- Inhale, move back to center.

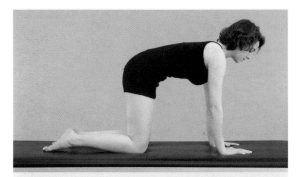

Figure 3.4
Anterior hip movement: curled spine

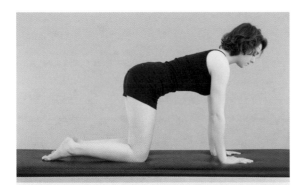

Figure 3.6
Medial and lateral hip movement: side to side

- Sway the pelvis to the left.

- Move back to center.

- Notice which side has difficulty in staying level in the pelvis; this is an indication of a limitation in the spinning side to side action of the hip.

Diagonal movement

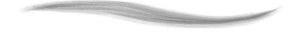

- Start in the neutral position (see Fig. 3.3 A).

- Sit back into hip flexion but direct the right sits bones past the right heel (Fig. 3.7).

- Again, the pelvis may not change its position.

- Stop if the pelvis and lumbar spine move into flexion.

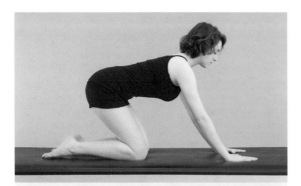

Figure 3.7
Diagonal hip movement

- Return to the center.

- Repeat on the left side.

- Choose to alternate diagonals or repeat one side several times before switching.

- It may be that one side is easy while on the other it is more difficult to maintain the pelvic position; repeat the more challenging side several times.

- Add a whole circle motion, moving from right diagonal back, to right side, to right front diagonal, through center forward (anterior), over to the opposite side left diagonal front, to left side, to left back diagonal, to center side (basically connecting all of the motions into one smooth circle glide) (Figs 3.8 and 3.9).

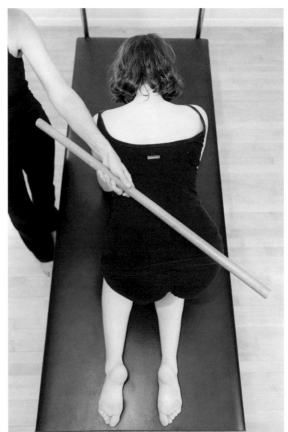

Figure 3.8
Circle hip movement

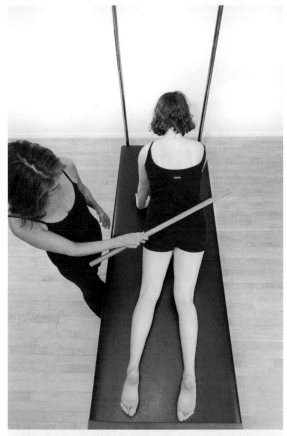

Figure 3.9
Circle quadruped

Rotation movement: the Tail Wag

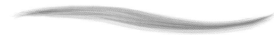

- Start in the neutral position, as above, and inhale.

- Exhale slowly as the tail initiates a side bending to the right (Fig. 3.10).

- The pelvis will unlevel, and the lower spine will side bend toward the side moving toward the lower ribs (hip hiking).

- Be precise and do not move the lowest ribs.

- Inhale and return to the center.

- Exhale and repeat to the other side.

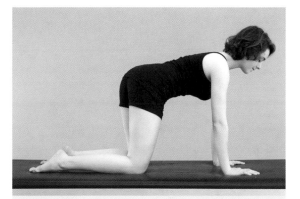

Figure 3.10
Tail Wag

Practitioner note

"Tail Wag" is an excellent movement to cue for the client to self-correct their position. When a person performs his or her own movement corrections rather than being placed manually, the brain imprints the new position more readily. The Tail Wag is also a great assessment tool for hip rotation and especially the lumbar side bending balance right to left.

Balancing the hip joint

In whole body movement, the hips are moving in a three-dimensional way. If the hip joints are in an off-balance position as a starting point, then movement will be altered and limited. For example, standing in a hip sway (a lateral translation of the hip joint) changes the alignment from the feet through the spine. It can cause one hip to be positioned in hip adduction and the other in abduction along with femoral rotation and anterior/posterior positioning of the femoral heads. When the hip joints are shifted to one side, the pelvis will be unleveled, with one side higher than the other, causing a pelvic rotation (see below, Fig. 3.11 B). The whole spinal chain above is compensating for the imbalance and the chain below is a misalignment of the legs into the feet, with most likely a leg length discrepancy. This is a common stance; it is often due to fatigue but it can be deliberately adopted, particularly by young women, because of a feeling that it is attractive or flirtatious. A long-term habit of standing this way may begin to develop restrictions in movement of the spine. Bring awareness of the benefits of standing equally on both legs.

Balancing the hip joint allows for the pelvis to sit more level on the femoral heads. Working in one range of motion, for example the medial and lateral spin, will subsequently improve hip flexion and extension. If a client is having difficulty in hip flexion, try the medial and lateral movements below followed by hip flexion movements and see if there is more ease in flexion.

> **Try it!**
> **Hip Sway Test**
>
> - Stand with the legs straight, putting equal weight on both feet.
>
> - Place your hands on the side of the pelvis at the place where the leg meets the pelvis over the greater trochanter (GT), not on the pelvis (Fig. 3.11 A).
>
> - Sway the hips from side to side, feeling for ease of movement.
>
> - The GT on one side will move into one hand (laterally) and other side moves away from the hand (medially); feel the dimple on the side of the hip become deeper as it moves away from the hand (Fig. 3.11 B).
>
> - Observe which hip does not move, or does not move well.
>
>   The hip sway side-to-side (medial and lateral) movement is an important joint movement for abducting (moving the foot away from the body) and adducting (moving the foot across the body).

> **Practitioner note**
>
> Use the "Hip Sway Test" above to assess the client's medial and lateral balance. Place your hands over the GT then sway the client side to side. Ask the client to be passive and allow you to move them. Listen with your hands for the ease of movement, as in gliding quality, and when the hip stops. If a restriction is evident, then use the movements of "Medial Spin and Lifts" (below) to facilitate change of the hip joint motion. Re-test the hip sway after the exercises have been completed and observe the quality and range of the hip motion.

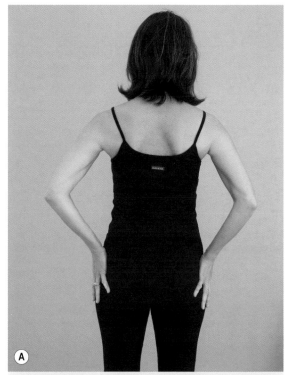

Figure 3.11 A
Hip Sway: start position

Exercises for medial spin and lifts

Improving the medial spin of the hip, and thereby its mobility, will encourage a reciprocal release of the inner thigh. A medial spin motion of the hip is limited by tightness of the inner thigh; the adductors, especially the adductor magnus, and subsequently the gluteus medius and minimus are inhibited. When the hip moves well in the medial spin, tone of the lateral hip musculature becomes functional. Working with restoring the hip joint accessory motion followed by strengthening the lateral hip is an intelligent sequence for encouraging the femurs to sit more central in the pelvis.

Adductor magnus MET and medial spin with trapeze

 Adductor MET on Cadillac
VIDEO LINK V 3.1

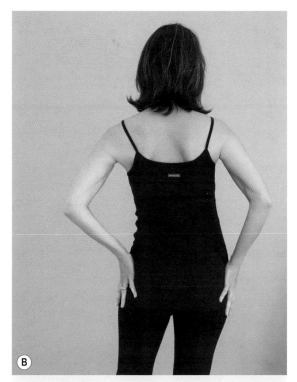

Figure 3.11 B
Swaying hips

This technique is done on the Pilates Cadillac using the trapeze to support the leg for isolation of the medial motion of the hip and as a barrier for resistance.

- Hang the trapeze of the Cadillac with two long heavy springs.
- The client side lies with the hip to be worked on top.
- Place the thigh through the lower strap of the trapeze at the point close to the pelvis; the knee is bent with the lower leg in alignment with the knee and hip (not externally or internally rotated) (Fig. 3.12).
- Stand behind the client to support the thigh with one hand reaching around to the front of the thigh.
- Support the knee by holding underneath the knee.
- Control the alignment of the leg, guiding it into the position desired.
- Cue the client to press into the strap, contracting and pulling the springs a very small amount.
- Hold the resistance for 5 seconds.

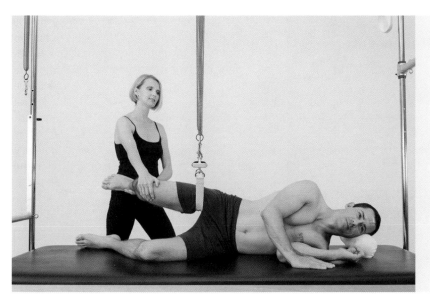

Figure 3.12
Adductor magnus MET Cadillac

- Release the contraction and allow the springs to recoil, creating a lengthening of the inner thigh.

- Assist with a slight inferior motion of the leg as it deepens into the socket.

- Repeat 3–5 times.

> **Practitioner note**
>
> Work with different degrees of hip flexion to access various lines of pull of the adductors; add a slight external rotation to access the posterior side (adductor magnus); also work with leg straight.

Leg Slide on the wall

It is recommended that the adductor magnus MET release be followed with movement to encourage integration of a new sensation of the hip.

- The client lies with the back against and along a wall and with the hip to be worked on top.

- Touching the wall: occiput, thorax, sacrum, heels (Fig. 3.13 A).

- Check the pelvis to be sure it is stacked and not rotated forward.

- The client or practitioner may hold the top of the pelvis with an intention of an inferior direction to maintain the pelvis level. NO HIP HIKING.

- Cue the client to slide the leg up the wall (Fig. 3.13 B).

- Repeat 10–15 times; stop at the point of first feeling a burn, rest, and repeat a second set.

> **Practitioner note**
> **Hands-on assisting the motion**
>
> Sit on the floor at the level of the pelvis and leg; reach the inferior arm under and around the upper to mid femur and use the superior forearm at the GT (Fig. 3.13 C). As the client slides the leg up, give a light traction out and press the forearm in and down (medial and inferior).

Femoral Glide with Magic Circle

- Stand sideways near a wall or side bar of the Cadillac; the side to be worked is away from the wall.

- Place the Magic Circle against the wall or bar and just above the GT on the ilium (Fig. 3.14).

- Stance is in optimal alignment with weight placed properly over the feet ("Standing On Pencils", Ch. 1) and small resistance into the Magic Circle.

- Reach the arms forward (>90° flexion) or fold the arms in front.

- Press the pelvis into the circle to compress it and slowly release.

- The hip joints are gliding to the side toward the wall, creating a medial glide and muscle engagement of the hip away from the wall.

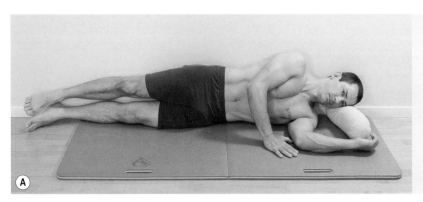

Figure 3.13 A
Leg Slide on wall: start position

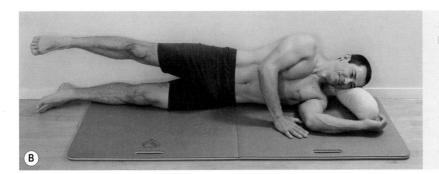

Figure 3.13 B
Leg sliding up the wall

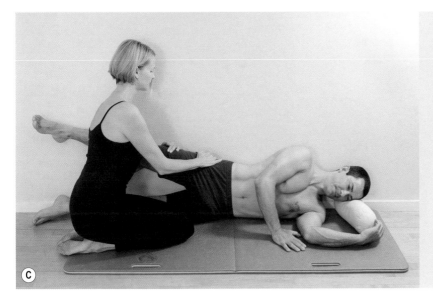

Figure 3.13 C
Hands-on Leg Slide

• Be precise in the movement; the whole body does not lean into the circle.

• No compensation of hip hiking or rib shifting.

> **Practitioner note**
> **Hands-on**
>
> Stand to the side of the client. Place one hand on the iliac crest and the opposite hand with a soft fist at the GT (see Fig. 3.14). As the client presses into the ring, assist gently to encourage a medial and inferior motion.

Femoral medial and lateral spin on Reformer ("Side Splits")

Performing the "Side Splits" on the Reformer is an excellent movement to encourage equal movement of the hips. The practitioner is able to enhance the movement, specifically the spin motion, while the client is moving. In any lateral and medial leg motion, whether standing, kneeling or lying down, the accessory motion of the hip is important to feel and see. Examples in Pilates include all the leg movements with long leg springs in abduction and adduction, and "Kneeling Side Kick"; examples in yoga are Utthita Trikonasana or Prasarita Padottanasana.

Set up the Reformer with a small standing platform and a light spring. A light spring allows for accessing the accessory motion of medial spin of the hip. If the spring is heavy, then the movement is changed from accessory to global motion. When the client lacks the accessory motion, working in a larger and heavier way will not give the body the opportunity to find the motion. The "Side Splits" exercise can be done standing

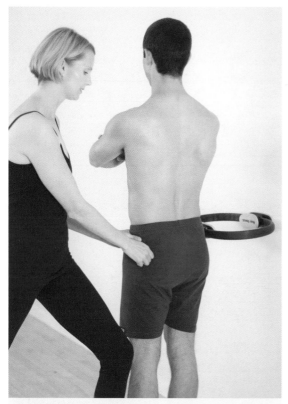

Figure 3.14
Magic Circle hip glide

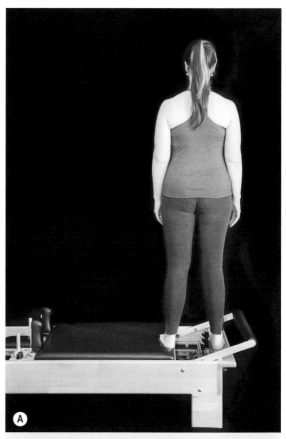

Ⓐ

Figure 3.15 A
Side Splits on Reformer

in the traditional form or kneeling, taking the feet out of the picture. The motion and hands-on are the same.

- Stand or kneel (pad the knee joints) with one limb on the platform and the opposite limb on the carriage (Fig. 3.15 A).

- Press the carriage away from the platform moving from both hips (Fig. 3.15 B). Observe how the spine remains centered throughout the movement. Try a cue to slightly shift the ribcage prior to pressing the carriage out.

- Return the carriage slowly and feel the elongation from the inner line of the legs up through the spine; observe how the body becomes taller as the carriage returns home.

- Repeat 10 times on both sides.

Practitioner note
Hands-on

Place the web space of both hands (between thumb and second finger) on top of the GT (Fig. 3.15 C). As the client presses the carriage out, follow the movement by gently drawing the hands closer together (medial) and feeling for the inferior motion and enhancing the downward movement. As the client returns the carriage slowly toward the platform, let up on the guidance. Repeat 2–3 times until the body has integrated the feel of a balanced hip movement; have the client repeat the movement without assistance several times; at this point changing the spring from light to medium is a choice.

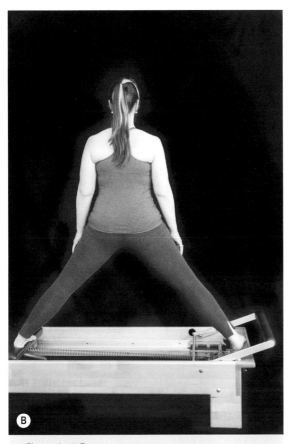

Figure 3.15 B
Pressing carriage away

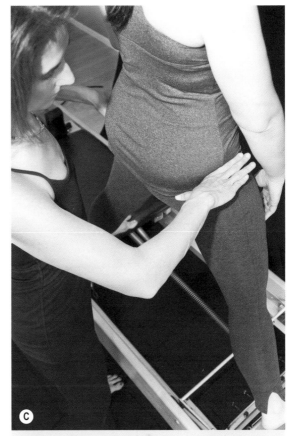

Figure 3.15 C
Hands-on

Hip flexion motion and spine stability

Both actions of moving the leg into flexion or rotating the pelvis anteriorly include the movement of hip flexion and therefore the micromovement of spin. This is easily felt while lying supine with the knees bent and folding at the hip (flexion) as the knee moves toward the chest, a Pilates fundamental movement called "Knee Folds." Gravity assists the motion of the hip dropping into the hip socket. Minimal thigh muscles are necessary to move the thigh into hip flexion in this position while the leg is dangling. If the spine is stable and the pelvis does not anteriorly rotate as the hip flexes, the work is more proximal, coming from the trunk. The initiation of hip flexion begins with the engagement of the iliopsoas that provides room to pull the head of

the femur into the socket and stabilizes the joint. Its longitudinal action is to pull the head of the femur in and create a stiffness to stabilize the spine (Hu et al., 2011). The elongation of the posterior hip capsule creates the room for the femoral head to drop back. For many people, the posterior hip capsule may be tight and restricting the ability for the femur to move posteriorly. Releasing the deep posterior hip assists a better spin of the femoral head and helps activate the psoas and multifidus for stability.

Windshield Wiper Legs: release for posterior hip

This release technique creates a softening of the posterior area of the hip, specifically visualizing the effect occurring at the level of the posterior capsule. This assists in increasing mobility and allows for improved posterior/inferior movement of the femoral head.

- Lie on the back, with both knees bent, feet on the mat.

- Place two small balls underneath the buttock, one at each side of a point about 2 in (5 cm) below the PSIS (posterior superior iliac spine) and about 1 in (2.5 cm) away (lateral) (Fig. 3.16).

- Move the bent knee like a windshield wiper, outward and inward, slowly.

- Maintain the pelvis in neutral (facing the ceiling) throughout the movement.

- Repeat several times; perform the movement on the other hip if necessary.

The ilioposas engagement stimulates a chain effect of turning on the psoas that originates at T12/L1 and runs downward along the spine, merging with the iliacus to attach at the femur (Fig. 3.17). The psoas

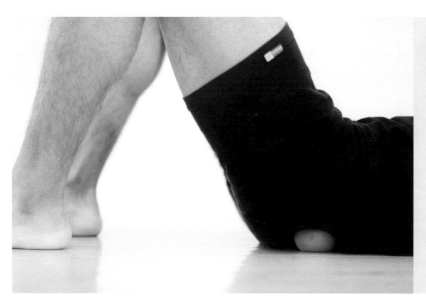

Figure 3.16
Small Ball posterior hip capsule release

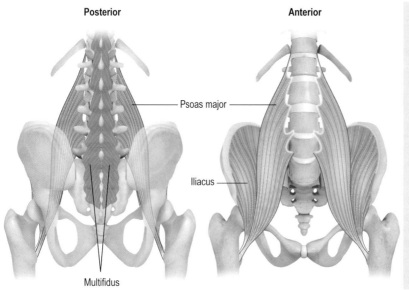

Posterior

Anterior

Psoas major

Iliacus

Multifidus

Figure 3.17
Front and back relationship of psoas major, iliacus, and multifidus

major has the ability to activate along its long body, the largest at the lower levels of the lumbar (McGill et al., 1988) in any position of the trunk.

Imagine the psoas and multifidus as airbags for the spine. Before beginning hip flexion movement (aka "Knee Folds"), visualize and feel a softening of the back hip and the dropping of the ball (head of the femur) into the socket. This will "inflate" the psoas and multifidus as airbags for the spine, providing the stiffness necessary to prevent a rotation of the lower spine as the leg begins to move. The power of thinking about the direction of movement stimulates the mind-to-body connection, turning on the local muscles for preparation to move globally. The anticipatory timing pattern of the psoas is similar to that seen in other local stability muscles (Gibbons, 2007).

> **Practitioner note**
> **Visual image**
>
> To provide an anticipatory response (turning on) of the psoas, imagine a puppet string running from the inner side of the thigh bone up through the pelvis, passing close to the spine up to the diaphragm. A puppeteer would be standing at the head to pull that string. When the puppeteer pulls the string, the tension begins at the top of the psoas at the diaphragm, and moves down the leg to initiate the thigh movement toward the chest as the foot lifts off the floor. The pulling tension of the string is the anticipatory action of the psoas to engage, the head of the femur pulling back and in to float the leg up.

Feeling the psoas activate: remember the "puppeteer's string"

Thigh Circles to set the head of the femur in the socket

To activate the "airbags" well, the femur needs to be sitting in the joint as well as possible.

- Lie on the back with the knees bent, feet flat on the floor.
- Bring the left knee toward the chest with the sacrum anchored into the mat.
- Place the left hand on top of the knee and straighten the arm; the lower leg is dangling and heavy (Fig. 3.18).
- Gently press the femur down deeper into the socket.
- Maintain a gentle pressure down and circle the femur deep into the socket (remember the mortar and pestle image but not crushing, just stirring).
- Circle in both directions, feeling the center of the joint and an even circle around it (the tendency is to miss the inner part of the circle).
- Repeat with the other leg.
- The pelvis stays facing the ceiling as the thigh circles; a low threshold of effort is present to stabilize

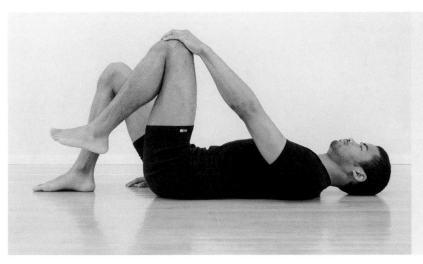

Figure 3.18
Thigh Circles

the pelvis so the hip may move without disturbing the pelvis.

- This is femur on pelvis motion versus the above exercise of pelvis on femur.

Activating the psoas

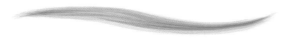

- With the left knee still up and the leg dangling, place the right hand on the top/front near the inner side of the knee (on the inferior, anterior, medial femur) and the left hand over the tissue near the crease of the right groin (Fig. 3.19).

- With the arm straight, press the knee into the hand and resist with the arm to bring up the tone of the iliopsoas and surrounding tissues. The psoas works with the internal oblique to stabilize the pelvis. Feel the area under the left hand for any quality of tissue change.

- Repeat on the other side.

- This provides a connection for the body to feel the activation. Using the feeling and puppet string imagery, when the client performs hip flexion or Pilates Knee Folds, the iliopsoas and the local muscles of stabilization kick in to stabilize before a larger movement occurs, such as "Single Leg Stretch " in Pilates or Navasana in yoga.

Practitioner note
Hands-on

 Hands-on activating psoas
VIDEO LINK V 3.2

- The client is lying on a table or Cadillac table, near the edge of the table.

- Stand on the right side of the client, facing their head (superiorly).

- Rest the client's right thigh against your chest and place the right hand on the inner top area of the femur to provide gentle resistance to hip flexion.

- Use the left hand on psoas to facilitate psoas contraction.

- Rest the base of the palm of your left hand over the ilium at the ASIS (anterior superior iliac spine) with the fingers facing toward the midline on the tissue near the groin to access the area of the psoas line of pull.

- Use the right hand to guide the femur slightly toward the midline, aligning with the insertion point of the iliopsoas on the femur (the lesser trochanter); no overpressure; the hip joint is still capable of micromovement within the joint.

- Ask the client to press the knee into your right hand and give resistance to the movement ("meet my resistance"); the client presses with an equal force to the amount of resistance you place on the knee.

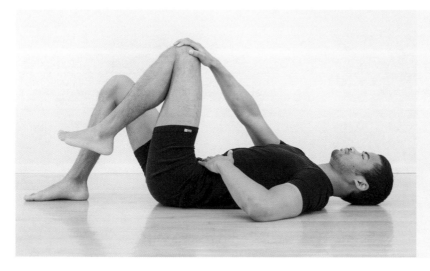

Figure 3.19
Activating psoas

- As the resistance begins, indicate the puppet string by moving the finger pads in a superior direction towards the line of pull.

- The tactile cueing helps the client's nervous system to register how to feel and turn on this area.

- The client repeats the hip folding (flexion with dangling leg, also called Knee Folds) without hands-on; repeat several times to imprint the feeling.

After teaching the felt sense, follow with a series of Knee Folds marching movement to challenge the core connection with hip flexion. Progress the challenge of recruiting globally and into more complex movements such as "Double Straight Leg Stretch" or Navasana.

"Psoas" Hip Circles on Cadillac

- Lie on the back (supine) on the Cadillac as in long leg spring series; use two heavy long leg springs (Fig. 3.20 A).

- Place the loop around and above the knee so that both hips are flexed and supported by the springs; lower legs are dangling.

- As in thigh circles, the pelvis is facing the ceiling and remains stable during the movement.

- Move the thighs in small circles (mortar and pestle):

  - begin in the down direction, toes toward the table (extension direction) (Fig. 3.20 B)

  - circle outwards in the range of hip extension (abduction)

  - slowly move in the flexion direction with the hips abducted

  - return to start position by bringing the thighs together (adduction).

- Reverse the direction: from flexion into abduction, abduction into extension, extension into adduction and adduction into flexion.

- Repeat 3–5 times in each direction.

- Figure eight motion: one leg moving clockwise and the other counterclockwise (Fig. 3.20 C).

- Time the figure eight movement with the thighs always moving opposing one another.

Cadillac long springs provide enough support for the legs so the motion deep in the hip socket is activating the psoas to do its "airbag" job of stabilizing the spine. The hip joint local muscles are challenged both eccentrically and concentrically. Lying on the back gives

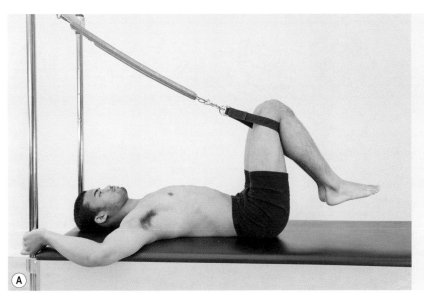

Figure 3.20 A
Thigh Circles on Cadillac:
start position

A

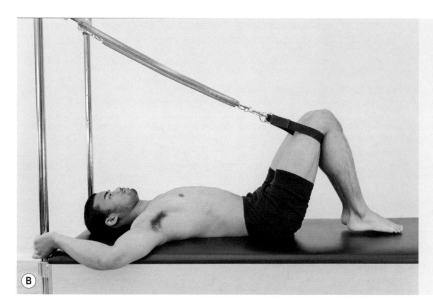

Figure 3.20 B
Pressing toward extension prior to abduction direction

B

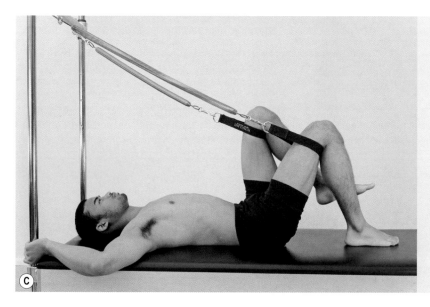

Figure 3.20 C
Alternating Thigh Circles

C

the spinal muscles support so the work is not inhibited in the front of the spine. The circling in the joint is also stimulating the joint surface for blood flow and nourishment of the joint.

Developing the consciousness of feeling the "psoas" during movements lying, sitting, standing, and walking gives a person a sense of support, a physical ease and grace. It is an integrated feeling. Moving in any movement from this sensation is a prerequisite for more complex movement patterning and challenges in global musculature.

Hip extension and spinal spiral in gait

Muscle strength of the legs is necessary in order to walk or run. The hips primarily drive the alternating leg movements, the pulling and pushing action. The combination of the eccentric work of the hamstrings and gluteals to decelerate the forward leg and the push-off of the opposite back foot releases energy, propelling the body forward. An integrated and coordinated action of the legs is a complex pattern. Training the strength of the hip joint in all planes will improve gait patterning. The spine is winding up and unwinding, moving the pelvis and legs along. Understanding the lumbopelvic and sacral motions in relation to hip joint movement is part of working with the whole dynamic of movement.

Posteriorly, the hip is directed to the spine via these continuous connections:

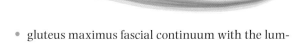

- gluteus maximus fascial continuum with the lumbodorsal fascia crossing over to the latissimus dorsi to the upper extremity

- gluteus maximus fascial continuum downward through iliotibial band to fibulas (Ch. 2, Fig. 2.8)

- biceps femoris to sacrotuberous ligament (consider the ligament as the long tendon of the hamstring)

- sacrotuberous ligament crossing over the PSIS to lumbar intermuscular aponeurosis

- lumbar intermuscular aponeurosis linked to the transverse process of lumbar spine through the iliocostalis lumborum, longissimus lumborum and the spinous processes via the multifidus

- lumbodorsal fascia mechanically linked to the fibulas through the sacrotuberous ligament and biceps femoris (Mitchell, 2001) (Fig. 3.21).

Weakness of the posterior hip is usually an inhibition of the posterior hip as a result of the anterior hip tightness, specifically the anterior joint capsule and the iliopsoas (Yerys et al., 2002). The anterior hip restriction creates a barrier in hip extension. The anterior hip tightness and lack of heel lift prior to toe-off is facilitating a central nervous system response to protect the hip from moving beyond its restrictive range. In addition, if the foot is unable to spiral and resupinate as the heel lifts, it inhibits the soleus and gastrocnemius work (posterior compartment of the lower leg) to switch from the decelerator to the knee flexion movement carrying the leg forward for the next step.

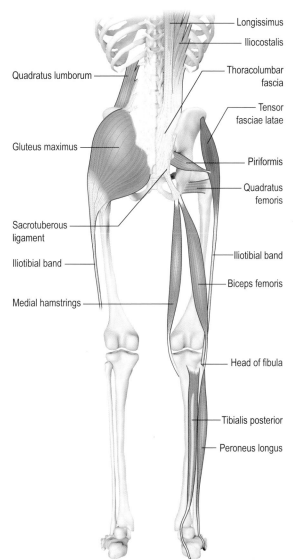

Figure 3.21
Mechanical link between lumbodorsal fascia and fibulas through sacrotuberous ligament and biceps femoris

Prior to strengthening the posterior hip, a release of the tight anterior hip structures will eliminate the protection response and allow an increased range in the hip to become available. With improved range, the posterior hip musculature will be able to engage properly. Note that it is also important to observe and work the foot and ankle when training the hip.

*Anterior hip release on Reformer or physioball:
lunge with hip drop*

 Lunge with hip drop
VIDEO LINK V 3.3

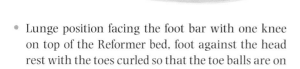

- Lunge position facing the foot bar with one knee on top of the Reformer bed, foot against the head rest with the toes curled so that the toe balls are on the carriage and heel pressing against the shoulder rest; the other leg is placed close to the front leg of the Reformer (Fig. 3.22 A).

- Hold onto a foot bar in the high position, with one medium spring.

- Be sure the pelvis is level (a small bolster or prop may be used under the knee to level the pelvis).

- Standing leg alignment is knee bent with the knee over the ankle, tibia vertical.

- Place about 75% of your body weight onto the knee on the Reformer carriage.

- Two actions to slide the carriage back occur at the same time:

  - pressing the foot firmly into the shoulder rest to press back

  - standing leg action lowering the pelvis downward by deepening the bend in the hip (hip flexion) with an elongation of the standing thigh (increasing hip flexion without the knee moving forward or back).

- Stop the carriage movement when the pelvis begins to unlevel or rotate (Fig. 3.22 B).

- Inhale in the pause.

- Exhale and purposefully lower the ilium of the carriage leg downward, away from the rib of the same side; it is a small side bending movement of the lumbar spine (Fig. 3.22 C).

- The hip is no longer level but elongating between the one side of rib and hip.

- Gently come up out of the position.

- Repeat 3 times.

- On the physioball, hold onto a table or counter top and try to simulate the angle of the trunk as shown.

- In the lunge stance, the moving leg is on top of the ball with the shin resting on the ball (Fig. 3.22 D).

- About 75% of the body weight is on the ball or Reformer – IMPORTANT!

- Movement for the physioball is the same as the Reformer action described.

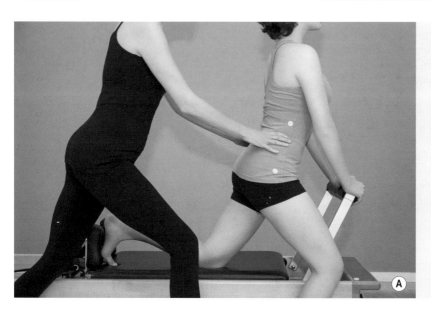

Figure 3.22 A
Anterior hip release lunge on Reformer: start position

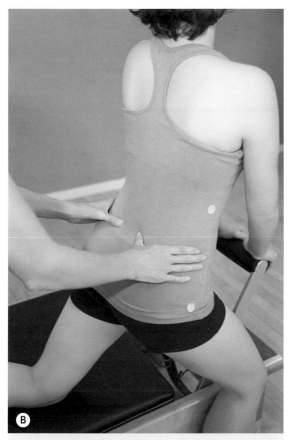

Figure 3.22 B
Moving carriage away

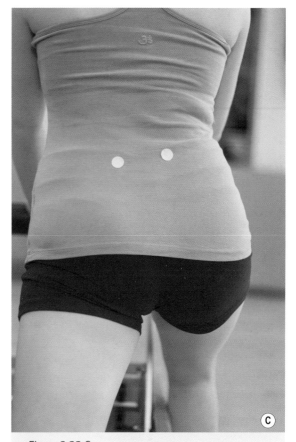

Figure 3.22 C
Unleveling the pelvis

Practitioner note

Stand behind the client to monitor the alignment of the pelvis. Place your hands at the rim of the pelvis to give a felt sense of a level pelvis (Fig. 3.22 E). The first repetition is usually not well executed. The second and third repetitions will be significantly better. The pelvis movement is small, only enough to allow lumbar side bending. Place your hands at the thoracolumbar junction (lowest ribs) to stabilize this area of the spine, to allow the lumbar spine to move, and to inhibit the ribcage from shifting.

Rotators of the hip

Posterior hip function is not only the work of the gluteus maximus, hamstrings, and its lines of fascial connections but the muscles attaching close to the top of the femur that control the alignment and motion of the femur in the acetabulum. One significant group, the lateral rotators, lies under the gluteus maximus. It is a fan of muscles directly connecting the femur to the spine via the iliopsoas and the pelvic floor via the obturator internus.

In traditional studies of anatomy and kinesiology, the deep hip muscles are known as the lateral rotators, or "deep six." However, the term "lateral rotator" is not a clear description of the many actions of this group. The orientation of the leg and pelvis in space will change the rotators' movement. The alignment of the femur and motion of the hip joint determines how the lines of the fan pull the limb, creating the desired movement. It becomes a paradoxical group of muscles.

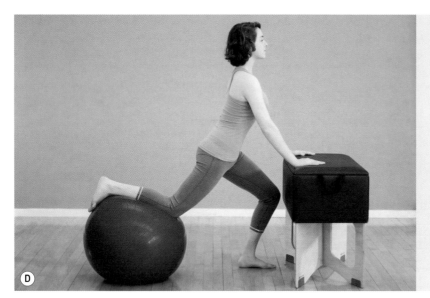

Figure 3.22 D
Lunge on physioball

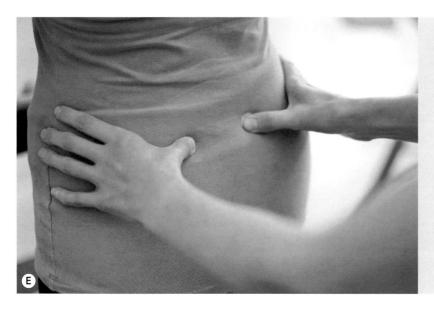

Figure 3.22 E
Hands-on

The "six" lateral rotators are, from the top of the fan to the bottom:

- piriformis: also abducts the hip above 60°

- superior gemelli: steadies the femoral head, assists in extension and abduction

- obturator internus: attaches to the levator ani pelvic floor group

- inferior gemelli: steadies the femoral head, assists in extension and abduction

- obturator externus: also a medial rotator

- quadratus femoris: also adducts and participates in hip extension or flexion

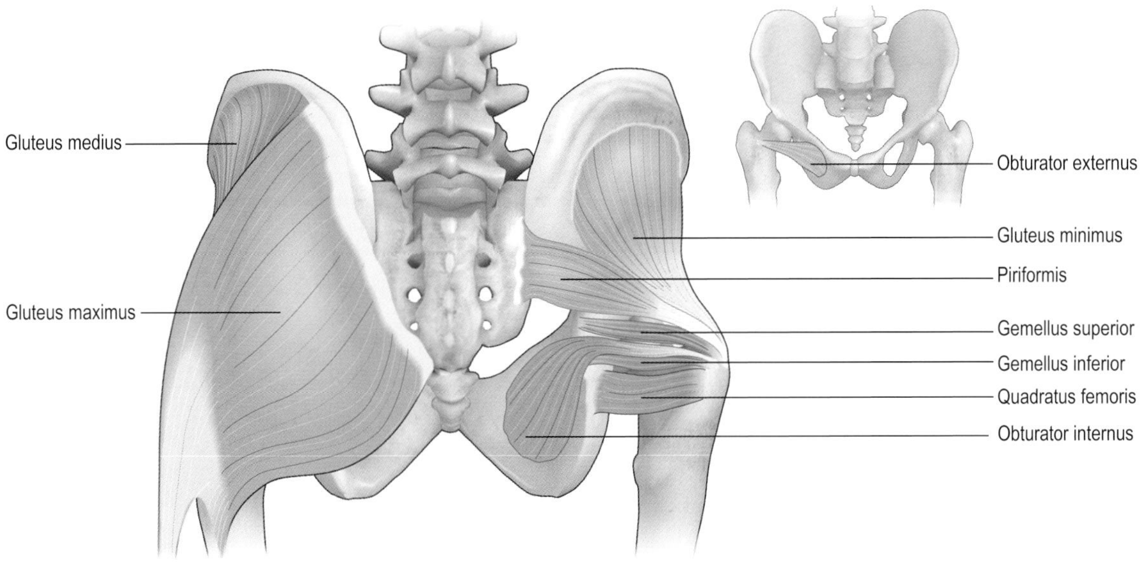

Figure 3.23
Lateral rotators of hip

Labels on figure: Gluteus medius, Gluteus maximus, Obturator externus, Gluteus minimus, Piriformis, Gemellus superior, Gemellus inferior, Quadratus femoris, Obturator internus

- as a new addition to the group, now called the "Seven," consider gluteus minimus (Fig. 3.23).

Practitioner note

In the relationship of the deep fascia and the fan of tissue of the posterior hip, clearly the gluteus minimus participates in lateral rotation, medial rotation, and abduction. The line of the leg in space determines the path that the line will pull. For example, when the leg is in abduction and a small degree of flexion and internal rotation, the line is working the rectus femoris, TFL, gluteus medius and minimus up to the internal oblique. The body does not function in isolated muscles, but as a whole unit working together through various lines of tension.

Medial rotators are less numerous than the lateral rotators and the range of motion between external rotation and internal rotation of the hip is not equal. The normal range is approximately 40–60° in lateral rotation and 30–40° in medial rotation. However, there are many variations in the shape of the joint and the angle of the neck of the femur that will increase or restrict the range. In addition, the strong ligaments around the head of the femur can be very tightly held, in contrast to those of people with hypermobility, who may have longer, looser ligaments, allowing greater ranges of movement. The degree of a person's range of motion is relative to their structure, training, and movement habits in life.

The muscles that play a role in medial rotation are:

- tensor fasciae latae
- gluteus medius and minimus
- if the range of the medial rotation is increased beyond 30° then the pectineus and obturator externus become medial rotators.

Hip relationship with spine and sacrum: connecting attachments of hip

There is a balance between the sacrum and the lumbar spine through the relationship between the piriformis, other rotators, iliacus, and psoas. Together they create a continuous supportive web connecting the spine to the femurs. Imagine a structure whose front is too long and whose back is too short. The guide wires are taken off and the structure will tip forward.

Front to back:

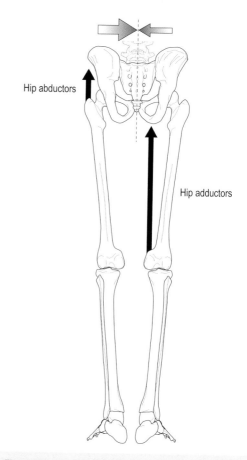

- back from sacrum to femur (piriformis, and other lateral rotators) at the greater trochanter (see Fig. 3.23)

- front from spine to femur (iliacus and psoas) at the lesser trochanter (see Fig. 3.17).

Side to side:

- lateral side ilium to femur of one leg (hip abductors: gluteus medius and minimus)

- medial side pubic ramus of ilium to femur of opposite leg (hip adductors: adductor magnus, gracilis, longus and pectinus) (Fig. 3.24; see also Fig. 3.11).

Hip myofascia

The hip myofascia is intimate with the pelvic bowl, specifically the lower area, called the pelvic inlet or pelvic diaphragm. The fascia covers the sides and bottom of the bowl (visualize wallpaper inside the wings of the pelvis) and is continuous with the pelvic musculature. The "wallpaper" is made up of the obturator membrane, the obturator internus muscle and its fascia, which is continuous with the levator ani. The sacrotuberous and sacrospinous ligaments are also part of the internal surface of the pelvis (Snell, 2012). The tissues are merging from the sides in toward the center of the pelvic floor, the inferior or lower wall (Fig. 3.25).

The leg fascia is more superficial until the femur enters the pelvis and then merges into the deep pelvis, becoming part of the pelvic floor. Visualize how the legs continue to reach upward following the path of the psoas to its origin at the thoracic diaphragm. Thus, the legs do not end at the bony joint but remain continuous into the thorax. The legs end or begin at the diaphragm, and are longer than imagined (Fig. 3.26)!

The movements of the medial/lateral motions and working with hip extension directly improve the rotators of the hip. Moving in various ranges and positions of the hip improves function.

Figure 3.24
Posterior view of side to side relationship of the abductors and adductors when standing with a right hip sway

Moving in hip extension

It is impossible to move the hip into extension by leg alone. The pelvis and sacral motions are integral to the movement. Read through the pelvis and sacrum sections prior to practicing the following movements to thoroughly understand the movement relationships for healthy extension.

Spiral of femurs prone

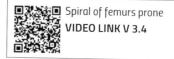

Spiral of femurs prone
VIDEO LINK V 3.4

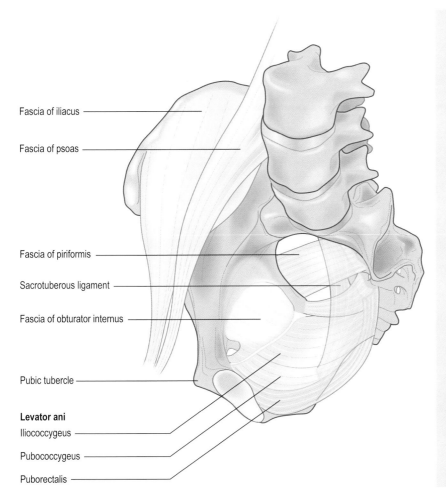

Fascia of iliacus

Fascia of psoas

Fascia of piriformis

Sacrotuberous ligament

Fascia of obturator internus

Pubic tubercle

Levator ani
Iliococcygeus

Pubococcygeus

Puborectalis

Figure 3.25
Hip myofascia connections to the pelvic diaphragm

Whether you are lying on your stomach to lift the trunk and legs or bridging or standing to drop back into Setu Bandhasana (backbends), the pelvis and sacrum move together, and the hip joints extend, thus creating the openness in the front of the body. The internal spiraling of the femurs as the hip extends moves the ilia, creating a narrowing across the front of the pelvis and widening of the sits bones, allowing for hip movement. The ascending motion through the spine into backward bending is emphasized in the upper thorax lifting and contrasting the direction of the pelvis. For each individual, it is necessary to explore how to find the "sweet spot" of hip action, sacral and pelvic motion with the contrast of the spine lengthening. In larger, whole body movements, finding the contrast of the force with the balance of letting go is within a personal practice.

Finding the internal spiral with sacral nutation

- Lie prone (on the stomach).

- Align the body; spiral femurs inward, allowing the heels to move outward (Fig. 3.27 A).

- Place a wood block between the upper thighs.

- Move the heel slowly inward until the heel is pointing straight up to the ceiling, neither in nor out.

- The thighs will move slightly and closer to the block; thigh bones move into the block.

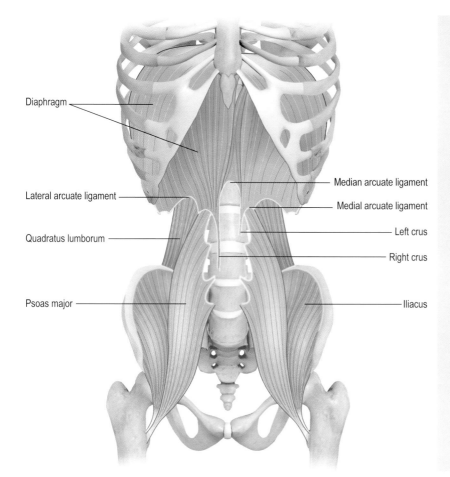

Figure 3.26
Leg connections to the thoracic diaphragm via the psoas

Diaphragm

Lateral arcuate ligament

Quadratus lumborum

Psoas major

Median arcuate ligament

Medial arcuate ligament

Left crus

Right crus

Iliacus

- The sits bones stay wide as the heel moves in toward the midline (Fig. 3.27 B).

- Feel the connection from the inner heel up the inner leg and at the same time the deep outer hip (abductors) engaging, causing a pressure into the block, not a squeezing of the block.

- Imprint this feeling and activity of the legs from the inner heel up and around the thigh.

Working on the spirals of the femurs will move the pelvis into a more neutral position naturally. However, it is common to experience the thoracolumbar junction moving too far into extension. The person has lost the action of the elongation of the trunk, especially the side body (waist). Cue the lower ribcage angle (costal angle) backward (posteriorly) just enough to match the lengthening of the waist.

The contrast of work here is to maintain the spiral feeling of the femurs and the anchor (weight) of the pelvis with connection into the lower ribs.

Practitioner note

To increase the activation from the inner heel to the hip, cue the roll of the heel by placing your hands on the inner heels (Fig. 3.27 C). Ask the client to slowly roll their heels into your hands to align the heels with the ischial tuberosities. Verbally cue that the heels are moving in toward the midline but the sits bones (ischial tuberosities) stay wide. Add a single or double leg lift maintaining this active alignment of the femurs and pelvis. Be observant that releasing the anterior hips prior to this exercise may be necessary in order to spiral the thighs and maintain the trunk integrity.

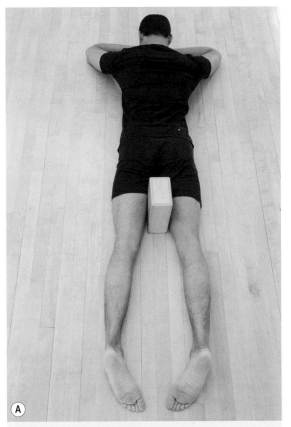

Figure 3.27 A
Spiral of the femurs prone: start position

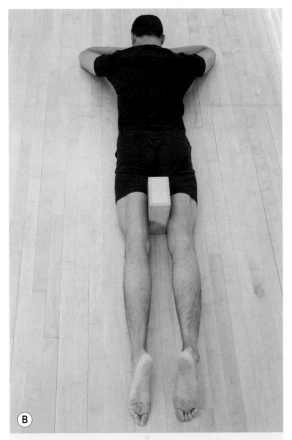

Figure 3.27 B
Aligned position

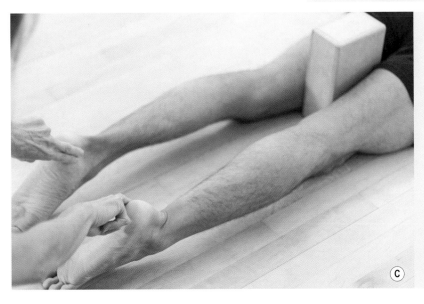

Figure 3.27 C
Hands-on

Push-off hip extension

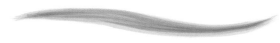

- The client lies prone with the femurs aligned and active as in the inward spiral of femurs above.

- Rest the forehead on hands that are stacked.

- Soften the left knee and tuck the toes under so that the foot is weighted on the metatarsals (toe balls) (Fig. 3.28 A).

- The weight is distributed across the metatarsal arch with more weight on the first toe ball (metatarsophalangeal or MP joint).

- Place a finger at the center of the heel and ask the client to press into the finger to push it away.

- The client extends the knee by flexing in the ankle and extending the hip.

- Observe for:

  - the spiral alignment of the leg

  - recruitment of the hamstrings–gluteals–opposite lumbar–bilateral lumbar area

  - pelvic maintaining nutated position and pelvis in neutral.

- Repeat 5–8 times until the pattern is established and coordinated.

- Perform on the other side.

- Ask the client to repeat the movement without the tactile cue.

- When the pattern is apparent, add holding the leg extended with the toe on the mat.

- Without the femur moving, point the toe (plantarflexion with movement of the femur) (Fig. 3.28 B).

- Dorsiflex the ankle to place the toe on the mat with the leg holding the hip extension.

- Soften the knee to finish.

- Repeat 10–15 times.

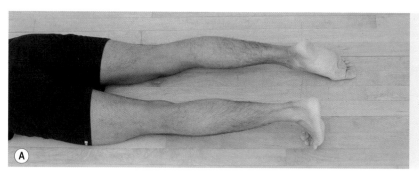

Figure 3.28 A
Push-off hip extension

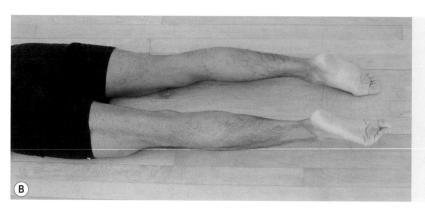

Figure 3.28 B
Lifting the leg

Hip extension prep on box

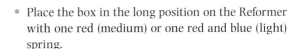

- Lie prone on a Reformer box or the edge of a table where the box or edge of the table is at the crease of the hip and the knee hangs down in knee flexion with the top of the foot resting on the floor (Fig. 3.29 A).
- Create elongation of the spine and feel the knee heavy toward the floor.
- Reach the knee down without changing the pelvic position.
- Slide the foot away from the box as the knee straightens (Fig. 3.29 B).
- When the leg reaches full knee extension, raise the thigh up maintaining the spiral inward position (Fig. 3.29 C).
- The pelvis maintains its position on the box but the sacrum moves into the direction of nutation.

- Observe where in the space the leg moves (the tendency is to abduct the leg out of alignment of the center of the hip joint).
- Repeat this 10–15 times.
- Once the movement is consistent in good form, add an ankle weight.

Swan on the Reformer using the box

This exercise is integrating the felt sense of proper alignment, healthy hip engagement, and full body extension. The feet are fixed on the frame of the Reformer and the motion of the hip will now be pelvis on hip rather than as in the prep exercise above, hip on pelvis.

- Place the box in the long position on the Reformer with one red (medium) or one red and blue (light) spring.

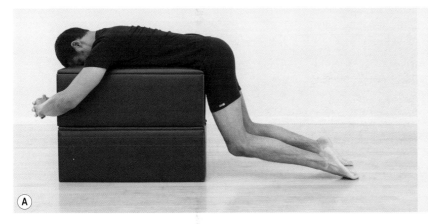

Figure 3.29 A
Hip extension prep on the box: start position

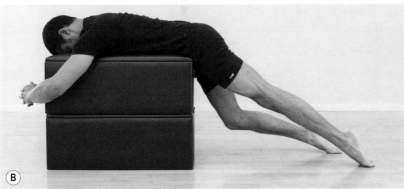

Figure 3.29 B
Extending the leg

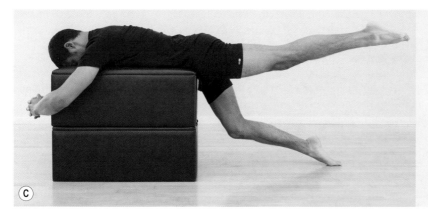

Figure 3.29 C
Lifting the leg

- Lie on the box prone facing the straps; the position on the box is the same as the hip extension prep on the box exercise above; the feet are placed inside the wood frame with the toe balls firmly planted on the wood (Fig. 3.30 A).

- Begin with the carriage at rest, the spine elongated on the box.

- The ankle joint remains in the available range of dorsiflexion, knees reaching toward the floor and active spinal elongation; cue "keep your Achilles long."

- First practice pressing the carriage out, keeping the Achilles long; the spine maintains its elongated position on the box.

- Returning the carriage in, cue "first soften the knees before the hip bends more, then reach the knees to the floor as you slowly bring the carriage home."

- When the movement timings of the ankle, knee, and hips are established, then add the spinal extension (Fig. 3.30 B).

- Press the carriage with good leg movement; with the legs extended, lift the trunk long off the box (Fig. 3.30 C).

- In one smooth movement, soften the knees, and reach the knees to the floor as the trunk lowers back onto the box.

- Repeat 5–10 times.

Hip rotation in extension movement

The movement from the "Kneeling Pelvic Press" exercise in Chapter 2 is excellent for improving the knee rotational micromovement, in addition to opening the front of the hip and its diagonal fibers. It benefits the knee and hip at the same time.

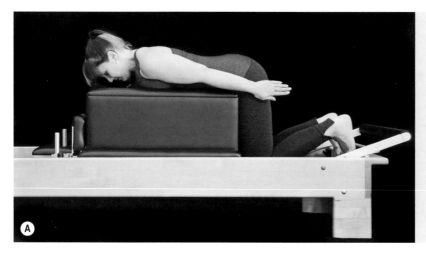

Figure 3.30 A
Swan on the Reformer using the box

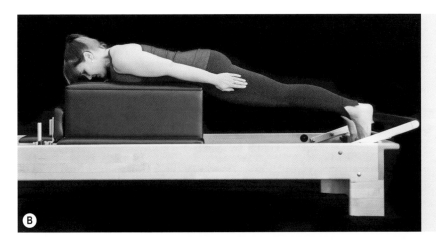

Figure 3.30 B
Adding elongation of spine

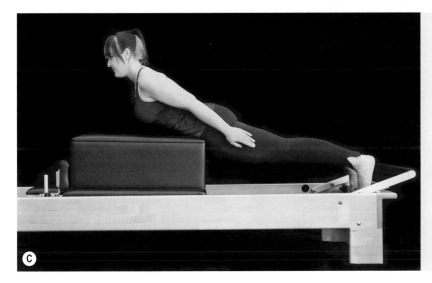

Figure 3.30 C
Lift of trunk

Bridging with hip rotation

In Chapter 2 "Bridging," adding pelvic rotations in the bridge works the rotation movement aspects of the hip. The movement is occurring primarily in the hip joint and the spine is maintaining its relationship with the pelvis (see Fig. 2.24 B). Simply cue the bridge movement: "face the pelvis to the right (rotating pelvis to the right), move back to center, face the pelvis to the left (rotate pelvis to the left), return to center."

Hovering Bridge on Reformer

In all foot and leg work or standing postures, the practitioner may observe the movement initiating from foot to spine or from spine to foot. In this exercise, the recruitment is hip motivated not foot motivated.

"Hovering Bridge" is a variation of a full bridge where the position requires integrating the strength of the local back stabilizers, pelvic stability (especially "psoas" activation), local hip muscles, and hamstrings. It teaches the client the muscle sequencing of controlling the carriage return.

- Begin lying on the Reformer prepared for foot and leg work, with one light spring.

- Place the rear to mid-foot area (heel) on the bar, where the cuboid and calcaneus meet.

- The pelvis will float slightly off the carriage, unweighting the sacrum but not changing the nutation of the sacrum and neutral pelvis (Fig. 3.31 A).

- Cue: " the fabric of your tights (or pants) is still on the carriage but there is no weight on the sacrum; float the sacrum."

- The carriage remains in the home position while floating the pelvis.

- Maintaining the pelvic position of floating, press the carriage out (Fig. 3.31 B). Motion occurring from hip extension, not pressing through the feet.

- Legs almost lengthen fully but do not straighten completely.

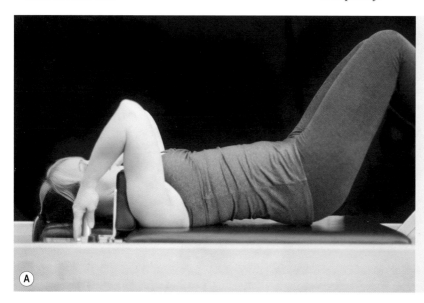

Figure 3.31A
Hovering Bridge: start position

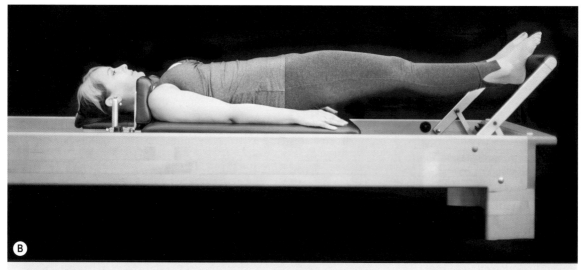

Figure 3.31 B
Pressing out

- Resist by pulling the carriage in, still floating the pelvis.

- Repeat 5–10 times.

Practitioner hands-on

Place one hand near the sacrum on the posterior side; cue the client to "float off" your hand (Fig. 3.31 C). Practice the floating until the body has a felt sense of the sacral position and no carriage movement. Many people will push on the bar and move the carriage. Once they find the floating pelvis, then cue to move the carriage out and in.

Integrated hip–pelvis–spine

A fully functioning hip allows for balance while standing on one leg, ease in walking, the ability to squat and stand up, and a sense of stability. Training the body with precise tools for addressing a restriction such as a hip micromovement opens the possibility of the whole body realigning itself toward the center. The second part of this chapter brings together the integral merging to center with the legs, the pelvis, sacrum and spine.

MERGING INTO THE CENTER: PART 2
Walking and falling

With every step the body takes it is adjusting and adapting, and this process continues throughout the

full sequencing of movement. Factors such as the surface we walk on, the shoes we wear and our neuromuscular patterning will all play a part in determining our physical response to movement. When we observe someone walking we can glean a wealth of information about that person's ability to move well. Contact with the ground, called heel strike, is the moment the spine prepares itself for the impact by changing its contour via lateral and rotational motions (Gracovetsky, 1988). The pelvis rotates to bring the hip joint forward and above the leg, to filter the impact of this contact. This is where the movement changes the hip joint from supporting a free swinging leg (mobility) to a stance leg (stability). The righting reflex of the nervous system, in conjunction with the tissue responses, is all about maintaining the body's equilibrium, about being centered.

Walking requires balancing on one leg while, on the opposite side, the leg swings free. In one step, as the weight is transferred to one leg, the pelvis tilts laterally slightly, with 5° of hip adduction of the stance leg, and the vertebral column bends toward the stance leg (Sahrmann, 2002) (Fig. 3.32). In a balanced one-legged stance when not walking, however, a stable pelvis will remain level. If the pelvis drops, it is an indication that there is weakness and instability of both the pelvis and the standing hip muscles down through the foot (Fig. 3.33). Normally the trunk shifts the weight over the leg for balance. This requires strength and

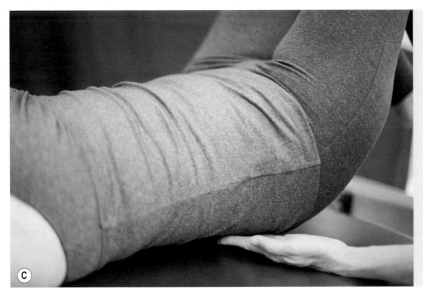

Figure 3.31 C
Hands-on

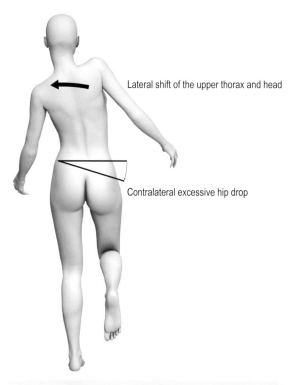

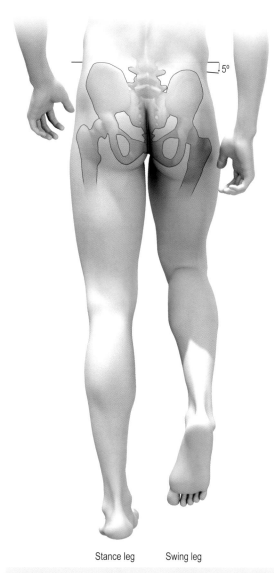

Lateral shift of the upper thorax and head

Contralateral excessive hip drop

Figure 3.33
Lateral shift of the upper thorax and head;
contralateral excessive hip drop

Stance leg   Swing leg

Figure 3.32
Degree of hip drop during normal gait

co-contractions of the hip joint, the abductors, the deep rotators, the adductors, and iliopsoas (bilaterally, both sides), which activates the whole myofascial core (trunk) for support. In addition, the rotatory motion of the thorax in opposition to the pelvic motion is a major component of good walking dynamics. The body is not well supported when the dynamic relationship of hip and trunk is compromised.

Try it!

Test your ability to balance on one leg. Stand with the weight equal on both feet (remember "Standing on Pencils" in Ch. 1) (Fig. 3.34). Place the hands on the upper rim of the pelvis, with the fingers facing toward the midline. Shift the weight slightly over to the left leg as the right knee bends and lifts up. Did the pelvis remain level? How was the balance? Did the weight shift on to the standing foot and lose contact of the big toe ball to outer heel connection? Practice standing on one leg and having awareness of the alignment of the foot, a level pelvis, and an elongation of the spine. Balance is a *whole body* action, not the isolated action of a few muscles.

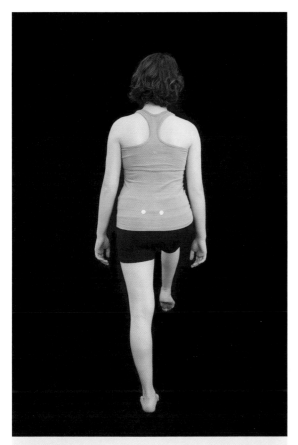

Figure 3.34
Standing on one leg

Pelvis and sacrum

The pelvis can be said to be the bridge of the body. It supports the weight of the trunk from above and rests on the lower limbs. The weight of the spinal column is set upon the sacrum, which acts as the keystone of the bridge. In standing erect, the weight is distributed through the arch of the bridge (sacrum and pelvis) and then transferred through the hip joints, where the heads of the femur receive it, and transmitted down the legs to the feet. In sitting, the transmission of weight moves through the pelvis in line with the hip joint (acetabula) to the lowest part of the pelvis (ischia), the sits bones, and then into the chair, while the force moves from the sits bones through the ilium to the sacrum. Standing, the ground forces move up from the femurs through the

ilium to the sacrum. Thus, both in standing and sitting, the pelvis and sacrum are the weight-bearing bones. A centered alignment distributes weight evenly through the bones, generating less stress and fatigue on the body. The orientation of the pelvis is important to the distribution of the force vectors moving through the tissues of the body.

> **Practitioner note**
>
> "Force vector" is a term often used in the physical training and bodywork fields. Force is a basic component of biomechanics. Force equals mass times acceleration. It has a vector quantity, meaning the force has a particular direction or point of application, a magnitude, and a direction. When introducing a force to the body, whether from a piece of Pilates apparatus, weights or manual resistance, the movement stimulated is the force moving in the body in a particular direction with a particular speed. The energy of the force vector moves through the body's tissues as it creates movement. One can follow the force vector in the tissue's resilience in movement.

Spiral movement

Spiral movement is a three-dimensional curve around a central axis crossing with oppositional paths. In order to twist, one area of the body moves in one direction as the opposite end contrasts the direction, moving away. This is evident in the motion of the spine and pelvis. To begin the ascending torque of the spine that creates walking, the pelvis and thorax will move in opposite directions. To move the body well, coordinated and oppositional rotations are necessary in the spine, specifically in the thorax.

In walking the pelvis spirals by moving the right innominate (ilia) forward (anterior) while the left side moves backward (posterior), causing the pelvis and sacrum to face toward the left. The pelvic rotation to the left places the hip joint rotated inwardly on the left and outwardly on the right. The lumbar spine will then begin spiraling toward the right (Fig. 3.35). From the base of the rotated position, the spine adjusts for the rotation segmentally all the way up to the head.

The spine rotates in the opposite direction multiple times in different segments of the spine, these

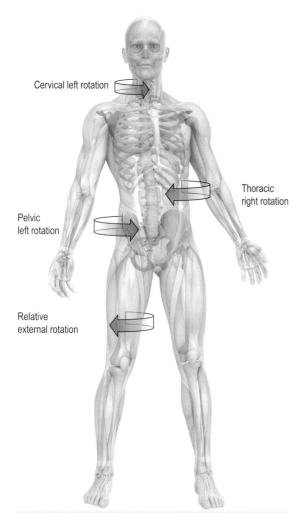

Cervical left rotation

Thoracic
right rotation

Pelvic
left rotation

Relative
external rotation

Figure 3.35
Pelvis rotation with oppositional rotational
movements of the spine and hip

transitions commonly occurring at the junctions
between the segments of the spine, namely:

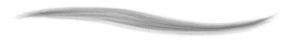

- L4/L5 and S1
- T12 and L1
- T1/T2 and C7
- O/A, C1 and C2.

Meanwhile, we accommodate our eyes' desire to
maintain a horizontal orientation, a level ground, in
order to feel centered, by means of the upper cervical spine adjusting the balance of the head on top of
the spine.

Taking a step

When taking a step, notice the lateral and rotational
movements from the hip through the spine in opposition to one another. Taking a step can be seen in the
following:

- Moving from a left stance leg toward the right leg,
  with the left arm swinging forward, the pelvic rotation is left with a right thorax rotation.

- Next, in the step of the left foot moving forward
  from the right stance leg, with the right arm swinging forward, the pelvic rotation is toward the right
  with a left thorax rotation.

- A balanced gait is the shifting of weight from the
  right leg to the left leg, with a centering during
  each phase.

- Observe for equal trunk rotation, stride length, and
  arm swing (Fig. 3.36). Most people favor one direction of trunk rotation over the other (the equivalent
  to walking in a circle rather than moving straight
  forward).

Working with the rotations of the segments in relation to one another will animate the cross-pattern-
ing necessary for evening out the dominant rotation.
Below is a series of seated movements designed to
recalibrate the rotations.

> **Try it!**
>
> If you have an opportunity to be in a place where
> walking with the eyes closed is safe and there is a
> surface that can track footprints (such as snow or
> sand), try walking straight ahead with eyes shut.
> Walk for a good distance, then open the eyes and
> look back at the path of your footprints. It may sur-
> prise you!

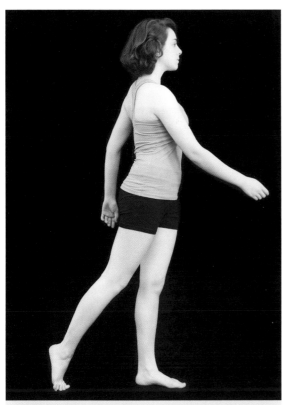

Figure 3.36
One step

Sacred bone center connection

"Sacrum" derives from the Latin *os sacrum*, meaning "sacred bone." The sacrum is the keystone to the pelvis and the intermediary between the lower and upper body. It can be a place of great bliss and great pain, and is the sacred place where life begins. Pelvic and sacral movements assist in the flow of fluids, both in the spine and in the organs that sit in front of it. Both structure and organ function play a role in the alignment and ability to move this area.

> **Practitioner note**
>
> The sacrum lives between the two "wings" of the pelvis. Each wing is made up of three bones, the ilium, ischium, and pubis, which, fused together, make up the *innominate* bone (a right and a left). The word "innominate" means "no name" (see Fig. 3.1). Most bones were named after their similarity to known objects but the shape of the pelvic bone bore no likeness to any well-known item – hence "no name."

Lines and layers of connection from the sacrum

The significance of the lines and layers extending from the sacrum is that they create stability for the sacroiliac joint (SIJ). Support for the SIJ and pelvis comes from the tensile force of the ilia and sacrum

CLIENT STORY

A client came in for her regular session after having spent a week at a yoga retreat in Mexico. As she walked in, I noticed she was not rotating well and her pelvis seemed stiff. I asked her how she was feeling and if there was anything about her body she wanted me to know. It was her awareness I was interested in because I had already noticed a change in her normal movement. Her response was that she felt tight because there had been an outbreak of food poisoning at the retreat, so it had not been possible to practice any physical yoga for the entire week she was there. She had recovered from the food poisoning but her pelvis seemed to be held tightly, as if compressed. Her hip joints were shifted to one side, the pelvis in a torsion facing the sigmoid colon (end of the large intestine) (which is to the left). The

spiral continued upward, back and forth, all the way to her head. Her internal organs, the gastrointestinal tract, had been subjected to violent movements as a result of the food poisoning and the body's posture and movement pattern had changed. Working with her specific spiral posture and moving her into the direction of restriction followed by the direction of ease allowed the movements of the hip, pelvis, and lowest part of the spine to balance the spiral into a centered place. The sequencing incorporated the hip spins and the lumbopelvic mobility exercises below and from Chapter 4, 'Resetting the Trunk." These movements allowed her to find the freedom to move more evenly, with less tightness, and internally, easing the tension of the pelvis, which allowed better movement of her organs.

through the contraction and pull from myofascial connections that stem from the sacrum (van Wingerden et al., 2004).

- Thoracolumbar fascia (TLF) transfers forces between the pelvis, spine, legs, and arms.

- Superficially, the TLF is continuous with the latissimus dorsi and the gluteus maximus at sacral level connecting to the iliotibial band (see Fig. 2.8).

- A deep layer of the thoracolumbar fascia ensheathes the spinous processes of the spine (center of the bone) and encases the erector spinae muscles to form part of the lateral weave (raphe) which the internal oblique is attached to along with the middle layer connection of the transversus abdominis (Fig. 3.37) (Vleeming, 2012).

- At sacral level, underneath the overlying erector spinae group lies the multifidus muscle, with its sheath, as part of the deep layer of fascia; when both groups contract together, it reduces the slack in the fascial envelope, producing stability (Fig. 3.38).

- Inferiorly, the lateral raphe is continuous with the sacrotuberous ligament and biceps femoris (see Fig. 2.8) (Vleeming, 2012).

- Anterior side of the sacrum and inside the pelvic bowl, the parietal fascia is continuous with the piriformis and coccygeus muscles (see Fig. 3.25).

- From the anterior sacrum to the leg via piriformis (Fig. 3.39).

The complexity of layers and lines of force at the sacral level upward to the spine and downward through the legs produces movement and stability of the spine and SIJ. Training for strength and balanced engagement of these myofascial relationships provides increased movement potential and better function. Movement of the hip joint influences the TLF tension, producing stability or external movement of the pelvis. The sacral position relative to the ilium is important to pelvic stability because of the dynamic tensile action of the muscles mentioned above, the connective tissue, including TFL, and the ligaments. The myofascial core engagement occurs through the sacral,

pelvic, and hip joint positioning (Ch. 4). Training for connecting and strengthening this support of the pelvis and spine through sound bone movements will improve stability and functional movement. (This topic is discussed further in Ch. 4.)

Sacroiliac movement: nutation and counternutation

The sacroiliac joints (SIJ) are intrinsic joints (smaller movement potential) of the pelvis and sacrum rather than extrinsic joints (larger movement potential) like the lumbar spine and hip joints. The micromovements of the SIJ are responsive to movement of the spine along with the pelvis, allowing for the rotational drive and normal spine bending.

The SIJ is shaped like a boomerang. It lies on the side of the sacrum, at the point where it meets the ilium. It has a vertical arm where it slides upward/downward and a horizontal arm where it moves forward/back. The motion of the sacrum occurs along the SIJ, where the sacrum slides forward (horizontally) and up (vertically) or down (vertically) and out (horizontally). Nutation is the nodding motion of the sacrum moving down and out. Imagine the sacrum as a head. The top of the head is the shelf of the sacrum (on top of which sits the spine), and the chin is the tail bone. The face is looking toward the front of the pelvis at the pubic bone. When the sacrum nutates, imagine the head nods downward, looking down and moving the chin (tail bone) away from the front of the pelvis (the pubic bone); this is a down and out movement (Fig. 3.40). As the tail bone moves away from the pubic bone, the sits bones (ischial tuberosities) widen, lengthening the pelvic floor and tipping the tops of the innominate bones in toward the center, approximating the PSIS.

The nodding upward motion (forward and up) of the sacrum is called counternutation (Fig. 3.41). The sacrum slides forward and up, moving the shelf of the sacrum backward and widening the top of the sacrum as the tail bone moves toward the pubis, and the ischial tuberosities moving inward, narrowing the pelvic floor space in the rear. This position of the sacrum is considered to place the back at risk for injury when transferring heavy loads. The terms nutation and

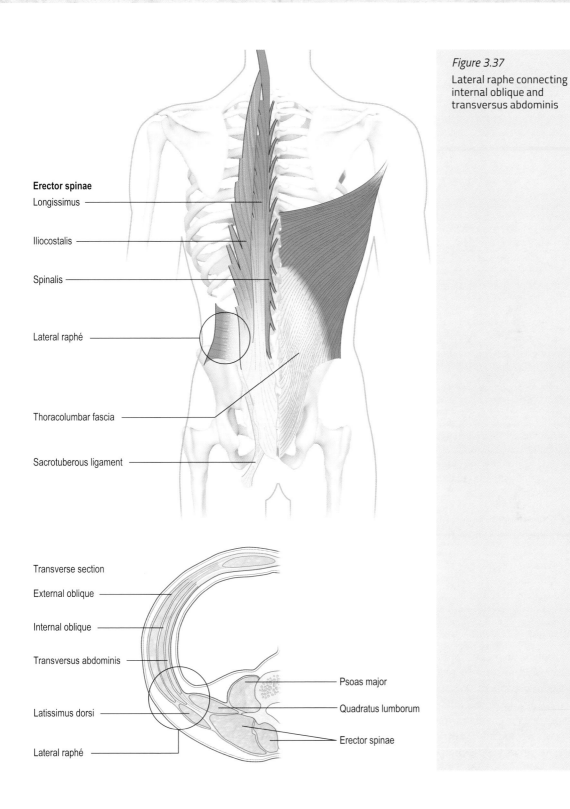

Erector spinae
Longissimus

Iliocostalis

Spinalis

Lateral raphé

Thoracolumbar fascia

Sacrotuberous ligament

Transverse section
External oblique

Internal oblique

Transversus abdominis

Latissimus dorsi

Lateral raphé

Psoas major

Quadratus lumborum

Erector spinae

Figure 3.37
Lateral raphe connecting
internal oblique and
transversus abdominis

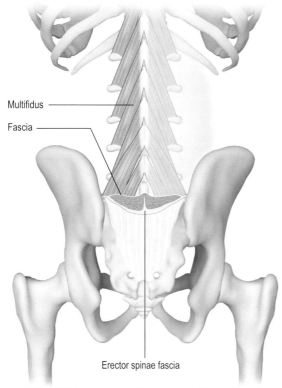

Multifidus

Fascia

Erector spinae fascia

Figure 3.38
Deep layer of thoracolumbar fascia on the sacral
level; multifidus sheath and erector spinae fascia

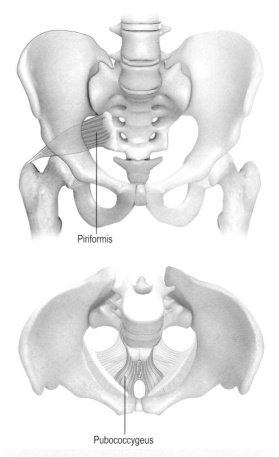

Piriformis

Pubococcygeus

Figure 3.39
Connections from the anterior sacrum: piriformis,
pubococcygeus

counternutation apply to describing the motion of the
sacrum relative to the innominate (Lee, 2011).

> **Note**
>
> *Nutation* means to nod.

Neutral pelvis

"Neutral pelvis" or "neutral spine" are two of the most
frequently used phrases in physical training across
all models of movement. What does "neutral" really
mean in theory, however, and what does it look like
on a body? A good metaphor for neutral is thinking
about a car "in neutral." Neutral is a place where the
body can move easily (less compensated) in any direction from a starting point. Our bodies are more like
a stick shift car, which is taken out of gear to be idle.
Neutral for the body is being in a position in which the

least amount of muscular effort is needed to be idle.
If the body is orientated in a particular direction, for
example a rotation to the right, then more effort will
be needed to rotate to the left but little engagement
required for the body to rotate right. In other words,
there is a movement bias for a right rotation.

In health, the body is in constant movement and
so the idea of observing a fixed neutral is impracti-
cal. Humans walk, they have limbs that move independently, and they are not symmetrical. The pelvic
bowl position in standing relies on balancing the pelvis
on the femoral heads. Since hip joints vary from person to person, an individual approach toward training needs to combine observation of the pelvic bowl's

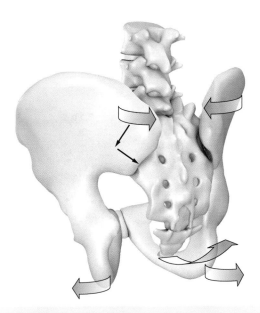

Figure 3.40
Sacral nutation bone movements

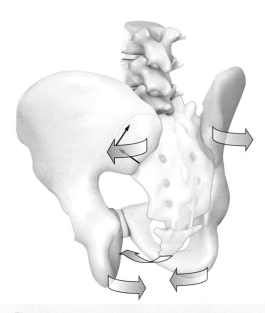

Figure 3.41
Sacral counternutation bone movements

orientation on the femurs with an awareness of sacral nutation. The nutation of the sacrum is in an idling place, not completely at its end range (closed pack position) (Lee, 2011). Finding an individual's neutral pelvic position is optimal for stability of the spine, core activation, and the cornerstone of overall alignment.

What is equally important is finding the whole body alignment to activate the postural muscles to support the structure. There is fine-tuning involved in this feeling. In Chapter 1, we described "Standing on Pencils" (p. 21). This is the place to begin aligning the pelvis. First, find the center of the hip joint and place the feet directly underneath. Shift the body weight over the point in the foot that is the center for bearing weight. Adjust the pelvic position by finding a neutral pelvis with the sacral micromovement of nutation, which creates stability for balanced standing.

> **Try it!**
>
> *To find the center of the hip joint,* draw a line from the top of the wing (ilium) of the pelvis (at the ASIS) on a diagonal to the pubic bone. This is called the inguinal line. Half way between the landmarks is the center of the hip joint (Fig. 3.42).
>
> *To find the neutral pelvis,* place your hands at the wings of the pelvis with the fingers pointing toward the midline (Fig. 3.43). Rotate your pelvis so that the tops of the wings are in a flat plane with the pubic bone (a posterior rotation). Hold this pelvic position. Visualize (remember this is a micromovement) the tail moving away from the pubic bone and sits bones (ischial tuberosities). The top of the pelvis does not move anteriorly. Hold this position. Notice that it created a narrow feeling of the pelvis, changing the tone of the lower abdominal area under the fingers. Imagine a myofascial ring between the lower ribs and pelvis, drawing inward and wrapping around to the back. Sitting is an easier place to feel the pelvis position with this subtle sacral movement. It also brings the attention to where the weight falls on the sits bones. Try this lying on the mat too.

In healthy standing or sitting, the sacrum is in nutation. Whenever the body is vertical, the sacrum sits in nutation relative to the innominate. While lying down (supine) with the legs straight, the traction of the anterior (flexor) region causes the pelvis to anteriorly tilt. Lying down with the knees bent, gravity will posteriorly

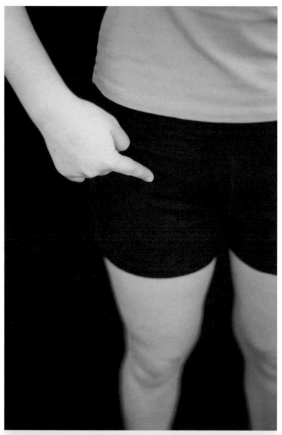

Figure 3.42
Center point of hip joint

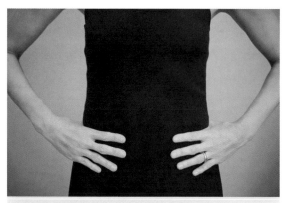

Figure 3.43
Holding pelvis at ASIS

tilt the pelvis. If there is a balance of tissue tensions in the front of the body (flexor region) and the posterior body (extensor area), there will be a smaller amount of tilt. If the pelvis has stability, the sacrum remains in its nutated position relative to the ilia. This may not always be the situation, though, since variations and discrepancies abound across the vast variety of human bodies.

Sacral and pelvic movement is complex and paradoxical due to so many factors, including the shape of the bones and, more importantly, the tensile nature of the ligament system surrounding the SIJ. According to Fred L. Mitchell Jr. D.O., "sacral movement is the result of gravitational, inertial, and elastic forces secondary to spinal movements" (Mitchell, 2001). His work emphasizes that muscles do not directly influence the movement of the sacrum between the ilia. The position of the body in relationship to gravity, how L5 is positioned in relation to the sacrum, and the elastic forces from the legs (which vary from individual to individual) are factors of the movement and stability of the pelvis and spine. When training, how the load transfers through the body is important. The load is transferred optimally with the nutated position during movement of the pelvis, hips, and spine, and the loading equal on right and left sides. Imagine lying on the Reformer or simply standing to do a squat. If one moves from a squat position to standing by pressing on one leg more than the other, an unequal loading causes a lateral translation that has a cascading effect up the spine (see the notes on movement patterning for foot and leg work on the Reformer in Ch. 1).

Try it!

Feel if your SIJ is moving well for load transfer. Sit on a stool or a chair, with your sits bones on the edge of the chair and feet on the floor; place your hands on the sides of your pelvic bones with your thumbs on the back and fingers pointing inward toward the midline (Fig. 3.44 A). Turn to the right as if you are looking at a friend sitting behind you (Fig. 3.44 B). Do you feel your pelvic bone on the right move back and on the left side move forward? If so, your SIJ moved well. Try it on the other side and see if it moves too. If only your neck and shoulders moved, then your SIJ is not moving well to allow for a full spiral and good load transfer.

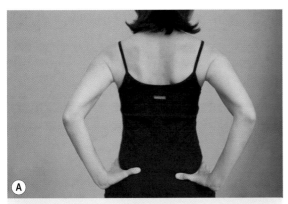

Figure 3.44 A
Feeling for movement of the sacrum and pelvis

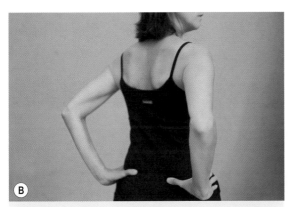

Figure 3.44 B
Rotating pelvis

Practitioner note

With a partner, palpate the iliac crest from the front around to the back until you feel the prominent bony end of the crest (the posterior superior iliac spine, PSIS). Position the thumbs horizontally and place the upper edge below the PSIS. Slide the thumbs upward until the thumbs meet the bottom edge of the PSIS. Move the thumbs wider to the lateral side of the PSIS. Place the whole thumb flat across this area to approximate having contact with the sacrum and pelvis (Fig. 3.45).

Sit upright on top of the sits bones. Slowly roll the sits bones under the pelvis, tail curling under and

pelvis rounding the back (posterior tilt of the pelvis) (Fig. 3.46). Do not move the thoracolumbar junction and above. Rock the pelvis back to the upright position. Tip the pelvis forward in an anterior tilt (Fig. 3.47). Observe the lumbopelvic rhythm. The excursion forward and back is smooth and balanced in healthy movement. Restoring balanced movement at the SIJ, pelvis, and spine enhances the spine's capability to roll up, bend forward and back, and twist.

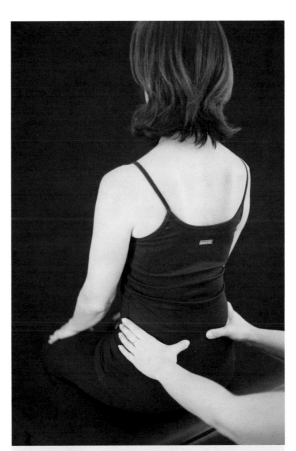

Figure 3.45
Practitioner note: hands-on for seated Sacral Rocks

Action of forward bending and backward bending

In a normal, healthy, and uncompensated forward bending movement of the trunk while standing, the spine flexes from the top of the head, down through the whole spinal chain until it reaches the lower

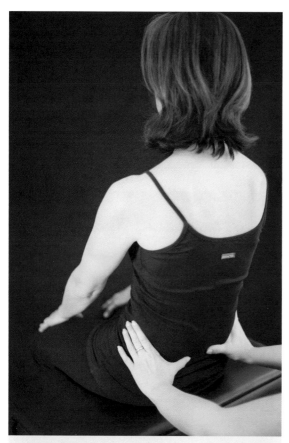

Figure 3.46
Seated Sacral Rocks: flexion

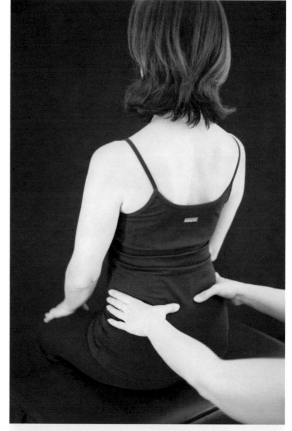

Figure 3.47
Extension

segment of the lumbar vertebrae. The pelvic girdle follows the forward spinal motion, rotating anteriorly with hip flexion, allowing the person to touch the floor (Figs 3.48 A & B). The sacral nutation is increased to the point of a close packed position. Observing or palpating the posterior iliac spines (PSIS) (see Fig. 3.45) during forward bending, there will be equal distance traveled in a superior direction as the pelvic girdle flexes on the femoral heads (Lee, 2011). There is a smooth lumbar curve relative to the thorax when the flexion of the spine is optimal. No side bending or rotation is evident. Rolling the spine back to upright, the pelvis posteriorly rotates and the sacrum slightly counternutates to return to its idling nutated position.

There are common limitations to a healthy forward bend. Once the limit of extensibility of the biceps

femoris, sacrotuberous ligament, and deep lamina of the posterior layer of the thoracodorsal fascia has been reached, the flexibility of the sacrum becomes less than the innominates. The pelvis continues to move forward (anteriorly rotate) on the femoral heads, flexing at the hip joint, but the sacrum no longer moves forward with the pelvis but reverses, going backward (counternutation).

As a movement teacher, when you see the shift of the body behind the feet prior to the completion of spinal flexion in the lower lumbar area, it indicates the person has reached the end of spinal motion and the length of the posterior hip and leg. The reversal motion of the sacrum from nutation to counternutation creates a potential for instability of the pelvis due to the decrease in compression of the joint of the ilium and sacrum.

However, if the sacrum remains nutated throughout forward bending, the SIJ retains integrity and loads can be more effectively transferred through the pelvic girdle to the lower extremities, thus moving the force and energy through the body into the ground. The elasticity of the biceps femoris and sacrotuberous ligaments is key to the ability to rotate around the femoral joints to touch the floor. To release the pulling and reversing of the sacral movement, a wise modification is to bend the knees to touch the floor.

Backward bending of the trunk from standing is a forward (anterior) shift of the pelvic girdle and the center of gravity moves toward the feet. As the spine segmentally extends up and back, the joints (facet joints) of the spine are sliding in an inferior and anterior direction with extension of the hip joints (the forward shift) (Fig. 3.49). Both PSISs should travel an equal distance in an inferior direction as the pelvis extends on the femoral heads. The sacrum remains nutated as the pelvis posteriorly rotates around the femoral joints. At the end range of extension, when L5 shifts more posteriorly, the sacral base will slide inferiorly.

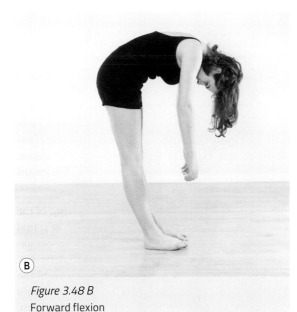

Ⓐ

Figure 3.48 A
Standing to roll down

Ⓑ

Figure 3.48 B
Forward flexion

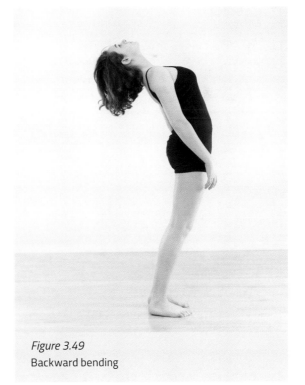

Figure 3.49
Backward bending

The sacrum now becomes the lowest segment of the extension or lordotic curve (Mitchell, 2001). In backward bends such as the Pilates "Swan," it is important to feel the sacrum moving downward in an inferior direction, staying in nutation as the spine lifts up and back, with the power of the legs to drive the hip extension increasing the lift of the spine. When working with all of the exercises in the section "Moving in Hip Extension" (see above), be focused on the nutation of the sacrum as described.

Balanced side bending and twists

There is a coupled motion of rotation in both the spine and SIJ when the lumbar spine side bends. If the side bending is balanced, the weight transmitted to the sacral base creates a passive side bending by the lateral shift of the load. The sacrum moves and rotates out from under the load by side bending and rotating to the opposite side of the side bending of the spine (Fig. 3.50).

In a rotation, the pelvis moves forward and the sacrum nutates on one side while the opposite side moves back, and counternutates the sacrum. Traveling up the spine, the vertebrae and ribs are translating to one side and the rotation occurs to the opposite side.

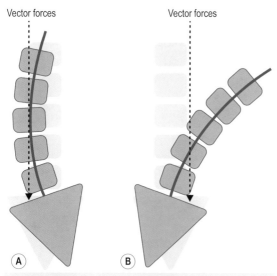

Vector forces   Vector forces

(A)   (B)

Figure 3.50
Balanced side bending of lumbar and sacrum; imbalanced side bending

The movement example of testing the SIJ and pelvis rotation above in "Try it!" (p. 116) demonstrates this motion. For many people, the pelvis and sacrum will be held in this rotation no matter what movement is being performed. Or a restriction may occur anywhere along the chain, which makes performing a twisting movement to one side easier than the other.

Pelvis in motion: exercises for integration of the lumbopelvic complex

These exercises continue after the anterior hip has been released and mobilized through the quadruped glides practiced in the first part of this chapter, allowing for ease in the hip joint. The lumbar and pelvic motions are significantly improved when the hip joint movement has been freed up and a felt sense of the nutated sacrum within the pelvis that activates the tone of the pelvic musculature for support has been established. Following this work, the movement of the pelvis and lower spine becomes more integrated in a whole body way, building from a submaximal recruitment into larger movements of Pilates, yoga or Gyrotonic®.

Lumbosacral mobility on the Reformer

This series balances by moving the lumbosacral complex (hips, pelvis, sacrum, and spine) in a specific direction with assistance and resistance.

Seated Sacral Rocks

 Seated Sacral Rocks, side and rotation
VIDEO LINK V 3.5

The client sits on the front edge of the Reformer carriage facing the foot bar, with the feet placed on the floor (Fig. 3.51 A). The foot bar has no springs attached. The practitioner stands to the side of the client to view the action of the pelvis and spine and to be prepared for tactile cues. (If the Reformer is not available, another option for Seated Sacral Rocks and Hip Hike is to sit on a physioball or a slide board.)

- Inhale to prepare the body with elongation; begin to curl the coccyx (Fig. 3.51 B).

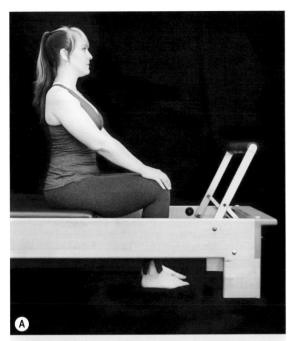

Figure 3.51 A
Seated Sacral Rocks on Reformer: start position

- Slowly exhale as the sits bone move under and forward, dragging the carriage underneath the body toward the foot bar or toward the shins. This action is the same movement as the anterior hip glide in "Quadruped Hip Movements" earlier in this chapter (p. 78), but seated.

- Be precise and only curl the pelvis and lower spine; the ribcage is stable.

- Inhale to reverse the movement; beginning at the pelvis wings, move them forward.

- Exhale, pushing the sits bones back and moving the carriage away from the bar (Fig. 3.51 C). This action is the same movement as the posterior hip glide in "Quadruped Hip Movements," but seated.

- Return to a fully idling nutated position.

- Be precise and move through the hip joints, pelvis, and lower spine; do not allow the lower ribcage to translate in any direction.

- Repeat the motion of curling and arching the pelvis and lower spine several times to allow the body to smooth out the movement.

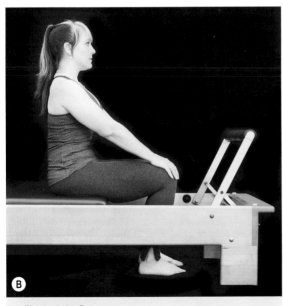

Figure 3.51 B
Curl

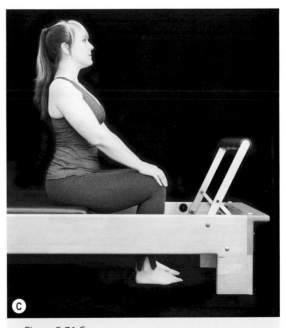

Figure 3.51 C
Arch

- Once the movement is embodied, adding a foam roller on the floor, under the feet, challenges the posterior hip as the pelvis curls and arches; it also challenges the stability of the lower legs and feet.

> **Practitioner note**
>
> Hold the client's lowest ribs to assist in their ability to understand the stability of the thoracolumbar junction while accessing the motion of the hip joint, pelvis, and lower spine. Observe for symmetrical nutation of sacrum as the spine arches and symmetrical counternutation of the sacrum as the spine curls. Watch for overworking, a shortening tension rather than an elongation engagement of the gluteus maximus and erector spinae muscles.

The Seated Sacral Rocks exercise is excellent for training core activation in both flexion and extension; coaching proper movement timing of hip joint to pelvis and spine motions in flexion and extension; observing sacral mechanics of nutation and counternutation; and finding a seated neutral position of the pelvis, giving the client a felt sense of how to sit on the bones for support.

Side seated Hip Hike

 Seated Sacral Rocks, side and rotation
VIDEO LINK V 3.5

The purpose of the Seated Hip Hike exercise is to free up the waist. It elongates and contracts the side muscles, such as the abdominal oblique muscles and quadratus lumborum, enhances lateral and medial glide of the hip joint, and articulates the spinal segments.

- The client sits sideways (left side toward the foot bar) on the Reformer carriage (no springs attached) (Fig. 3.52 A).
- Inhale to prepare the body with elongation.
- Slowly exhale and slide the carriage toward the foot bar by sinking your weight into the right sits bone

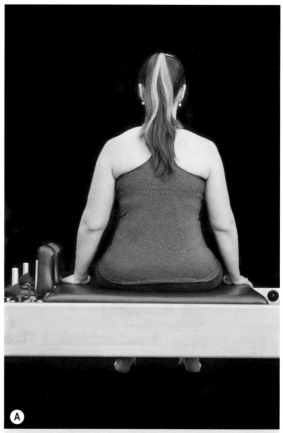

Ⓐ

Figure 3.52 A
Seated Hip Hike on Reformer: start position

(the one away from foot bar), allowing a slight hip hike of the left side and feeling a small unweighting of the left sits bone (Fig. 3.52 B).

- The ribcage will translate or move a small amount toward the right.
- Inhale to return the carriage with equal weighted sits bones.
- Exhale to repeat the Hip Hike to the other side, moving the carriage away from the foot bar.
- Since there is no resistance added (though a light spring may be added once the movement skill is fully learned), the client does not need to turn around to sit facing the other side for the second half of the exercise. If resistance is added, then turn to face the other side for the second hip hike.

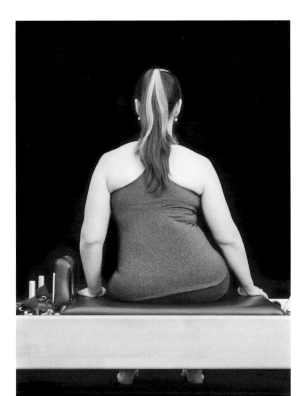

(B)

Figure 3.52 B
Hiking hip

Practitioner note

Observe whether, as the lumbar spine side bends, the innominates maintain their frontal position. Encourage the client to move without a forward or backward rotation of the ilium. Keep the range of movement small in order to access the lumbar and sacral movement with ease.

Oppositional ilium mobility

 Seated Sacral Rocks, side and rotation
VIDEO LINK V 3.5

Oppositional ilium movement linked with stability of ribcage movement is training a balance within the diagonal musculature and the whole cylinder of the waist. Breathing and movement quality may become restricted if the waist is too stiff. Since the waist is the mediator of forces through the soft tissues, however, it needs a degree of both resilience and stiffness at different times as the body moves and takes different life actions (Feldenkrais, 1944). In addition, the rotational movement of the exercise is mobilizing the ilium and sacrum, freeing up the ability to move well in the pelvis and SIJ.

Equipment needed: one 12 inch (30.5 cm) or BAC Disc; two wooden dowels. The feet are supported on the floor or on a box.

> **Note**
>
> The BAC (Biomechanical Asymmetry Corrector) disc was invented by Jean Claude West in collaboration with Katy Keller. The aim is to work on functional side bending of the spine, utilizing the discs to create translation and side bending in order to adjust the facet joints of the spine and engage the intrinsic muscles of the spine.

- Place the disc on top of the Reformer carriage with springs attached, or on top of a table or in a non-moveable place where the client is stable.

- The client sits on the disc holding the two dowels, one in front of the torso and the other behind the back, with the elbows hooked over the dowel at the back (the dowels are parallel and level) (Fig. 3.53 A).

- The dowels remain still while the client begins to rotate the disc.

- All the movement occurs in the hip joint, pelvis and sacrum.

- The motion is to rotate the right hip and knee forward while the other side moves backward; the thighs stay in line with the hip joint, not allowing the knee to move in toward the midline (adduction) or away from the midline (abduction).

- The movement is to rotate back and forth without allowing the dowels to move so that all the motion is in the hip joint, SIJ, and lumbar spine to the thoracolumbar junction (Fig. 3.53 B).

- Breathe easily throughout the movement.

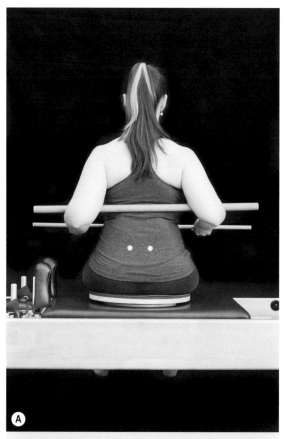

Figure 3.53 A
Opposition ilium mobility with rotational disc and poles

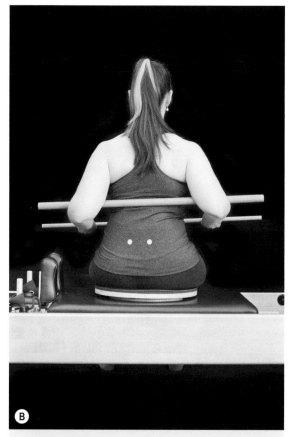

Figure 3.53 B
In rotation

Practitioner note

Observe for the specific ilium and sacral movement of sacral nutation and counternutation on one side and compare with opposite side. If the observation is that one side is not moving well, then repeat that side several times in succession or add a resistance component such as a MET to release the holding and enhance the movement.

Oppositional ilium MET on disc

Seated Sacral Rocks, side and rotation
VIDEO LINK V 3.5

- Ask the client to move into the restricted direction and pause at the point of the restriction.

- Freeze this position (let's say it is right side forward and left side back).

- Place your hand on the disc (right side) and say "I am going to pull the disc back but do not let me do it, meet my resistance" (Fig. 3.53 C).

- Pull the right side back and the client resists and creates an isometric contraction by trying to rotate the right side forward, but no movement of the disc occurs.

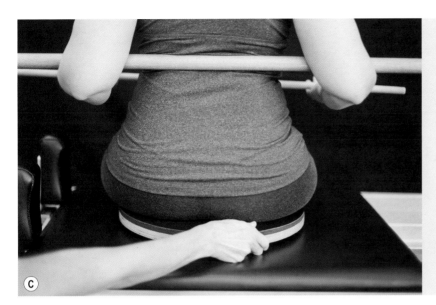

Figure 3.53 C
MET hands-on

- Hold for a slow count of 5.

- Stop the resistance and ask the client to move just a little into the direction of restriction (forward on the right).

- Repeat the resistance pattern at the new range 3–4 times.

- Perform the movement back and forth and see the increased ease of motion.

Bridging to Chapter 4

Understanding and observing the "normal" motion of the body will provide clues to the presence of a restriction that is inhibiting movement. Remember that there are macromovements and micromovements throughout the body and if the micromovements are missing, then the flow of force will be redirected or held. Restoring the movement capability to balance the spiral motion allows the body the freedom to distribute forces more evenly, thereby reducing or eliminating stress in the structure. This exploration continues further in Chapter 4, delving deep into the trunk.

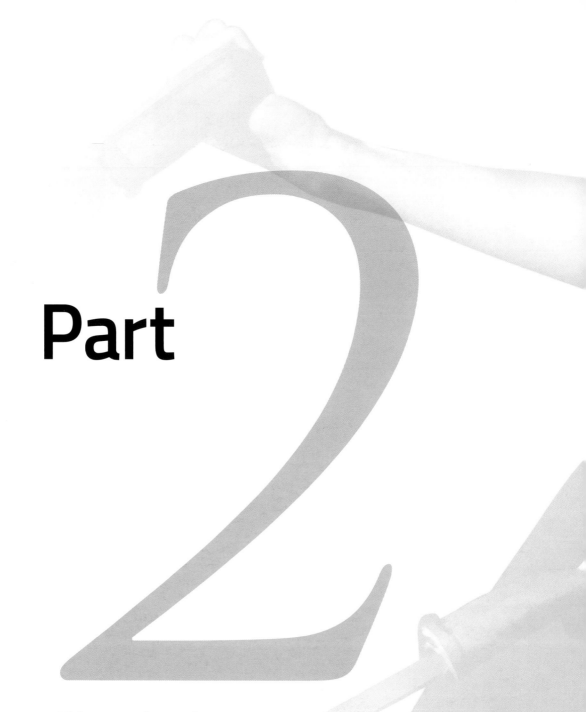

Part 2

Pivotal point:
where the ribs meet the lower spine

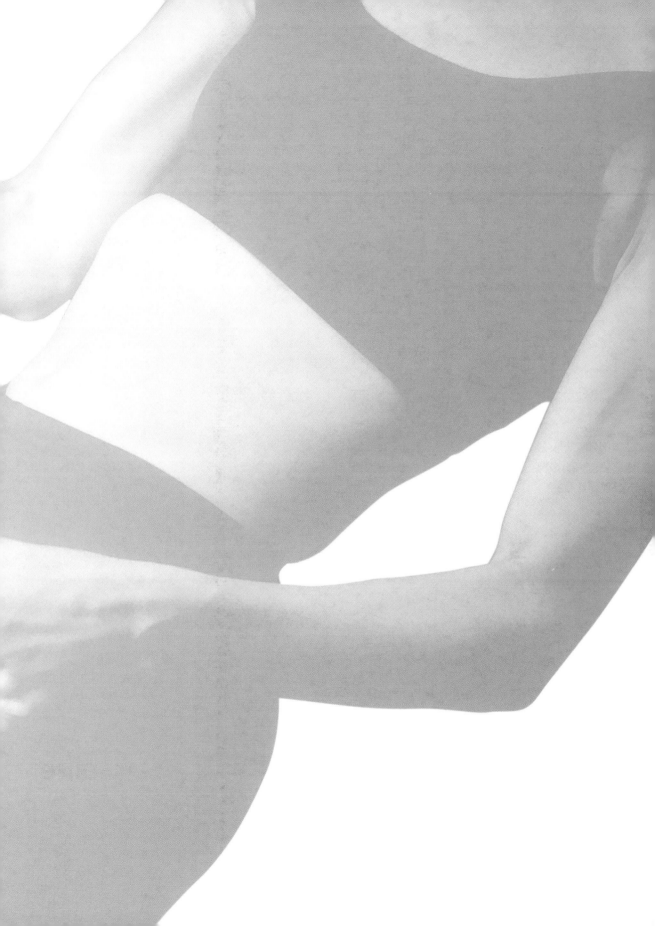

4

Trunk connection

> "The primary function of the lumbopelvic complex is to transfer loads safely while fulfilling the movement and control requirements of any task in a way that ensures the objects of the task are met, musculoskeletal structures are not injured, either in the short or long term, and that the organs are supported/protected in concert with optimal respiration."
>
> Diane Lee, *The Thorax*

Contemplative awareness: connectivity

The trunk is the powerhouse of all movement. It is the central superstructure of the body, housing life-sustaining systems that are interdependent and function as a whole, and this connectivity influences how we move, breathe, and maintain equilibrium.

Imagine looking inside the body without dissecting the torso: we would see that the inside is intertwined with the "underneath side" of the outside, that the contours of the body change in depth and field according to the interweaving of the tissues. Besides the tissues, though, we must consider the spaces between them, for space in the body is as much a part of function as the solid parts. As the body bends or twists, the tissues move into the spaces, which provide a place for the solid body to move into and around. The spaces (cavities) inside the trunk play an important role in shaping the torso as it shifts. From the outside, the skin, superficial fascia, and myofascia provide the shape of the trunk and at the same time support the inside.

Trunk connections: core

Core

Core training involves three-dimensional movement of the trunk with its connective tissues that move and support the spine. Imagine the trunk as a container shaped like a cylinder. Superficially, a cylinder has a top, sides that wrap around, and a bottom. A body cylinder has the base of the neck and along the shoulders as the top; the circular mid-section includes the sides from armpits to outer hips; the base of the pelvis is the bottom of the cylinder. For our purposes, the core of the trunk is this whole cylinder, together with the breath. Specifically, the non-bony ring between the ribs and pelvis, the myofascial ring, is the area one needs to activate for whole trunk support (Fig. 4.1).

Defining the body's core is a topic that has been much debated and there are numerous viewpoints concerning what structures are recruited and how to effectively train the core. New research is unfolding possibilities for yet more differing opinions and beliefs around this complex subject. The discussion is focused on lumbar spine stabilization by recruiting co-contraction of the diaphragm, abdominal transversus abdominis, and pelvic diaphragm, increasing intra-abdominal pressure (Lee, 2011). (More about intra-abdominal pressure can be found in Ch. 5.) A second perspective focuses on recruiting full co-contraction of the abdominals for bracing and stiffening (Grenier and McGill, 2007). These perspectives are arrived at through scientific studies and clinical practice. It is important to keep in mind the relevance of current and past research, with all its variables and clinical observations, and integrate the information that matches the movement practice methodology. Most important, however, is to first consider the individual person being coached.

Are we looking to stabilize the lumbar spine in isolation or do we want to allow for good grounding through the legs into the pelvis, with a strong spine

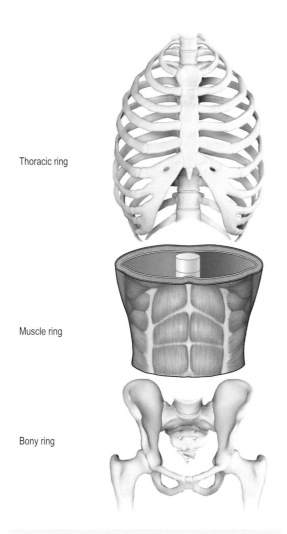

Thoracic ring

Muscle ring

Bony ring

Figure 4.1
Rib rings, myofascial ring, and pelvic bowl

that articulates well? Pelvis and hip strength is part of the whole trunk support as well as spinal muscles. When choosing a mechanism for training the core, keep in mind that the movement of the trunk varies from person to person. It is important to be observant of how each body moves in all planes of motion, optimizing trunk and hip strength, and also to match the amount of effort needed for the movement tasks to what is required by the person's life and goals. Are they training for an athletic event such as a marathon or do they simply want to garden without back pain? Movements in different spatial orientation (standing, inverted, or lying down) require recruiting a variety

of muscle patterns synergies. The variety strengthens the core in all potential ways of moving. In everyday life, the core is dynamic, supporting the spine through a healthy nervous system response to the body in space. Training the core requires multidirectional movements, challenges to the nervous system's righting reflex, and matching the skill level of the person to improve core resilient strength.

Superficial and deep

The trunk myofascia weave together as the fascia courses across the surface of the body and invests itself deeply into connections below the surface. It travels from superficial to deep, from wide to narrow, and wraps the trunk like a corset from the lowest part of the pelvic bowl right up to the head. All the planes of motion – rotation, flexion/extension, lateral bending, and elongation – combined create the whole body movement.

The weave of trunk rotation

Rotation of the lower body in one direction and the head in the opposite direction in the context of the nervous system response is gait patterning. The trunk muscles travel from the back of the pelvis to the side, and diagonally upward to the front of the body, the neck, and the back of the head (Fig. 4.2).

The weave of rotational movement is described below, beginning with the quadratus lumborum and finishing at the back of the head:

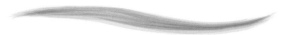

- Quadratus lumborum (QL) lies deep in the back (dorsal) body wall, with two oblique fibers:

  - lateral fibers arise from the transverse processes (TPs) of L5, the iliolumbar ligament and iliac crest, ascending to the spine, to the TPs of lumbar vertebrae above L5

  - medial fibers run from the back (posterior) of the iliac crest to the 12th rib

  - fibers are also found running obliquely from each TP to the 12th rib (Bogduk, 2005).

- Start the rotational movement from the QL fibers on right side; these run from the pelvis medially

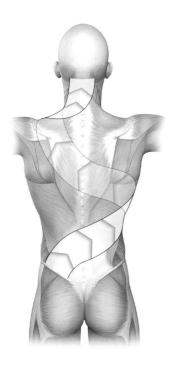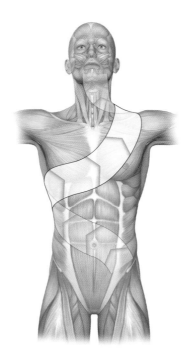

Figure 4.2
Weave of trunk rotation: superficial and deep

into the deep layer of the thoracolumbar fascia (TLF) toward the TPs as a continuation with intertransversarii and multifidus across the midline to the opposite (left) side of the spine connecting to the serratus posterior inferior (Vleeming, 2012).

- From the serratus posterior inferior the weave continues with the left side QL fiber running from the pelvis to the ribs, merging into the middle layer of the transverse abdominal fascia (Breul, 2012).

- The middle layer of the transverse abdominal fascia attaches the internal oblique to internal intercostals, around to the front of the body, crossing the midline again to join the superficial abdominal fascia layer of the external oblique and the middle layer of transverse abdominal fascia (Breul, 2012).

The external oblique merges with the external intercostals that continue upward and deep to the posterior scalenes, with the fibers upward to the suboccipital region (Beach, 2010).

Flexion and extension continuum of the trunk

The movements involved in flexing and extending the trunk take place in the fields of the ventral (front) and dorsal (back) sides of the body. The front and the back are not separate, however, but form a continuous loop that runs up the front and down the back of the trunk and head. There are certain points (at the nose and just above the pubic bone) where the movement changes from flexion to extension (Beach, 2010).

The following lists link landmarks, fascia, and muscles in relation to the nervous system reflex:

Extension reflex path (Fig. 4.3):

- This starts at the nose, goes up through the inner eye, over the crown of the head to the occiput (occipitofrontalis) (Beach, 2010), connecting with

- the suboccipital muscles, specifically the superior rectus in the deep posterior cervical fascial layer, continuous with

- the erector spinae (Myers, 2001); this muscle group lies under the trapezius and runs downward, becoming superficial at the T6–T8 region before changing depth into the TLF, passing through the transverse fascia into

- the superficial lamina of the TLF (Lee, 2011), at the

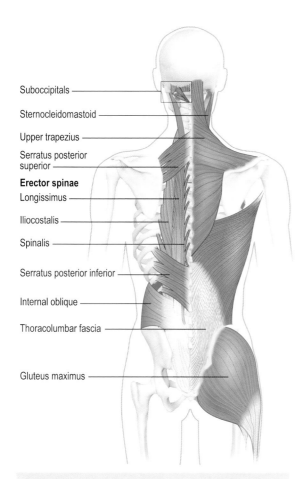

Figure 4.3
Extension continuum of trunk

- lateral raphe, the fascial melding of the abdominal fascia TLF, where the internal oblique attaches then fuses with the fascia of the erector spinae, which

- surface onto the sacrum and continue fascially to the tip of the coccyx, forming part of the pelvic diaphragm (see Fig. 5.3); in addition

- a spiral of the pelvic diaphragm muscles, specifically the pubococcygeus muscle to the pubis, merges with lower fibers of the rectus abdominis

- medial fibers of the rectus abdominis cross at the pubis (see Fig. 4.3)

- transversus abdominis surfaces, constructing the anterior sheath of rectus abdominis

- rectus abdominis attaches to the linea alba, a tendinous raphe formed by fascial sheets of all the abdominal muscles (see Fig. 4.4) and

- pyramidalis inserts on the linea alba over the rectus abdominis up to

- the lower portion of the rectus abdominis to below the navel (Beach, 2010).

Flexion reflex path (Fig. 4.4):

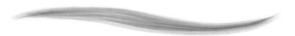

- The path continues upward at the front of the rectus abdominis to the ribcage.

- The rectus does not attach to the sternum but extends high up onto the ribs.

- Rectus abdominis is fixed in position by a very strong tendinous connective tissue sheath; the

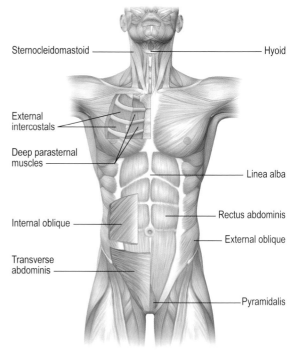

Figure 4.4
Flexion path

lateral side is called the linea semilunaris (named for its half moon shape).

- It runs for two rib segments on each side (known as the "six pack" when contracted into the sheath).

- The rectus abdominis merges with the external intercostals and connects through the lowest, deep pectoralis fascia into the external parasternal interchondral membrane at the soft joint of the ribs to sternum, called the interchondral joints (Lee, 2001), continuing upward.

- The path continues with the sternocleidomastoids (SCM), hyoid muscles, anterior deep cervical muscles, and root of the tongue up to the massester (jaw) and temporals (Beach, 2010).

Healthy movement synergy comes from the organized use of tensile oppositional force in space. Movement in the body initiates from a stable place but at the same time moves away, giving movement a polar quality. When throwing a ball, for example, the feet (or foot) are placed for stability as the torso winds up and releases the arm away. In the trunk, the poles (the nose and just above the pubis), moving in flexion and extension, are the points of transition from the front to the back. These poles, at the two ends of the trunk, curl in toward each other in flexion and move away from one another for arching back extension.

The initiation of flexion from the head, the curling in from the cheek bones and an opposing movement of the occiput spiraling upward and back, prevents the head from falling forward and stimulates a flexor response in the body, turning on the lower area of the abdominals just above the pubic bone. The spinal curve is supported both on the inside (concavity side, in the front) and on the outside (convexity side, in the back), creating a fully engaged trunk in flexion. When lying supine, to begin lifting the head up, the occiput sphere rolls forward as C1 slides back in the opposing direction and initiates the engagement of the deep cervical muscles and the erectors, along with the lower segment of the abdominals, to support the extended curve. Coaching with the concept of these movement borders, and using specific cueing (see below), signals the nervous system to turn on a sequence of muscle firing patterns throughout the body.

Try it!

Lie supine (on the back) with the legs straight. Touch underneath your nose with one hand and place the other just above the pubic bone, using the flat of your hand on the tissue. Listening with the lower hand, notice if there is any tissue change when the head moves. Nod the nose down as if dipping your nose down into a wine glass to sniff the "nose" of the wine. Allow the head to curl off the floor (Fig. 4.5). Did you feel any engagement in the lower abdominal area? Did the tissue change? You have not made a large curl-up motion, as you would, say, in a crunch sit-up; nevertheless, the abdominals have automatically engaged.

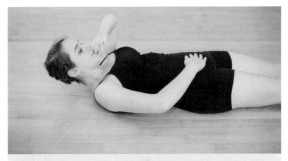

Figure 4.5
Try it! Feeling the initial engagement of the trunk flexors

Lateral bending of the trunk

A whole torso side bend includes the whole length of the body, from the head to the tail and the legs (abduction and adduction). For the sake of defining the direction of trunk movement only, the legs will not be included. The section in Chapter 3 entitled "Balancing the Hip Joint" (p. 81) presented the hip spinning motions of abduction and adduction and this is relevant to add to the trunk side bending.

Starting at the head (Fig. 4.6) and proceeding downward:

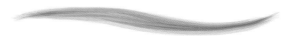

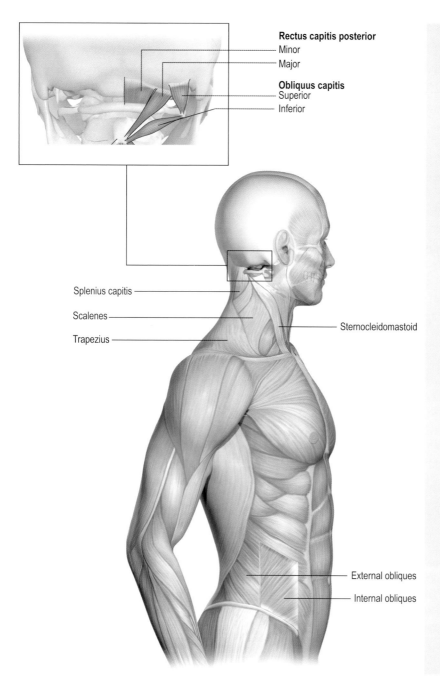

Rectus capitis posterior
- Minor
- Major

Obliquus capitis
- Superior
- Inferior

Splenius capitis

Scalenes

Trapezius

Sternocleidomastoid

External obliques

Internal obliques

Figure 4.6
Lateral movers of the trunk

- There is lateral movement of the eye, ear, jaw, and side of the tongue; the response of hearing evokes the side bending of the head (Beach, 2010).

- The SCM, trapezius, and suboccipitals, specifically the rectus capitis lateralis, superior and oblique,

and splenius capitis all work together to side bend the head toward the direction of the trunk in side bending; alternatively, in balancing toward the center, the head side bends in opposition to the direction of torso's side bending, in a righting reflex.

- Pure side bending involves an equal pull from the external and internal obliques.

- The ribs on the concave side of the torso approximate while those on the opposite side open to expand.

- Typically, there is a flexion or extension component to side bending (see below).

- The movement extends deep into the pelvic bowl, to coccygeus, iliococcygeus and the perineal body.

- At the perineal body, the right and left sides merge and spiral to continue onward to the other side (Beach, 2010) (see Fig. 4.3).

Once the degree of side bending displaces the center of gravity of the trunk, the lateral flexors initiate and direct the movement. The opposite (contralateral) side is more active against gravity, in order to balance the load (otherwise one would fall to the ground). The contralateral lateral flexors balance the action of the gravity and control the rate and extent of the movement (Bogduk, 2005).

Elongation: narrowing of the body

Elongation of the trunk with any movement is one aspect of stability necessary for support of the spine. Core stability is an important function for controlling a body's position and motion to transfer and control force in physical activities or posture. Narrowing the trunk to feel elongation is an anti-buckling mechanism for the spine. The integrated core naturally enables an upright posture without effort. And with physical exertion, a rotatory stiffening action of the core will protect the spine from strain or injury.

When the body resists a force from above and below (head and feet or, if seated, head and lower pelvic bones), the internal action is one of drawing the body inward to go outward against the force in both directions. The synergistic action of the psoas, internal obliques, and multifidus engaging by filling up the area around the spine (remember the airbag imagery in Ch. 3) is reinforcement for the spine. The effect is an elongation and longitudinal reinforcement of the spine allowing for dynamic stability.

Try it!

Sit upright in a chair with the feet on the floor. Arms can hang by the side (Fig. 4.7). Feeling the feet and sits bones moving downward and the crown of the head moving upward, exhale, and feel the elongation as a contrast between the movement of the trunk upward through the head and downward through the feet and pelvis. Use mental imagery for the trunk, imagining it as a tube of toothpaste. Exhale, and evenly squeeze the tube from the sides and feel the surfaces of the trunk draw in and the toothpaste streaming out at the top of the head and the feet. On the inhale, feel the tube filling out to its original width. Practice this action for recruitment to elongate.

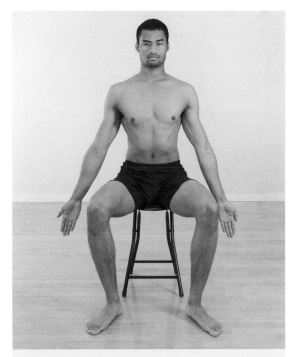

Figure 4.7
Try it! Elongation

The coiling feeling around the trunk in elongation engages (Fig. 4.8):

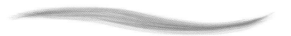

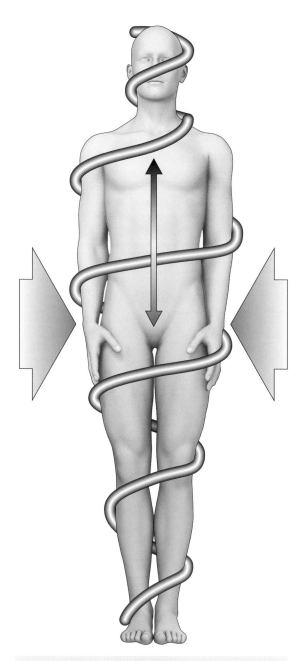

Figure 4.8
Elongation imagery

- TrA (transversus abdominis), which spans the whole abdominal area between the ribcage and the pelvis, wrapping around like a corset, forming a myofascial ring:

  - starting at the back from the lateral edge of the quadratus lumborum to iliac crest with

  - internal oblique merging from the lateral raphe of the thoracolumbar fascia, moving toward the front along the

  - inguinal ligament and anterior two-thirds of the inner lip of the iliac crest

  - blends and constructs the anterior sheath of the rectus abdominis, reaching

  - the linea alba in the midline

  - internal aspects of the lower six costal cartilages (ribs) interdigitating with the costal fibers of the diaphragm

- the ribcage, the external and internal intercostals along with the external and internal oblique muscles

- scalenes, specifically anterior scalenes

- the throat internally and the platysma as it blends with the mouth (Beach, 2010).

The TrA is interdigitating with the diaphragm and lies deep under the rectus abdominis. However, the TrA surfaces more superficial in the lower pelvic area as it weaves into the rectus abdominis sheath. On an exhalation, the action of drawing the abdominal wall inward moves the organs back toward the spine, eliminating overpressure on the pelvic floor. The TrA and the pelvic diaphragm are dynamically connected and coordinated throughout breathing. During the exhalation, the TrA contracts concentrically and the diaphragm is eccentrically contracting to facilitate the upward motion of the diaphragm (Richardson et al., 2004). A feeling of narrowing and elongation occurs with the TrA/diaphragm movement along with the pelvic bones drawing closer together, creating stability for the pelvis. The ribcage narrows as the intercostals and external obliques participate in the funneling of the ribs inward and downward.

The action of elongation stimulates a whole trunk engagement through the intrinsic tone of the

- the pelvic diaphragm plus the hip joint muscles, which are continuous with the pelvic floor (Ch. 3, "Hip Myofascia")

- psoas, multifidus, the paraspinal muscles, and

myofascial network. The inward pulling tension against the spine, which is a more rigid structure, will push out against the tension coming in; this creates stability in the structure, allowing the joints of the spine to move freely. In practicing a whole body narrowing, the only observable movement is one of elongation.

Trunk spiral movements

In everyday life, the spine is moving in all dimensions. All movement evolves around a combination of flexion/extension, side bending, and rotation. It is the overall shape of the vertebrae in each region of the spine that dictates its motion (Fig. 4.9). The cervical

Figure 4.9
Curves of the spine and facet joints

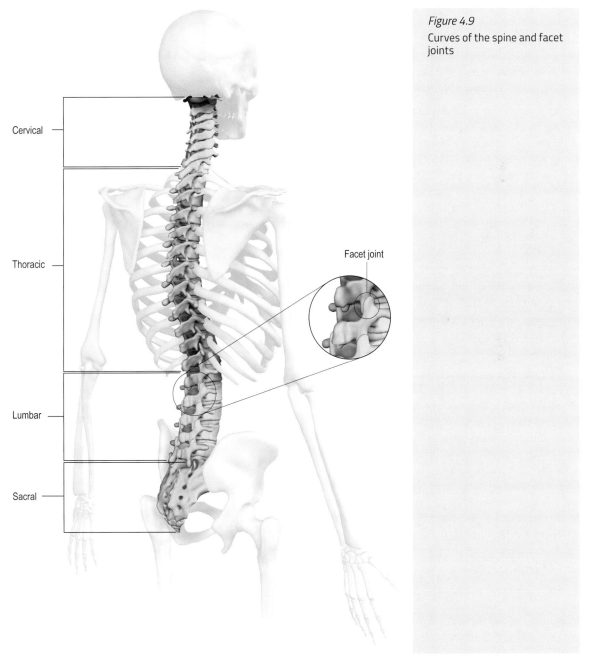

Cervical

Thoracic

Facet joint

Lumbar

Sacral

spine has a convexity in the front and a concavity in the back, in the same way as the lumbar spine. Both of these regions extend well; however, although flexion is possible it is not as available. The thorax has the reverse curve, with concavity in the front and convexity in the back. In addition, the thorax has ribs attached to the vertebrae and these also influence the range of flexion and extension (see Ch. 5, "Motion of Breathing"). The shape of the bones of the sacrum is convex in the back and concave in the front but by the age of 22–25 the parts have fused together to form one bone that moves at the sacroiliac joint with the pelvis (Ch. 3, "Sacroiliac Movement").

In the study of movement mechanics, the analysis and definitions of coupling spinal motions are varied and complex. In flexion and extension there is no coupling per se unless one's spine is in a significant twist, as in scoliosis (review Ch. 3, part 2, "Action of Forward and Backward Bending"). When side bending and rotating the spine, the design of the joints at each region lends itself to a slightly different motion (Lundon and Bolton, 2001). The size of the vertebral body and the orientation of the facets change how that segment will move (see Fig. 4.9). The cervical vertebrae are smaller, with facet joints orientated in a flatter coronal plane (side to side) below C2 so that the motion available in the lower cervical vertebrae is greater for head turning movements (Ch. 8, "Characteristics and Movements of Cervical Spine") (Kapandji, 1974).

The typical thoracic vertebra's articular facet orientation allows a sliding of the bones relative to each other, producing flexion, extension, and rotation. In rotation, there is an oppositional translation motion. Also, when rotation occurs in the thoracic spine, the movement occurs at each corresponding rib at every segment. Segmental movement, rotation and translation of the thoracic vertebrae allows for the whole spinal column movement. It is common to see minimal to no movement in the thoracic spine and excessive movement in the lumbar and cervical spines.

Unlike in the thorax, the shape of each lumbar bone varies from the top down, from smaller to larger, and rotation occurs as the upper vertebra slides over the lower one. Instead of a rotation and translation motion, as in the thorax, a shearing motion is present (Kapandji, 1974). In a healthy person, the torsion

of the disc provides a resistance to the torque and the facet joints protect the spine from excessive strain (Lundon and Bolton, 2001). As stated by Lundon and Bolton (2001), the disc provides little resistance to side bending at the first few degrees of movement. Moving beyond the range available severely stretches the disc and increases the pressure. Adding an excessive load with side bending, the risk for a negative change of the basic disc structure is possible. Awareness of the movement of the spine as a whole structure, distributing the load throughout the central axis of the spine and balancing the spiral movement will improve the body's ability to respond to tensile forces.

> **Practitioner note**
>
> What is the difference between kinesiology and biomechanics? The definitions are that kinesiology is the study of motion while biomechanics is the study of the mechanics of life. Kinesiology therefore is inclusive of biomechanics. Understanding the mechanics of movement is fundamental in both fields. Biomechanics includes statics (the study of forces in equilibrium), and calculations and mechanics of any bodily function. It is more precise to use the word kinesiology in the setting of physical training.

Coupled movements

"Forward Saw" (Fig. 4.10) is a classic Pilates mat exercise; it is a perfect example of the spine's combined movement of rotation, flexion, and lateral bending. From an upright and seated position, the trunk spirals to the left, as shown, then unspirals to sit upright. Observe for the concentric rings of the thorax moving forward on the right and backward on the left. The ribs are opening on the right side and approximating on the left side. If the thorax is rotating and flexing well, there will be a translation of the vertebrae to the right. This spiral is the weave of trunk rotation motion (see Fig. 4.2), especially the connection of the right side oblique line from under the arm toward the left pelvis. These muscles move the thorax relative to the lumbar spine and pelvis. When the thorax is less mobile, the rotation will occur in the lumbar spine, inhibiting the local stabilizers of the lower spine and pelvis. The global muscles rotating the thorax are underworked.

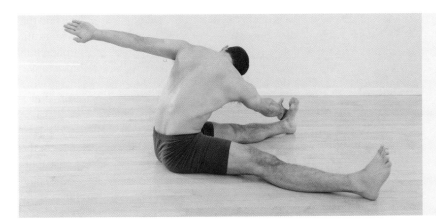

Figure 4.10
Forward Saw

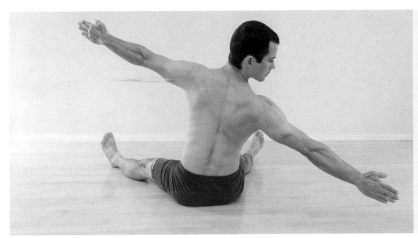

Figure 4.11
Backward Saw

"Backward Saw" (Fig. 4.11) is a variation of the "Saw", moving the spine in rotation and extension. Again, the thorax movement involves a similar rib-cage motion to that seen in the "Forward Saw". Moving into the rotation and extension engages the weave of rotational trunk muscles, specifically calling on the global muscles of the posterior thorax that span several ribs, iliocostalis, longissimus, and spinalis.

Rotation in the thorax is a functional movement that is necessary to train dynamic stabilization and eliminate stress in the lumbar spine. It is important to note the degree of flexion and extension in the spine prior to moving into the rotation. A normal kyphosis allows for well placed scapulae and greater potential for movement. Some postures are excessive in flexion or extension. A challenging posture for a movement teacher is scoliosis, which becomes very complex when observing an individual or a group of people in motion.

In promoting ease of rotation of the spine, look for a balance of the spine in all three motions. When stacking the movements, each one is smaller than the previous movement. The coupled motion is the body describing a spiral in space that feels expansive, not restricted.

Thorax regions

The thorax is complex, containing varied vertebral bone shapes and ribs; it can be divided into four regions (Fig. 4.12):

- Region 1: vertebromanubrium T1, T2, first rib, second rib, and manubrium
- Region 2: vertebrosternal T3–T7 with associated ribs

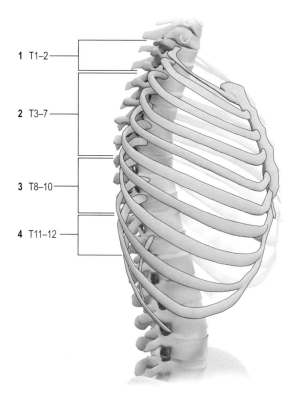

1 T1–2

2 T3–7

3 T8–10

4 T11–12

Figure 4.12
Regions of the thorax

- Region 3: vertebrochondral T8–T10 with associated ribs

- Region 4: thoracolumbar T11–T12 with floating ribs.

Region 1 is associated with arm, head, and neck movements. This region is also significant in breathing. The first rib is unique because it is a fibrous, and therefore a stable rib. The first and second ribs are less mobile than the adjoining thoracic vertebrae. In the thoracolumbar region (Region 4), the floating ribs do not hinder the ability to flex and extend the 11th and 12th vertebrae, so there is pure spin (Lee, 2001). Flexion in Region 2 is possible with the least amount of coupled movement and is augmented with an inhalation. The sternum has micromotion with breath and is able to move independently (Lee, 2001). In Region 3, the orientation of the facets allows for movement in an anterior and posterior rotation of the ribs. There

is more freedom in rotation and lateral flexion in the third region.

Movement of the trunk is variable between individuals, depending on the flexibility of the ribcage and spine, and it also varies with age. In the young, the ribcage is more mobile because the secondary ossification of the upper (superior) articulation of the rib on the vertebrae is not fully developed. In contrast, in the mature adult, the stiffness of the superior articulation restricts rotation in all three planes.

Ease in flexion depends on the motion available at the rib. There are three patterns for flexion and extension (Lee, 2001):

- Flexible thorax:

  - in flexion the motion has reached its limit in the spine (vertebrae stop moving forward) and the ribs continue to move anteriorly relative to the vertebrae

  - in extension the motion of the vertebre meets its end range moving posterior and the ribs continue to move posteriorly relative to the vertebrae.

- Stiff thorax:

  - in flexion the ribs are less flexible than the spine; when flexing, the ribs meet their limit first, followed by continued vertebral motion anterior and the vertebrae continue to move on stationary ribs

  - in extension the ribs meet their limit and the vertebrae continue to move posteriorly.

- Thorax and rib flexibility between the ribs and spine are the same with no apparent movement between the vertebrae and the ribs. When the motion is similar it reduces available motion and the quantity of movement is reduced.

Ease in side flexion of the thorax is when the ribs on one side approximate while those on the opposite side separate or open. The spine will translate in the opposite direction of the side bending. In both the mobile and stiff thorax, the ribs during side flexion stop moving before the vertebrae (Fig. 4.13).

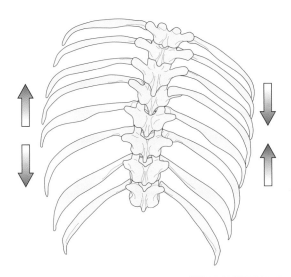

Figure 4.13
Approximation of ribs

Knowing the body's potential for flexible or stiff ribs is valuable information for the movement teacher. Some bodies are able to twist and bend more easily in the thorax than others. When a body is pushed past its barrier, a number of things may happen: the soft tissue in the area may become overstressed, a rib may dislodge, or the client may feel a sense of inadequacy due to being unable to move as far as is being asked. Teach the client to move within the available range by sensing when the movement of the ribcage ceases.

Helpful cueing is to visualize and describe the ribs as concentric rings. When moving into flexion the rings in the back move upward, sending the rings in the front downward. In rotation, move the right side of the rings back as the left side moves forward. When the mind sees the bones moving, naturally the movement will be within the range available. Paying attention to the body's barrier will allow the client to move with resilience and strength, eliminating over-movement.

Practitioner note

Understanding the skeletal movement potential enhances the ability to see, feel, and sense an individual's movement barrier. The practice is to meet the person where they are, offering a direction of movement into their barrier but not past it. The observation is asking whether the barrier is a skeletal barrier, an emotional barrier (fear), a connective tissue issue, or breath restriction. The teacher's sense of resistance from the client is read, honored, and, as by a loving parent, the client is encouraged to go just a little further, just outside of their comfort zone – "A comfortable challenge." Awareness of the barrier in a client comes from the mastery of one's own barriers and resistance.

Cueing

As movement practitioners, the art of cueing is a skill that we are continuously developing; it is an intuitive process. The listener is the person who is influenced by the cues and by understanding the words or images. One person may understand and execute a movement with a particular cue while another person fails to respond to it. Building up a repertoire of many possible cues allows more choices for describing the intent of the movement skill.

Typically in Pilates, when training the trunk, the movement begins either at the head/upper trunk or at the pelvis/lower trunk. There are two opposing movements occurring at the same time: the movement being executed and the countermovement of slowing it down or stabilizing it. Even when moving from the top there is a contrasting action occurring at the other end. This contrast is creating the stability of being anchored into the ground while extending in the opposite direction, for expanded stability. Be clear on the contrasting directions, on the areas of the body anchored, and on the movement of the bones.

Cueing bones

Movement cues which emphasize the bones rather than muscles promote moving the whole body functionally rather than isolating a single muscle. Using the intention of bone movement connects the mind to the body and stimulates a response in the body that shifts it into sensing internal movement. The visualization of a bone moving in opposing directions promotes a precise amount of effort needed to facilitate a felt sense of total engagement.

The cues are important in describing the direction of the bones in counter-direction to one another; for example: "Drop the head of the femur deep into the socket before floating the knee up." The direction of the bone, the head of the femur, is down and in, with an opposite upward action of the knee. This promotes the proper spin in the hip joint for hip. The action of the hip joint movement stimulates a support of the spinal column through the myofascia (psoas and multifidus, Ch. 3, "Hip Flexion Motion and Spine Stability").

Loops and Wheels

Beginning a movement from a place of best alignment enables the body to move with integrity. If the head is forward prior to moving forward, for example, then there is no movement available. Another example is that if the trunk is rounded over, the body is already in flexion, with no accessible spinal motion of flexion. An optimal place to begin movement is one of being centered. Imagine the loops moving in oppositional directions to facilitate feeling upright and balanced without stiffness (Fig. 4.14).

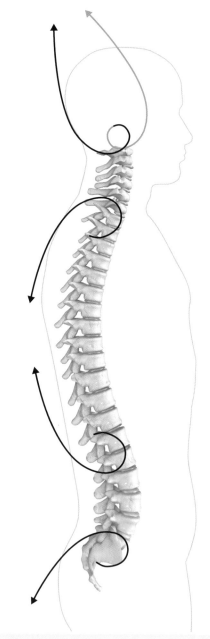

- Imagine the loop from the occiput that moves up and spins forward to balance the head.

- At the level of the shoulder girdle, clavicles, and manubrium, including the shoulder blades, the direction of the bones is to rotate the clavicles minimally (micromovement) backward, allowing for the shoulder blades to melt down the back and maintaining width across the chest.

- The kidneys in the back and the inverted V of the front ribs, as one loop, rolls forward.

- The pelvis rolls backward.

- The weight of the feet is "Standing on Pencils" (see Ch. 1).

Motion of flexion cues

Visualizing the rotational direction at these specific segments of the spine while moving into flexion or extension imprints the movement pattern. The purpose of these particular cues is to:

Figure 4.14
Loops and Wheels imagery

- perceive the segmental movement mentally to train the nervous system (Malouin et al., 2003)

- allow for the movement to be well distributed, thereby engaging the whole myofascial connections in the different planes

- learn to support the curves of the spine.

Top down

Moving the body into flexion from the top down requires the head to roll from the occiput on the first cervical vertebra (details in Ch. 8). Cueing is to imagine the ear as a wheel and the wheels rolling in a curved path moving from the back of the ears up, over the top, and forward (Fig. 4.15).

> **Tip**
>
> Visual cue: "You have eyes on the back of your head. Begin looking up with the eyes on the back of the head."

In standing moving into forward flexion, gravity takes a hold of the head and the sternum softens, moving into the body, not downward. Then the lower ribcage (Regions 3 and 4) on the back (posterior) side moves up, away from the back rim of the pelvis (posterior ilia), so that the lower front border of the ribcage, the inverted V angle of the ribcage, moves from the sides in an anterior rolling direction. (Note that to "soften" does not mean relax: the word evokes a sense of minimal effort, an amount of effort that is "just right.")

> **Tip**
>
> Verbal cue: "Imagine the kidneys [make sure clients know where kidneys are located – it is informative to ask them to touch the kidneys] and move them away from the spine and upward as the front ribs soften down." This important action creates a tension to elongate the waist to support the front of the curve through the eccentric length of the back.

The pelvis will rotate around the femoral heads as it moves anteriorly (refer to Ch. 3, "Action of Forward Bending and Backward Bending," for when the pelvis shifts behind the pedal base).

Curl-up from head cues: head float

In order to practice full torso flexion, as done in many of the Pilates mat work exercises, it is necessary to

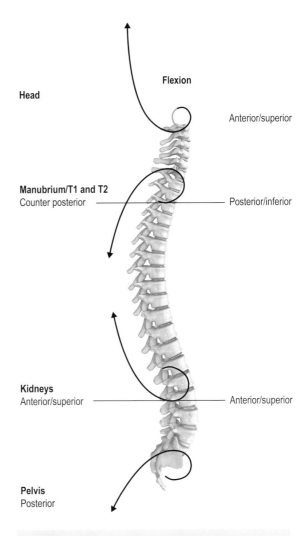

Figure 4.15
Flexion wheels

lift the head off the mat. Many people have tight and weak necks that inhibit the head rotation loop described above. Chapter 8 describes neck releases and strengthening exercises that may be performed prior to lifting and holding the head off the mat. The motion of the rotation loop begins at the occiput and atlas (O/A) joint where the skull meets the first vertebra. It is segmental motion following the initial O/A motion. Prior to movement at the O/A to begin cervical flexion, it is necessary to pre-engage the deep anterior cervical muscles. Practice the following cues:

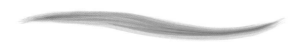

- Lie supine on the mat with the knees bent.

- Be sure the head rests on floor in alignment with the thorax; if a person has a head forward position it is necessary to place a small flat folded towel under the head (not under the neck) (Fig. 4.16 A).

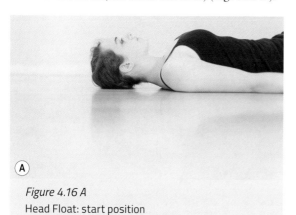

(A)

Figure 4.16 A
Head Float: start position

- "Look at the ceiling; on an inhale, slightly imagine floating the head so that the back of your head is unweighting but still in contact with the mat" (Fig. 4.16 B).

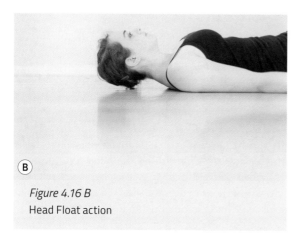

(B)

Figure 4.16 B
Head Float action

- Exhale and place the head on the mat.

Practice this micromovement, adjusting the awareness of the client's head alignment. No change of head position, either chin up or chin down, should be seen.

It is only an *intention* of moving the head to activate the deep anterior cervical muscles. Working from this feeling, follow the movement of the turning on of the anterior cervical muscles with an "eyes on the back of your head" cue to anteriorly rotate the head, and begin the segmental flexion through the trunk. (For more movement cues and exercises that can be used for the head to thorax regions, refer to Ch. 8.)

Small Curl-up

Coaching a person to flex their spine for core exercises is important for developing the segmental timing of the movement of the whole spine to stimulate the local muscle support with the global muscles action. This avoids compression of the spine, especially in flexion, and will strengthen the trunk without the risk of injury to the spine. In a class situation, the participants use their own hands to monitor the movement and timing of the curl-up.

- Lie supine with the knees bent.

- Place the tips of the fingers along the middle of the sternum and place one finger of the other hand under the nose (Fig. 4.17 A).

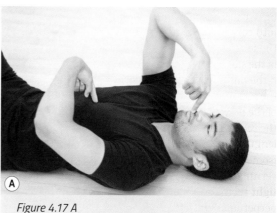

(A)

Figure 4.17 A
Small Curl-up: start position

- Using the cues above, inhale through the nose, float the head, and begin the loop of the occiput.

- Exhale slowly.

- Press gently on the sternum toward the floor and slightly toward the sacrum (Fig. 4.17 B).

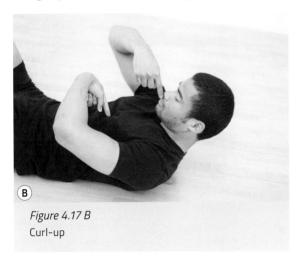

Figure 4.17 B
Curl-up

- Hold the position and breathe 2–3 cycles.
- Inhale lower down the base of the neck first, then the head.

The hands inform the body if the head position loses its occiput loop. The finger under the nose will feel an increase in pressure from O/A shifting forward. The amount of pressure on the finger does not change from the beginning to the end of the curl. The sternum cue assists in the mid-thoracic movement into flexion along with the inferior intention of connecting into the rectus abdominis. It is very important that the length or distance between the xiphoid (bottom of the sternum) and the pubic bone remains the same. If the pubic bone curls up, the pelvis is not stable and the abdominals are shortening. The mid-sacrum area of the pelvis is anchored into the mat, which requires the rectus abdominis to work in its functional muscle length, using a concentric contraction at first then an isometric to stabilize. (Ch. 5 goes into more detail concerning abdominal contraction patterns.) Short and tight rectus abdominis and fascia of the abdominals perpetuates the kyphotic posture and does not serve the person's strength for being upright. (See "MET for the Lat-Pectorals and Abdominals," below).

Bottom down

When rolling down from sitting, the initiation begins with elongation of the trunk (see the image of squeezing toothpaste, described above), followed by the coccyx curling and femoral movement. The erectors are part of this connection and therefore, a lengthening of the erector spinae group occurs as the coccyx begins to move and the hip joint extends. The pelvis moves posteriorly as the lower two regions of the thorax begin the kidney motion of up and anterior rotation, creating a lengthening "bow" of the back muscles in conjunction with the "engaged" concave curve of the front abdominals. Cue to "lengthen the waist." Again, the distance between the bottom of the sternum, at the xiphoid, and the pubic bone neither shortens nor lengthens but remains the same throughout the rest of the movement.

Moving into extension

The starting position of the body always sets up the potential for optimal movement.

Lying prone

The exact details involved in lying on one's stomach vary due to different body types and the varying size of frontal tissues (meaning breast size in women and everyone's abdominal girth). There will be no neutral position to begin with. First, align the body in the best form possible. Place a small rolled towel on the floor to rest the forehead, to breathe easier, and as comfort for the neck. This position is one that is engaged to place the body in the proper alignment before starting the exercises. Generally, the shoulders tend to fall forward toward the floor with gravity, creating too much width between the shoulder blades, and the legs will be either in external rotation or in internal rotation (each individual has a natural tendency for one position over the other).

Prone position alignment and activation (see "Prone Leg Spirals" in Ch. 3):

- The shoulder blades should be sitting on the ribs so that the inner border of one scapula is approximately 3 inches (7.62 cm) from the edge to the spine.
- The arms and humeral heads are lifted off the floor, with the arms long, the palms facing the thighs, and the thumbs to the floor.

- The front surface of the pelvis is in contact with the floor as best as possible, with the ASIS and pubic bone on the mat; it is important for the pubis to be in contact as well as the top of the thighs; there is no hip flexion.

- Legs are looking for balance of work in the hip with the inner and the outer upper thigh.

Cueing extension motion from the prone position, begin with cueing the eyes to look up (not the chin to lift up). The eyes stimulate the nervous system to engage the extensors. Lead the movement of the sternum forward and up as the clavicles rotate backward, as in standing upright loops. At this point the height of the trunk will depend on the movement being performed and the specificity of the level of the thorax being activated. The important movement is the sternum and clavicle motion in contrast to the pelvis anchoring and oppositional lengthening of the tail (Fig. 4.18).

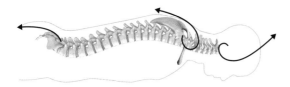

Figure 4.18
Prone extension loops

Pelvic diaphragm cues

The pelvic diaphragm (a more accurate name for the pelvic floor) responds best to movement and breathing when the pelvis and ribcage are in alignment. Commonly used pelvic floor cues are to perform a "Kegel" exercise or to hold back gas, but these cues are not optimal in terms of training for function because they promote gripping. In movement, the pelvic diaphragm co-contracts with the diaphragm, transversus abdominis, obturator internus (a hip external rotator muscle connected to the levator ani muscles), and small back muscles called multifidus. It is a dynamic system to develop a functioning and strong pelvic diaphragm, working with the core, breathing, and hip joint strength.

In a healthy normal body the pelvic diaphragm is "wired" with both the conscious (somatic) and unconscious (autonomic) parts of our central nervous system to work with movement and breathing. Imagery for pelvic floor co-contraction is helpful for clients to access feeling the dynamic system of the breath and activation of the deep hip and transversus abdominis muscles. Practicing the "Seated Elongation with Hips" (below) or "Narrowing of the Body" (above) exercises helps to engage these connections.

Describe the elongation process, adding attention to the pelvic area as a bowl with the inner pelvis space between the sits bones, pubis, and coccyx where a trampoline attaches to the edges of the space. If you jump on a real trampoline, the fabric elongates with tension as the body places its weight down onto it, then recoils as the body launches into the air. In the body, on the inhalation, the diaphragm lowers and the trampoline expands to support the organs and on the exhalation it rebounds, returning to its original position. Practicing the breathing and visualizing the depth changes of the pelvic diaphragm helps the nervous system make connections for better support.

Visually describe where the pelvic diaphragm is located along with its co-contraction partners. Practicing the timing of the breath with diaphragmatic movements of both thorax and pelvis is helpful to mindfully access healthy support. Acknowledge the feeling of a relaxed versus contracted pelvic diaphragm. The following are suggestions for effective visualizations:

- Imagine the deep pelvis bowl inside; a woven basket is sitting inside attached to the inner rim from the pubic bone, along the rim, toward the right inner hip, around to the tail bone, continuing around to the left inner hip and pubic bone (see Fig. 4.3).

- Think of slowly drawing the basket inward to make it smaller and lifting the whole basket up into the pelvis.

- Visualize a drawstring purse and the hole with the strings is in the center; imagine drawing the strings in and up into the bowl, closing the purse; relax and allow the strings to loosen.

- Using the mouth to mimic the contraction and relaxation is fun to try; drawing the pelvic diaphragm up into the bowl is the closing of the mouth; relax and open the mouth.

- Try working with imagery changing the breath: inhale–contract; inhale–relax; exhale–contract; exhale–relax; hold the breath in both contract and relax.

Having an understanding of the pelvic diaphragm and of the feeling of it contracting and relaxing is important neuromuscular patterning prior to challenging exercises. During this practice, there should not be any apparent movement of the bones. The contraction is slow. Encourage practice at home for those who need to develop better connection. Practice breath work in coordination with the feeling of the pelvic diaphragm movement (Ch. 5). All the pelvis and hip exercises in Chapter 3 are also recommended.

Once the pelvic diaphragm movement is embodied, challenge the body by moving in all directions. Strengthening the deep hip muscles and the trunk will effectively train the pelvic diaphragm. The simplest movement for improving pelvic function is a squat. Practicing squats will move the pelvis and sacrum into an optimal position structurally and strengthen the hip muscles. The squat balances out the pelvic floor areas that have tightness and lines up the weaker areas to connect into its functional whole.

Seated elongation with hip

The following is a good home program exercise for clients. During this exercise, the legs, hips, and spine are engaging as a unit – a full body movement.

- Sit on a stool or on the edge of a chair so that the hips are higher than the knees.

- The weight of the trunk is on the middle of the sits bones; the legs are open to a comfortably wide position of about 60–70° abduction, with the feet slightly in front of the knees; the knee is open a few degrees, the shin is at a slight angle, the arms are hanging down, and the spine is upright (Fig. 4.19).

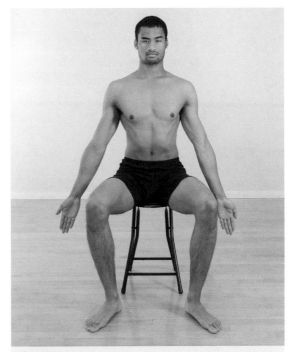

Figure 4.19
Seated elongation with hip

- Lift the toes so that the balls of the feet and heel can press into the floor.

- On the inhale press the feet into the floor and away, as if the feet will slide away, but do not actually move them; feel how the thigh bones engage in the hip.

- On the exhale, practice the toothpaste squeeze of the torso.

- Practice pressing the feet into the floor and pull the feet toward the stool, activating the posterior leg.

- Choose the intention of the feet sliding away or pulling in to match the alignment need of the pelvis; if sitting too far back, pull the feet in to move the sacrum and pelvis forward; press away to move the sacrum and pelvis back.

- A suggestion is to take a stiff belt (not elastic) and fasten it around the pelvis bones just below the ASIS. Tighten the belt as much as possible (Fig. 4.20). When the exhale and narrowing action occurs, the belt should feel looser.

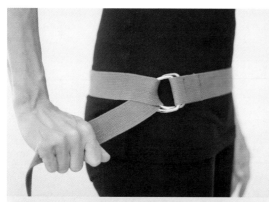

Figure 4.20
Belt around the pelvis for felt sense of pelvis stability

Practitioner note

Visual image for balanced sitting: the stacked diaphragms; feeling the pelvis weighted on the center, favoring front edge of the sits bones, with the thorax loop moving from the back to front, chest moving from front to back, and head rotating from the ears forward.

Rotation and side bending movement cues

Rotation and side bending cues are described in the "Trunk Spiral Movements" section above. An additional cue for side bending and rotation is "One Lung Breathing," a cue from Eve Gentry (1910–1994), an original Pilates teacher. It involves simply inhaling into one lung to facilitate the opening of the ribs on one side.

Note

Eve Gentry taught Mr. Pilates "Contrology" from 1936 to 1968, when she moved to Santa Fe, New Mexico, where she continued her work.

Try it!

Sit in good alignment; place one hand on the right side of the ribcage. Breathing through the nose, inhale slowly, sending the air into one lung.

A variation, to facilitate a clearer feel, is to turn the head 10° toward the lung being filled. Use the finger of one hand to close the opposite nostril (Fig. 4.21). If head is turned to the right, close off the left nostril. Inhale slowly, feeling the expansion of the right lung. Feel with the hand on the side of the ribcage for the expansion of the ribs.

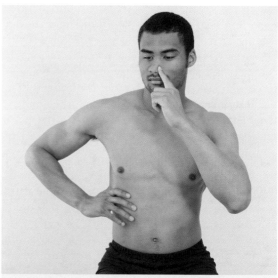

Figure 4.21
One Lung Breathing

The expansion of one side of the ribcage facilitates side bending. If breathing into the right side, the right rib cage opens and the spine side bends to the left (convexity of the curve on the right side). The left side bending translates the apex of the convex curve to the right. ("Translate" means to slide or change the position of an object without rotation.) Seeing the shape and movement of the spine as it side bends, the apex of the curve moves to the right. Cueing a right rotation with flexion (due to flexion and rotation the spine will side bend to the same side), as in the Pilates exercise "Saw" (see Fig. 4.10), the breath will fill the left side of the ribcage. Experiment with the one lung breathing while moving in and out of side bending and rotation of the spine.

Resetting the trunk

CLIENT STORY

A client with whom I have worked for over 10 years has a twist in her body that we work to keep as centered as possible. She is over 60, healthy, and moderately active in her life. Her program has been a combination of mat movements (not the traditional Pilates mat) specifically for her spinal rotation and traditional Pilates apparatus work twice a week. She was traveling in Europe when her back "went out" as she was getting into a cab. Her first reaction was to call me immediately. Back at the hotel, she chose to try moving for a remedy. Lying on the floor, she said to herself, "what movements would Madeline have me do?" She remembered the "Leg Reaches," "Rotating Hips," "Tom Swan," and pelvic tilt movements. In addition, when she felt "put together," she

followed up with the Quadruped series and Bridges. She was able to walk without discomfort, she could sit, though not for too long as stiffness crept in, and sleeping was fine with pillows supporting her spine. A well-trained client is one who embodies the simplest movements to retune her body back to her center.

The combination of "Leg Reaches" and "Rotating Hips" resets the spine that is stuck in a torque, lateral bending with the rotation. It may present as SIJ (sacroiliac joint) pain, sacral tension, lumbar stiffness or discomfort, and hip pain. Because it is a whole spine movement, the combination of the two relieves holding and tension in the thorax, shoulders, and neck.

Leg Reaches

Assessment:

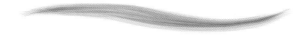

- Lie supine (on back) with the legs straight.

- Reach the right leg long as if someone was pulling it; only reach as far as you can keep your lower ribcage in contact with the mat (do not arch the back) (Fig. 4.22 A).

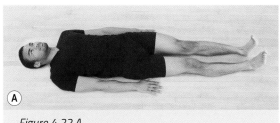

Figure 4.22 A
Reaching right leg

- Assess: does the right leg reach easily?

- Reach the left leg and compare it with the right side (Fig. 4.22 B).

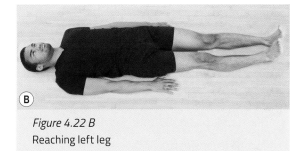

(B)

Figure 4.22 B
Reaching left leg

- Which leg is more difficult to lengthen? (As an example, let us say it is the left leg.)

Movement strategy:

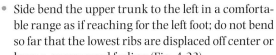

- Side bend the upper trunk to the left in a comfortable range as if reaching for the left foot; do not bend so far that the lowest ribs are displaced off center or have a compressed feeling (Fig. 4.23).

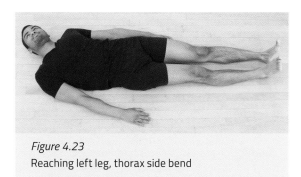

Figure 4.23
Reaching left leg, thorax side bend

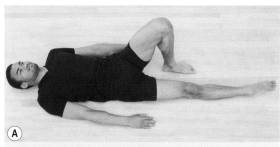

Ⓐ *Figure 4.24 A*
Rotating Hips: start position

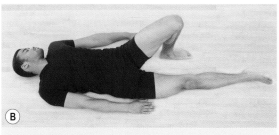

Ⓑ *Figure 4.24 B*
Rotation

- Perform the leg reaches with the left leg while in the left thorax side bend.

- Hold this position and repeat reaches with the left leg until you feel more ease of movement when reaching this leg.

- Perform the "Rotating Hips" exercise (below) with the left leg bent.

- Bring the spine back to the center, and reassess using the leg reaches; notice the ease of the left leg; if the right side feels comparatively stuck, repeat the movement on the right; if it feels good on both sides, finish.

Rotating Hips

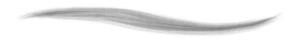

- After "Leg Reaches," lie centered again.

- Bend the left knee so the foot is on the floor (we are still using the left side as the example; it could be the right foot if the leg reaches were performed on the right) (Fig. 4.24 A).

- The right leg is straight; the arms are at the sides.

- Press into the foot of the bent knee, rotate the pelvis to face right and simultaneously look over the left shoulder (Fig. 4.24 B).

- The knee does not move; it remains upright; do not allow the left knee to follow the pelvis; there is no adduction of the thigh; the pelvis is rotating around the femur (remember the mortar and pestle in Ch. 3).

- The action is a spiral from the back around to the front, moving evenly from back to front; the tendency is to push from the back and not connect into the diagonal line of the internal oblique to the external oblique–serratus anterior continuum.

- Inhale on the rotation and exhale, returning to starting position.

- Repeat until you feel more movement in your spine.

- Reassess and feel for the change in your ability to reach the left leg.

Tom Swan: simple

The exercise called "Tom Swan" is named after two people named Tom, both of whom influenced this way of working with the body. The first, Tom Hendrickson DC, developed a unique system of realigning the connective tissue using his wave mobilization method, called the Hendrickson Method® of orthopedic massage. The second, Thomas Hanna, was the founder of Hanna Somatic Education® and developed the field named somatics. In Pilates, the "Swan" exercise is a back extension movement. In Tom Swan, which combines somatic ideas with the Pilates Swan, the spinal motion is extension and rotation with hip extension. It is important to balance the elongation, extension and rotation, feeling length in the extension.

- Lie prone with the head turned to the right (Fig. 4.25 A).

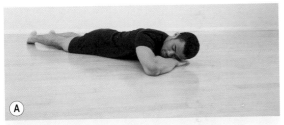

Figure 4.25 A
Tom Swan beginning

- Place the back of the right hand on the left cheekbone, resting it on the mat; look at the right elbow; the hand is attached to the cheekbone and moves with the trunk.
- On an inhale, elongate the body and float the chest with the hand on the cheekbone; the chest and arm lifts up and rotates to the right, looking over the right shoulder toward the left leg (Fig. 4.25 B).

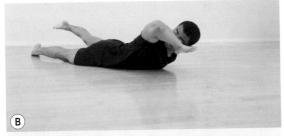

Figure 4.25 B
Lifting movement

- Simultaneously, the left leg extends off the mat.
- Lower and repeat 5 times; change to the left side.

Movement Flow with Tom Swan

- Lift into Tom Swan, rotating to the right (the right leg and left arm are on the mat, not moving in space but stabilizing).
- Look at the floor and extend the right arm overhead (one arm swimming) (Fig. 4.26 A).

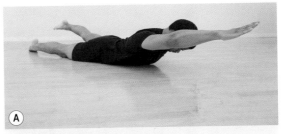

Figure 4.26 A
Movement Flow with Tom Swan: arm extend out for flow

- Lift both legs and move the arms into a T position (now only the trunk is on the mat, with the upper thorax lifted) (Fig. 4.26 B).

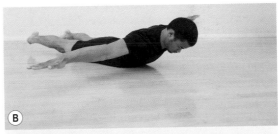

Figure 4.26 B
Arms in T with leg up

- Move the left arm over the head, right arm to side, and lower the left leg to the floor (one arm swimming on the other side) (Fig. 4.26 C).
- Bring the left hand to the right cheekbone, turning the head to the left, looking over the left shoulder at the back right leg (Fig. 4.26 D).
- Lower down; now the body is on the other side to start the movement on the left.

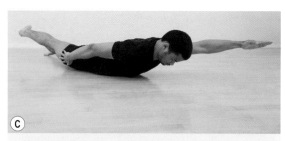

Figure 4.26 C
Left arm up, right leg up, one arm swimming

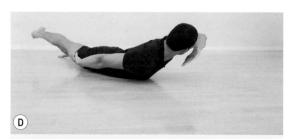

Figure 4.26 D
Rotation to the left

Release techniques for the trunk

The densification of fascia in the body is caused by a lack of gliding between the layers (Stecco, 2014). This alters the ability to extend the arm well or curl the spine smoothly. In the trunk, the thoracolumbar fascia (TLF) and the pectoral fascia continuous with the abdominal fascia are the areas that tend to lack glide. On the side body, the lateral posterior waist area is where the lateral raphe of the TLF wraps toward the front. Many people refer to this particular place as being the area of their QL tightness, resulting in restriction of side bending.

Movements that can be restricted in this situation include the following:

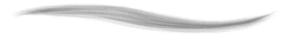

- TLF gliding can be compromised, restricting movement of the shoulder girdle and arm, causing stiffness in the lumbar spine, lack of flexion and bilateral side bending of the trunk.

- The pectoral fascia is continuous with the TLF so it restricts shoulder movement; it can also hold the upper trunk in flexion, pulling on the neck.

- Abdominal fascia holds the trunk in a flexed position, with a posterior tilt of the pelvis that places the sacrum in a counternutated position that inhibits the necessary motion of the SIJ, and affects the pelvic floor muscles by poor pelvic position; the myofascial core ring is unbalanced, with a shortened front and held long back muscles; there is also inhibition of the gluteus maximus.

MET release for the Lat-Pectorals and Abdominals

 MET for Lat-Pectorals and Abdominals
VIDEO LINK V 4.1

- Set the Pilates East Coast Barrel on the Cadillac table with the barrel side at the edge of the table underneath the push-through bar.

- The push-through bar is reversed top loaded (note that this is a dangerous position of the bar if the client lets go of the bar: therefore, ALWAYS keep one hand on the bar until completely finished).

- The body lies supine on the barrel with the head at the push-through bar end of the table (Fig. 4.27).

- The mid-sternum is over the apex of the arc.

- The head is arched over with a balanced lordotic curve; place a small prop under the head to support the head and curve.

- Begin with the knees bent on the table.

- Once the upper body is set into position, have the client lift the pelvis slightly and elongate the tail so that there is length at the waist and the pelvis is facing the ceiling.

- Straighten the legs and place the feet under the strap of the table.

- Using both hands, ask the client to hold the bar (ALWAYS hold the bar).

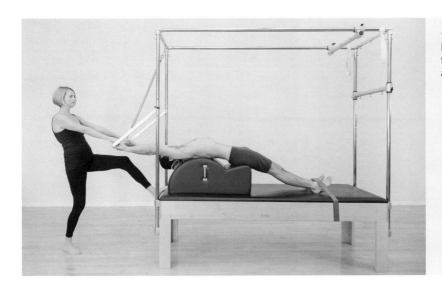

Figure 4.27
Release techniques for trunk: MET Lat-Pectorals and Abdominals set-up

- Align the client's arms slightly wider than shoulder width.

- Cue the client to keep the arms straight and pull the bar toward their head, as you hold the bar, not allowing the bar to move; cue "I am going to pull the bar away from you; do not let me do this."

- Look at the contractile quality of the latissimus dorsi and pectorals.

- The resistance of the client should match the effort of holding the bar; cue "Meet my resistance."

- Hold for 5 seconds.

- Be sure client is breathing continuously.

- Stop the resistance.

- Gently lean back to elongate the armpits (fascia, lats and pecs); do not pull the bar – a slight lean back is less disruptive and gives a nice sliding quality to the length rather than the client's nervous system reacting by tightening.

- Repeat 3 times.

- Finish with a reciprocal work: ask the client to push the bar away; hold the bar still.

Practitioner note

The push-through bar may be adjusted so that the arm flexion is minimized. If a client has a shoulder impingement or issue with pain, this is not recommended.

For the abdominals

- In the same position, keep the arms straight.

- Cue the client to bring the bottom of the sternum to the pubic bone and the pubic bone toward the sternum, contracting the anterior abdominal wall (Fig. 4.28 A).

- Hold for 5 seconds.

- Stop the resistance; no abdominal contracture (Fig. 4.28 B).

- Lean back again, creating the length.

- Repeat 3–4 times.

Getting the Client Upright

- The client bends the knees, feet on the table.

- Hold the bar and instruct the client to release the bar and cross the arms on the chest.

- Place one hand under the client's occiput and the other hand at the mid upper back, but not under it completely (Fig. 4.29 A).

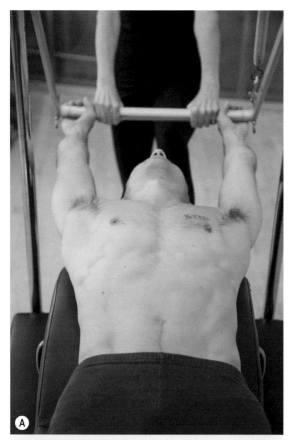

Figure 4.28 A
Contracting abdominals

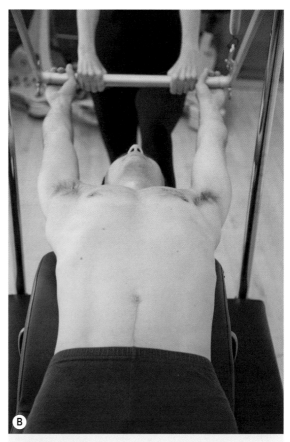

Figure 4.28 B
Not contracting abdominals

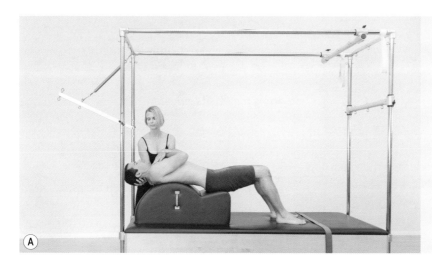

Figure 4.29 A
Getting the Client Upright:
set-up

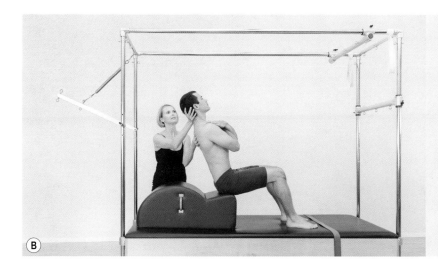

Figure 4.29 B
Lifting client

- Ask the client to press gently into the hand at the occiput and resist the action of lifting the head, matching the amount of pressure from the occiput hand.

- As the client presses back, this engages the extensors of the back, which stiffen the trunk; lift the trunk as one piece into sitting up with not a lot of effort (Fig. 4.29 B).

MET for lateral trunk

This contract release technique may be called a QL release. Through contracting the area from the iliac crest up toward the ribs posteriorly it allows for gliding of the TLF in this area. If there is a movement restriction of hip hiking and dropping, then the associated lumbar spine side bending is inhibited. This technique restores the pelvic motion and associated lumbar and hip movement.

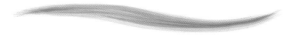

- The client lies on the side with the side to be worked up (Fig. 4.30 A).

- Place a bolster or rolled towel underneath the mid-thorax to support the spine in side lying and create a small amount of thoracic side bending.

- The underneath leg is bent for stability, while the top leg is straight.

- Align the pelvis so it is stacked and neither forward nor back.

- Hold the leg just above the ankle.

- Align the leg with the greater trochanter so the hip is in 0°; no flexion or extension, if possible.

- Cue the client " I am going to pull your leg and don't let me do it." Observe how the client moves. Where is the contraction occurring? Is it more anterior (the obliques) or posterior (the internal oblique, QL, portion of the erector spinae, specifically the iliocostalis)?

- To affect the posterior fibers, move the leg in the direction of extension.

- Contract at this line of pull.

- Hold for 5 seconds.

- Stop the resistance and lean back to feel the lengthening (do not pull).

- Repeat 3–4 times.

- End with a reciprocal contraction.

- Place the client's foot on the side of your iliac crest and ask the client to press into the pelvis; it lengthens the side worked and contracts the opposite side to set the new length (Fig. 4.30 B).

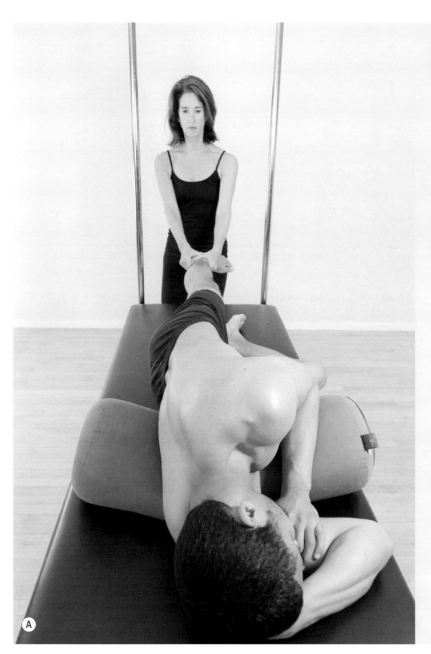

Figure 4.30 A
MET for lateral trunk
position

A

Exercises: trunk challenges

Magic Circle trunk

Once the "Small Curl-up" with all the cues and breathing is embodied, add resistance for strengthening the trunk through the full engagement of the trunk muscles with integrity and length.

Trunk flexion with Magic Circle

While holding the Magic Circle, the arms remain straight throughout the movement of the trunk. The Magic Circle moves because of the trunk motion, not the arm movement. Monitor the head and neck position in relation to the curve of the thorax. The length

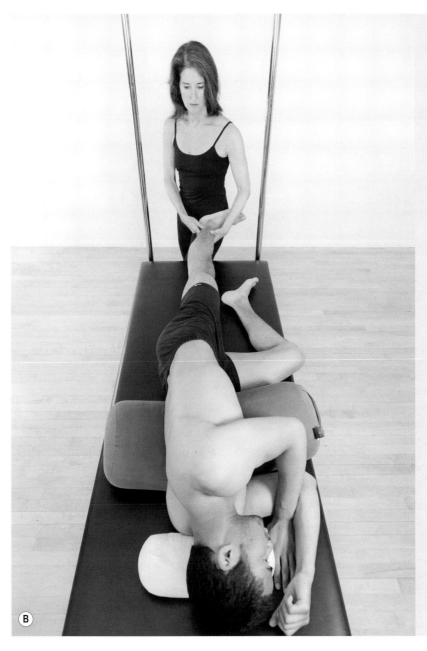

Figure 4.30 B
Reciprocal motion

B

between the xiphoid and the pubic bone remains constant.

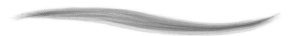

- Lie supine (on the back) with the knees bent, as in the "Small Curl-up" position.

- Hold the Magic Circle between the palms of flat hands; straight arms at 90° shoulder flexion, light compression of the ring (Fig. 4.31 A).

- On an inhalation, float the head (see Fig. 4.16).

- On an exhale, move the trunk into the "Small Curl" (Fig. 4.31 B).

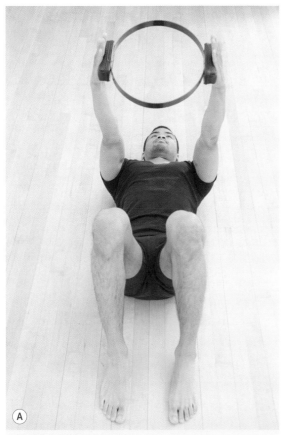

Figure 4.31 A
Magic Circle trunk flexion: start position

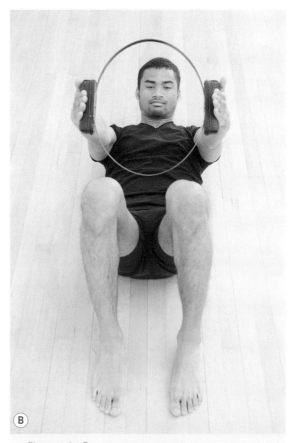

Figure 4.31 B
Curled up

- Magic Circle compression with straight arms emphasizes the intercostal action as the trunk curls.

- Hold the position for three cycles of breathing; release a small amount of tension on the ring (do not drop it) on the inhale, and on the exhale compress it lightly.

- Finish lowering the upper trunk down on an exhalation.

- Repeat 5 times.

Trunk flexion and rotation with Magic Circle

The circle is always hovering over the knee for the engagement of the oblique line from under the armpit to the opposite hip. If the circle is past the knee, then there is a rotation in the lower thoracic vertebrae without a strong connection of the oblique line.

Movement connections are for serratus anterior to the external oblique on one side, connecting to the internal oblique on the opposite side.

- Same position as above with both knees up.

- On an inhale, head float.

- On an exhale begin curl of trunk in center.

- Inhale a small amount (sniff).

- On an exhale rotate to the right with a light compression of the circle (Fig. 4.32).

- The Magic Circle will be hovering over the right knee.

- Inhale back to the center.

- On the exhale rotate to the left, with a slight compression hovering over the left knee.

- Inhale back to the center.

- Repeat the rotation–center–rotation, or rest the head down and repeat the whole sequence from the head float.

- Repeat 5 times on both sides.

Adding a challenge

The following is a variation incorporating the iliopsoas and isolating the trunk by removing the hands from the movement:

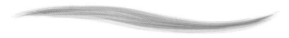

- Lie in the supine position with one knee up.

- Place the right hand behind the head and using your left hand, place the ring on the front of the right thigh.

- Stabilize the circle with pressure from the elbow and thigh.

- Both hands are behind the head.

- Curl up a small amount higher in the center, which compresses the circle between the thigh and the elbow (Fig. 4.33 A).

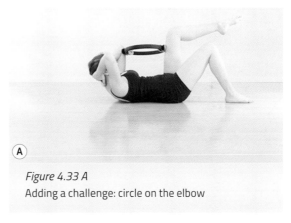

Figure 4.33 A
Adding a challenge: circle on the elbow

- Lower the curl only enough to release some compression of the circle.

- Repeat on both sides, 5 times each side.

- Add trunk rotation as the curl is increasing the height of the trunk and compression of the ring (Fig. 4.33 B).

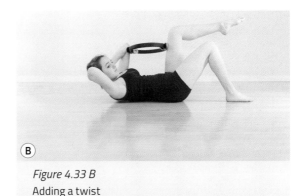

Figure 4.33 B
Adding a twist

- Look to the opposite knee.

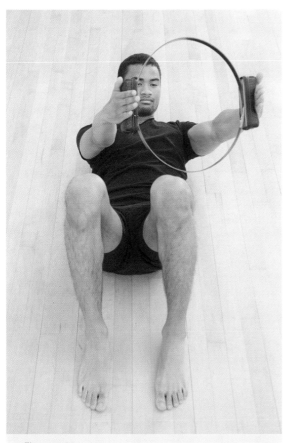

Figure 4.32
Oblique twist

Practitioner note

The compression resistance on the thigh sets the femur firmly into the socket, stabilizing it, which engages the iliopsoas line. The rib rotation is working the intercostals, obliques, and serratus anterior – the anterior sling line.

Lean Backs

"Lean Backs" can be practiced in any seated position. Sit with the spine upright on the front edge of the sits bones. It is preferable to start with the feet in contact with the floor. The arms can be resting on the thighs or hanging by the sides.

Practitioner note

Performing this movement can be tricky. The intention is to find the elongation of the spine, which requires the deep hip muscles, multifidus and transversus abdominis to be engaged as the trunk leans back. Without this prior engagement, the abdominal muscles will inhibit the back muscles and potentially cause sacroiliac joint discomfort or pain. The sacrum remains nutated, and the movement is a hip joint action moving toward extension with an elongated spine.

Lean back and forward

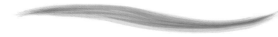

- Inhale and establish the elongation engagement of the body (Fig. 4.34 A).

- On an exhale, lean back without changing any curves of the spine; the movement occurs at the hip joint; the spine is a plank moving back (Fig. 4.34 B).

- Inhale in the back position; exhale to return to center.

- Repeat 10 times.

- Change to leaning forward, with the same breath pattern (Fig. 4.34 C).

- Repeat 10 times.

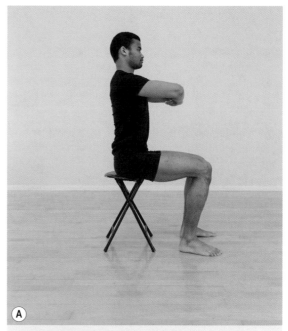

A

Figure 4.34 A
Lean Backs: seated position

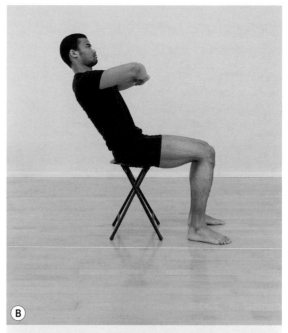

B

Figure 4.34 B
Leaning back

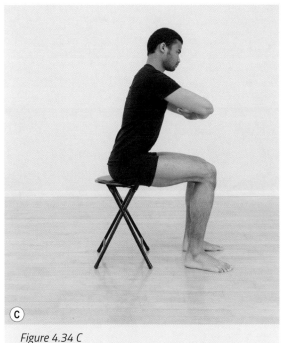

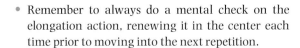

Figure 4.34 C
Leaning forward

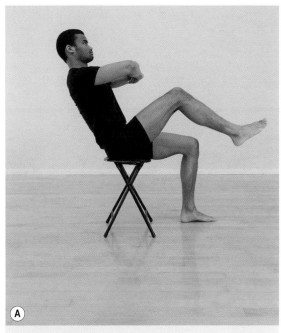

Figure 4.35 A
Leaning back with one leg

- Remember to always do a mental check on the elongation action, renewing it in the center each time prior to moving into the next repetition.

Lean Back with single leg lift

The spine does not change its curve or height while the legs are lifting. Mentally check the elongation engagement with each repetition. The abdominal wall remains fully engaged without bulging outward. The exhalation helps maintain the drawing in of the abdominal wall.

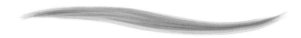

- Inhale in the center for elongation.

- On an exhale, lean back.

- Hold and take a small breath in.

- On the exhale, lift the thigh up with a dangling lower leg (remember psoas activation in Ch. 3 with the ball of the hip joint dropping down and back) (Fig. 4.35 A).

- On the inhale, lower the leg.

- Repeat on the other side.

- Repeat leg lifts 5–8 times on each side.

- Add lifting both legs up at the same time (Fig. 4.35 B).

Lean Backs with a twist

Hold a ball (preferably the width of your shoulders), a Pilates Magic Circle, or simply a stick. If holding a stick, another possibility for added resistance is to wrap an ankle weight around the center of the stick. Another option to avoid shoulder movement is to fold the arms in front of the chest as shown.

- Inhale for elongation engagement.

- On the exhale, lean back and lift the right thigh.

- Hold and inhale.

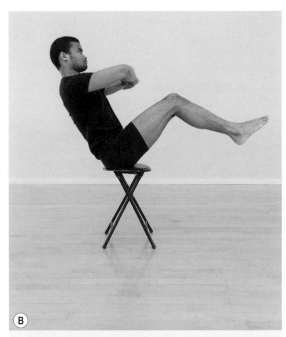

Figure 4.35 B
Leaning back with both legs

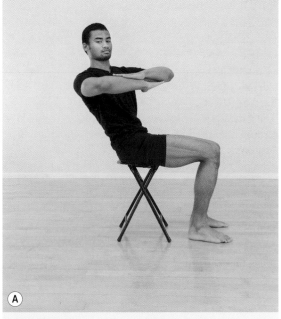

Figure 4.36 A
Leaning back with twist

- On the exhale, rotate the trunk to the right, moving back to center, rotate to the left, return to center.

- On the inhale, place the leg down.

- Repeat lifting the left leg, and the rotational movement occurs starting to the left, moving to center, then to the right, back to center.

- On the inhale, place the leg down.

- Repeat for 4 sets.

- Try lifting both legs and adding the rotational trunk movements as above (Fig. 4.36 A & B).

The difficult part of adding a spinal twist is to stabilize the pelvis and legs as the trunk rotates. If the leg moves, then it indicates that the pelvis was not stable. Mentally think of the oblique lines running from under the armpit toward the opposite hip from both sides, making an X on the front of the trunk. Move in a small range to begin with; when the movement feels controlled increase the range. The challenge is to perform this exercise on a large physioball, minus the double leg lifts!

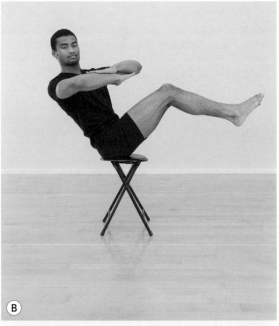

Figure 4.36 B
Leaning back with twist: both legs

Lateral lifts on the Small Barrel

Place the Pilates Small Barrel on the floor with a mat underneath or on top of the Pilates Cadillac. The Cadillac has a strap wrapped and fastened around one end of the table. The strap is useful to anchor one leg. Sit sideways, placing the right hip into the seat part of the barrel with the right knee bent and externally rotated. The left leg straightens out and slips the foot under the strap. The thigh is parallel with the inner edge of the foot on the table or mat. Lengthen the right waist and arch over the barrel. The hands are interclasped, with the palms holding the occiput. The whole arm is in a long spiral, creating a length tension from the tips of the elbows through the armpits and down the sides of the body. The spiral is outward but feels like inward because as the shoulder externally rotates, the elbows move in. Gently use the hands to pull upward on the occiput as if giving traction to the spine. Connect the length tension from the arms to the waist into the oblique system. Elongate the whole trunk as much as possible (Fig. 4.37 A).

- Inhale to feel the super length.
- On the exhale, lift the whole trunk off the barrel (Fig. 4.37 B).

- Inhale down, touch the barrel, and repeat right away.
- On the exhale, lift.
- Repeat 10 times.

The lift is not a side bend and compression of one side. The action is to lift the trunk with both sides in length. Cue to begin the movement by lifting the left ribs (the ones facing up), up toward the ceiling. Try to reverse the breathing where the lift is on the inhale. Cue Eve Gentry's "One Lung Breathing." Inhale into the left side as the left ribcage lifts up toward the ceiling.

Corkscrew

"Corkscrew" is one of the classic Pilates mat movements. There are a few variations of the Corkscrew in terms of range of motion. Here is a version that can be done in a small range, building into a large spiral. Using the ball or the Pilates Magic Circle is challenging and fun to do.

- Lie supine, legs straight at 90° or slightly less, with a ball or Pilates Magic Circle between the ankles. The lower the legs are, the harder it is to keep the spine anchored on the mat (Fig. 4.38 A).

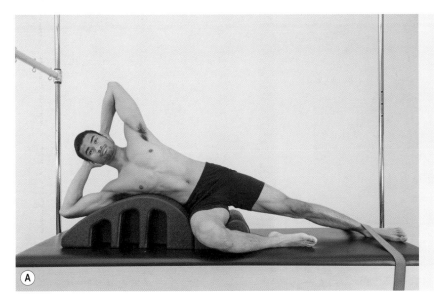

Figure 4.37 A
Lateral lifts on Small Barrel: start position

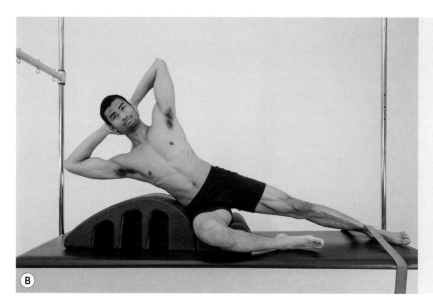

Figure 4.37 B
Lifted position

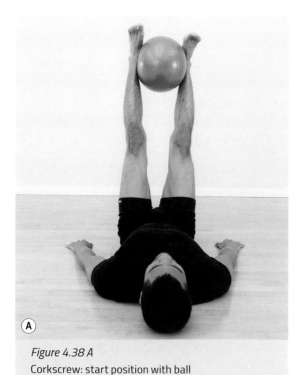

Figure 4.38 A
Corkscrew: start position with ball

- Anchor points of the body on the mat are the back of the head at the occiput, the shoulder blades, the lowest ribs, and the sacrum at the mid-point.

- Maintaining the stability of the anchor points, reach the legs up with the prop.

- The first movement is at the hips only (Fig. 4.38 B).

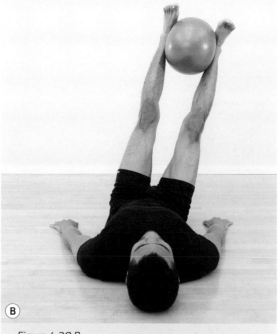

Figure 4.38 B
Motion of legs to the side

- Engage the ball or circle and sway the legs to the right, back to center, sway to the left, back to center, moving in adduction and abduction of the hips.

- Inhale on the legs moving away from center, and exhale returning to center.

- Be sure the pelvis does not face the direction the legs move.

- The work is stability of the pelvis with hip abduction and adduction.

- Practice this until the movement is clear and confident.

- Add a circling, sway right, stay to the right, circle down and toward the center (legs are anywhere from 70° to 45°), sway at the low point to the left and bring the legs up to the starting center position.

- Repeat swaying to the left and move around the circle.

- Repeat for 3–5 sets.

- The majority of the moving work is in the hip joint muscles and the core is stabilizing the trunk.

- The second movement is for the pelvis and lower back.

  - The pelvis will drive the circle. The legs are engaged but the hip joint is more stable. There is a slight movement of the hip joint toward hip extension and flexion. The primary action comes from the pelvis.

  - Begin in the up centered position of the legs with the prop or simply with the legs together.

  - Inhale, roll the pelvis to face right; the legs move with the pelvis as a unit (Fig. 4.39 A).

  - On an exhale circle the pelvis back toward the center as the legs move down toward the low position (Figs 4.39 B & C).

  - The pelvis rolls to face left and the legs return to the starting position (Fig. 4.39 D).

  - Repeat the circle to the other side.

  - Repeat for 3–5 sets.

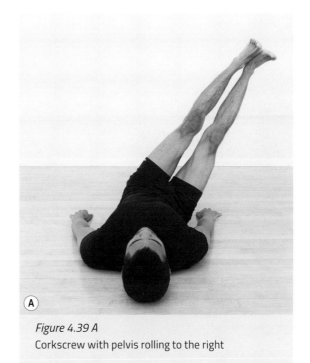

Ⓐ

Figure 4.39 A
Corkscrew with pelvis rolling to the right

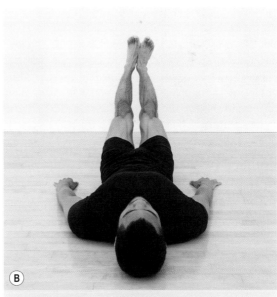

Ⓑ

Figure 4.39 B
Lowest point of circle

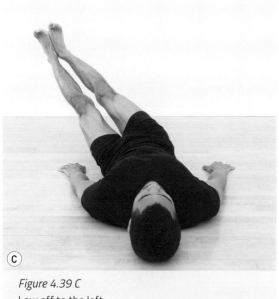

Figure 4.39 C
Low off to the left

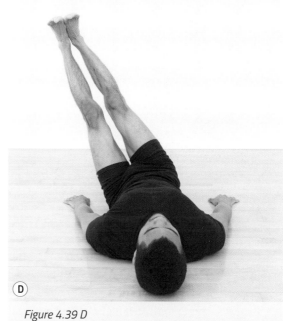

Figure 4.39 D
Over to the left side

The circling of the pelvis feels as if the weight on the sacrum is tracing the outer edges of the sacrum without losing the imprint of the sacrum into the mat. As the pelvis tips to the right, more weight is on the right side of the sacrum. The left side is lifted. As the legs lower and the pelvis is rolling toward the left side, the imagery is a tracing of the bottom of the sacrum without losing the contact of the top of the sacrum. Then the weight shifts to the left side of the sacrum with the right side lifted, followed by rolling the pelvis back to the center.

Bridging to Chapter 5

The Pilates Method was developed with the whole body–mind connection. The repertory of Pilates is extensive and offers movement choices for all levels of conditioning. The learning process for moving with intention to make changes in one's body is the first step, followed by the mental awareness of noticing the unconsciousness of personal movement habits, then becoming conscious of the habits in order to change them. With more practice, the habits do change, becoming permanent, an unconscious consciousness of good movement form. Training the body to elicit this nervous system response via the multidirectional movement of the body results in an improvement of strength with elasticity of movement. Fluidity and elasticity in any sport prevent injury and improve skills. In everyday activities, being flexible is living well. As we age, strength and elasticity become more important, as does breathing well. We take breathing for granted, only becoming aware of it when we are unable to breathe easily. The next chapter will cover the mechanics of the breath, movements for improving our capacity to breathe, and the deeper connections of the breath with form, function, and psyche.

Ribs inspired: the diaphragm as a breathing and postural muscle

> *"No matter how still a man may be, he is always adjusting to his respiratory needs, his circulatory needs, his perceptual needs, in an organic world, there is no such thing as complete lack of movement."*
>
> Ida Rolf, *Rolfing*

Contemplative awareness: cycles

Two truths in this life are that the first breath is taken at birth and the last one at death. Imagine if that first breath were to remain stored deep in the body and it was this breath that became the last breath expelled. This image creates an idea of the breath as a continuum of life and death. The act of breathing is a wondrous human life-sustaining movement and connector. It is at the magic moment when the first cells form in the womb that the movement of life, the breath of life, begins. The growing fetus breathes with the mother, feeling the waves of her movements and breath. The water surrounding the fetus is like an ocean, moving in tides that match the breath's rhythm. Once the first breath is taken, the entrance into a new world connects the body to the universe. The breath is the bridge between the internal and external worlds. It is a continuous relationship, mixing and diffusing into each cell and sustaining both worlds.

Breathing is an automatic cyclical motion of the trunk, stimulating waves of movement. The rhythm of the breath changes to meet the body's needs: it is impossible to separate the breath from the biological, psychological, and motor control of being human, for all elements affect each other. The way the body adapts is through changing fluctuations of the breath, changing tempos, and modifying the body posture. The breath is the vehicle for finding balance. Naturally, the body has protective mechanisms in place for maintaining homeostasis, for the normalization of health. However, protective mechanisms can develop compensatory habits in movement and breath patterns that, over time, may compromise health. Living life well for the whole lifetime requires paying attention to the breath as well as movement.

Joseph Pilates, the creator of the Pilates Method, placed great emphasis on the importance of breathing and was an avid promoter of improving health through movement and the mind–body connection. His philosophy of exercising the whole body with concentration on the mind and breath is still significant today. He considered that "A body free from nervous tension and fatigue is the ideal shelter provided by nature for housing a well balanced mind, fully capable of successfully meeting all the complex problems of modern living" (Pilates and Miller, 1945). The breath is the balancing force in both mental and physical well-being.

In this chapter, the focus will be on the mechanics of the breath, the influences on structure and function, posture, breathing techniques, re-education movements, imagery, and valuable tools to improve overall function. The work shared here will be applicable to any movement system being taught or practiced.

Function and structure

The first image of a breathing structure that comes to mind is the diaphragm. Thinking about how breath moves air from the atmosphere into our body and the body exchanges its gases then returns it back in a different form links our physical body with the world.

Christopher Gilbert (Chaitow et al., 2014) phrased it perfectly when he said "The diaphragm is the muscular equivalent of an umbilical cord linking us to the environment." The diaphragm, though, is more than just a breathing muscle. It is a postural muscle, and moves the abdominals and interacts with the cranial, cervical, thoracic, and perineal regions as well.

Normal breathing can be observed externally by watching the rise and fall of the tissues and the quality of the person's movement and posture. When there is faulty breathing, the dysfunction begins to shape the body's form, making movement noticeably restricted. The function of breath forms the body's structure and the structure serves the function. It can become difficult when the structure is compromised, which in turn reinforces faulty breathing. Both aspects, function and structure, are important to remember when attempting to facilitate movement re-education of the body. Awareness of the breath is a great source for change.

Structures of breathing

Now visualize the cylindrical container of the torso. Inside it there are two chambers, separated by the diaphragm. The upper chamber (the thorax) houses the heart and lungs. The lower chamber (the abdomen) contains the stomach, spleen, kidneys, liver, pancreas, the whole of the gastrointestinal tract, and the reproductive and sex organs. The spine in the back, with its associated ribs and the sternum, protects the upper chamber (Fig. 5.1). The lower chamber is mainly supported by the connective tissue of the pelvis and the lower spine.

On the inside of the body wall, stretching from the depths of the pelvic bowl up to the top of the upper chamber, there is fascia. Imagine wallpaper. It is not just stuck flat on the wall, however, but forms envelopes coming off of the wall that weave around and within the organs, the deep muscles and spine. As breath is taken in, it expands the upper chamber and compresses the lower, changing the space inside. Breathing stimulates the activation of the trunk muscles.

Breathing is controlled both in the somatic part of the central nervous system (meaning there is conscious control of the breath to a point) and the autonomic

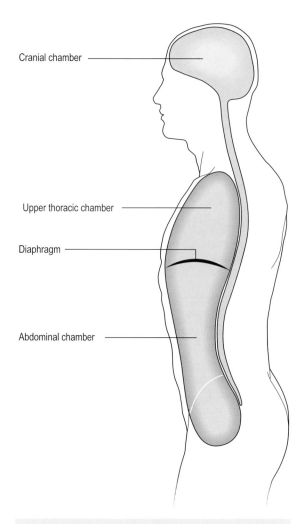

Cranial chamber

Upper thoracic chamber

Diaphragm

Abdominal chamber

Figure 5.1
Chambers of the trunk

nervous system, which responds to a stimulus, whether an emotion or a biochemical response in the body.

The movement of the diaphragm is described as a piston sliding inside a cylinder. The upper chamber's business is circulation and exchange of gases while the lower chamber is about metabolism and elimination. The two chambers are continuous to one another by way of the fascia and ligaments. The diaphragm arises from the whole internal circumference of the thorax. The back of the dome reaches down further than the front. The back area of the diaphragm is attached along the lowest ribs, and on the spine by means of the right and left crura. In the front, the diaphragm's fibers are on the internal surface of the cartilages and lower bony portion of the front ribs, interdigitating with the transversus abdominis. The central part of the diaphragm is a fibrous layer called the central tendon, which the inferior vena cava passes through. The tendon is multidirectional and multilayered to reduce the tension from exertion on the vertical vessels of the abdominal area. The muscular peripheral part spans the whole area of the ribcage (see Fig. 3.26).

Fascial continuum

Remember the image of the wallpaper with envelopes and folds coming off the wall of the trunk? There are important fascial articulations along the ribcage connecting the abdominal chamber to the chest chamber. The sternal fascia has fibers that interweave with fascia anteriorly inserting on the xiphoid process. The lateral fascia is found at the inside superior part of the last six ribs. Both of these peripheral fascia of the diaphragm are continuous with the fascia in the upper chamber, called the endothoracic fascia. The peripheral connections of the diaphragm also run continually with the transversalis fascia and transversus abdominis muscle of the abdominal chamber (Paoletti, 2012) (Fig. 5.2).

At the top of the endothoracic fascia are the lungs, sitting underneath the shoulder girdle and neck musculature and fascia. The endothoracic fascia runs along and upward into the cervicothoracic region, the fascia of the neck (Paoletti, 2012). The pleura of the lungs are connected to cervicothoracic fascia by suspensor ligaments and fascia of the neck. The endothoracic fascia, parietal pleura and the ligaments pull to suspend superiorly, filling the lungs and increasing the vertical space of the thorax.

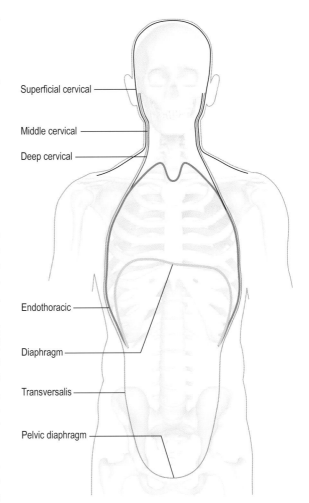

Superficial cervical

Middle cervical

Deep cervical

Endothoracic

Diaphragm

Transversalis

Pelvic diaphragm

Figure 5.2

Fascial continuation of the chambers of the trunk: cervical, thoracic and abdominal fasciae

On the posterior side of the abdominal chamber is the spine. The diaphragm has two significant attachments onto the anterior vertebral ligament, called crura. The ligament runs the length of the front of the spine forming a continuity of the crura (diaphragm) with the occiput and the sacrum. There are two other ligaments creating a fascial continuity, the medial and lateral arcuate ligaments. The medial arcuate ligament crosses over psoas major, connecting the diaphragm and the pelvic bowl. The lateral arcuate ligament is a lumbocostal arch that lies over the quadratus lumborum and merges with the

> **Try it!**
>
> Feel the domes of the lungs move by resting the hands on top of the shoulders near the base of the neck and breathing slowly in. The shoulder and neck tissue expands as the lungs expand and move into the top of the endothoracic fascia. Notice one side moves before the other.

abdominal transversalis fascia (see Fig. 3.26). Inferiorly, the transversalis fascia has a relationship with the pelvic bowl fascia.

There are many connections from the pelvic diaphragm to the thoracic diaphragm. Consider these lines:

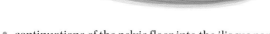

- continuations of the pelvic floor into the iliacus part of the iliopsoas, iliopsoas → diaphragm (Fig. 5.3) (Myers, 2001)

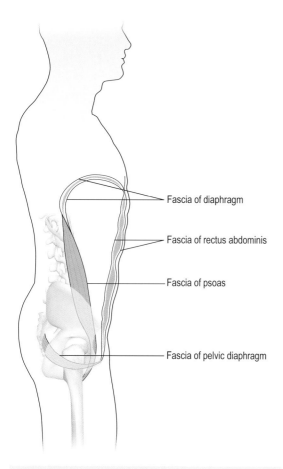

Fascia of diaphragm

Fascia of rectus abdominis

Fascia of psoas

Fascia of pelvic diaphragm

Figure 5.3
Pelvic diaphragm connections with the thoracic diaphragm

- rectus abdominis → pubococcygeus → anterior longitudinal ligament of the spine → posterior sternum → posterior fascial sheet of the rectus → pelvic floor (Myers, 2001)

- fascial connections from the pubococcygeus and the transverse abdominis to the diaphragm.

Three diaphragms

The diaphragm is the unifying tissue that gives function to both the upper and lower chambers of the torso (the thorax and the abdomen). The diaphragm is the floor for the upper chamber and the ceiling for the lower chamber. Beginning at the top, the cervicothoracic, endothoracic, and parietal fascia are separated from the abdominal chamber by the muscular dome of the diaphragm. Even though there is a separation, the upper chamber fascia nevertheless exchanges fibers with the transversalis fascia connected into the parietal peritoneum.

The parietal peritoneum is located at the bottom of the pelvis and called the pelvic diaphragm (pelvic floor). The pelvic diaphragm forms a similar dome shaped structure to the thoracic diaphragm but inverted, like a bowl.

The myofascia along the top of the shoulder area (such as the scalenes, pectoralis, and cervicothoracic fascia) is also considered to be a diaphragm, called the cerviocthoracic diaphragm. The two additional diaphragmatic structures complete the picture of the whole cylinder. The three diaphragms function synergistically on the inhalation to change the dimensions of the trunk.

On an inhalation, the uppermost (cervicothoracic) diaphragm elevates, the middle (thoracic) diaphragm flattens, and the lowest (pelvic) diaphragm pulls the bladder upward and supports the organs. The diaphragms function optimally together when stacked over one another in a vertical axis. Put simply, any misalignment moves the central tendon of the thoracic diaphragm off its vertical orientation, which inhibits the piston-like movement of the diaphragm (Kolár et al., 2014).

Postural alignment in any exercise position is crucial for optimal recruitment. Instead of cueing "shoulders down, pelvis lifted," use the three and add the fourth, the cranial diaphragm, as a description for alignment. Visualize four diaphragms, pelvic, thoracic, cervico-thoracic and cranial, stacked over one another for alignment. Breathe while maintaining this feeling of the three structures centered over one another. Try a rotation of the three, thinking of them as discs stacked one above the other. Rotate the spine, feeling the discs turning on each other but remaining stacked, as in a perfect golf swing (Fig. 5.4). It is useful to use the image coming out of flexion or extension when the client is centering the spine to be upright.

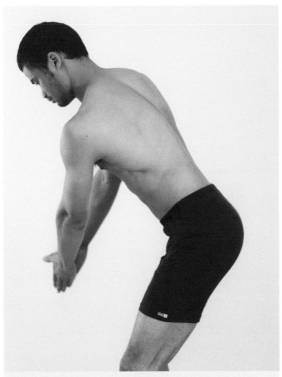

Figure 5.4
Diaphragms stacked during spinal rotation

Muscles of breathing

The external body, the trunk muscles, and fascia (see Ch. 4) are also an integral part of the structure for breathing. The transversalis fascia and thoracolumbar fascia are the structures that directly connect the inner body to the outer. Additional muscles of breathing that have not been discussed yet are the shoulder girdle, neck, and local muscles of the thorax. There are primary muscles of breathing and accessory muscles of breathing.

Inhalation primary muscles

Efficiency of breathing is achieved when the primary muscles of inhalation flatten the diaphragm as the ribs rise, expanding the thorax in vertical and transverse dimensions (Fig. 5.5) (Chaitow et al., 2014).

The primary muscles of inhalation are:

- diaphragm
- internal intercostals
- external intercostals (upper and lateral level)
- levatores costarum
- scalenes.

Inhalation secondary or accessory muscles

During increased demand of breathing from exertion or in dysfunctional breathing patterns is when the secondary muscles come into play over the primary muscles (Fig. 5.6) (Chaitow et al., 2014).

The accessory muscles of inhalation are:

- sternocleidomastoid
- upper trapezius
- pectoralis major and minor
- serratus anterior
- latissimus dorsi

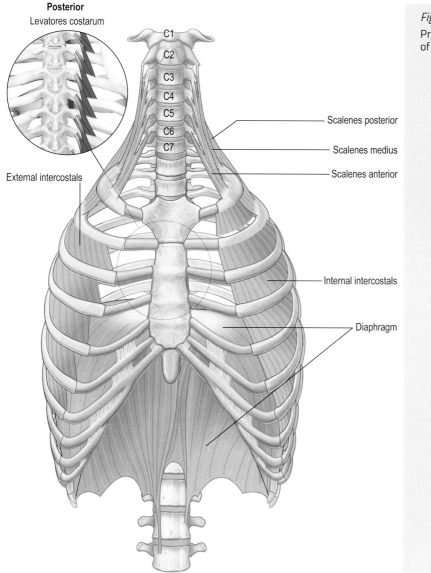

Posterior
Levatores costarum

C1
C2
C3
C4
C5
C6
C7

Scalenes posterior

Scalenes medius

Scalenes anterior

External intercostals

Internal intercostals

Diaphragm

Figure 5.5
Primary muscles
of breathing

- serratus posterior superior

- iliocostalis thoracis

- subclavian

- omohyoid.

Exhalation primary muscles

The action of the primary muscles of exhalation is an elastic recoil response to the end of the cascading inhalation. At the end of the exhalation the abdominal musculature is activated for expiratory airflow and regulation of the length of the diaphragm (Hodges, 1999).

The primary muscles of exhalation are:

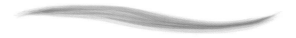

- diaphragm

- pleura

- costal cartilages.

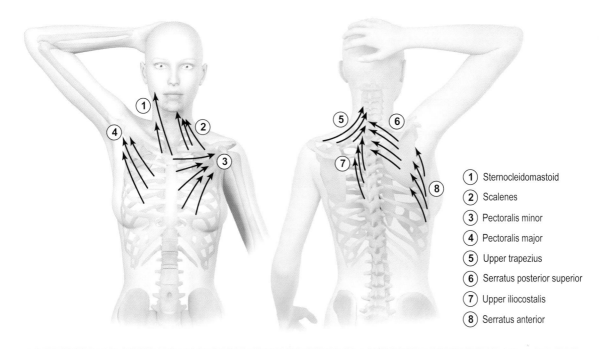

1. Sternocleidomastoid
2. Scalenes
3. Pectoralis minor
4. Pectoralis major
5. Upper trapezius
6. Serratus posterior superior
7. Upper iliocostalis
8. Serratus anterior

Figure 5.6
Secondary muscles of inhalation

Exhalation secondary or accessory muscles

Exhalation during quiet breathing activates the abdominals toward the end of the exhalation and the accessory muscles are predominately passive. If under stress and sensing air is being retrained in the lungs, then the accessory muscles are activated. A forced exhalation, whether by stress or conscious effort, uses the accessory muscles. If no pathology is present, a forceful exhalation activates these muscles (see below, "Oxygen Myth").

The accessory muscles of exhalation are:

- internal intercostals
- abdominal muscles
- transversus thoracis
- subcostales (infracostales)
- iliocostalis lumborum
- quadratus lumborum
- serratus posterior inferior
- latissimus dorsi.

Motion of breathing

During active inhalation, the air flows through the nose, where it is filtered and warmed before being drawn into the lungs by the downward movement of the diaphragm and expansion (outward) of the abdominal wall and lower intercostals. The secondary inhalation muscles provide upper chest expansion. When the expiration is effortless and not forced, the abdominal wall relaxes and the diaphragm ascends, returning to its domed position (Chaitow et al., 2014). The ascending movement of the dome is due to the elastic recoiling of the lungs and abdominal wall.

The ribs move into elevation on the inhalation, increasing the vertical dimension following the lift (anterior) of the sternum. During an exhalation, the ribs return to the original position, from elevation to downward. The ribs move in a cascading way which starts at one end and moves to the other, changing the shape of the thorax (Chaitow et al., 2014). On the inhalation, the cascade begins superior and moves down. The upper rib is responsible for stabilizing by way of the scalenes, which allows for the wave motion to move downward. On exhalation, the cascade moves from inferior to superior. The lower ribs require stabilization by the quadratus lumborum for the wave to move upward (Chaitow et al., 2014). The lowest ribs increase the transverse dimension by elevation and rotation, similar to a bucket handle moving up and down. During exertion, the lowest ribs increase lateral expansion due to the contraction of the diaphragm and increased abdominal pressure. The sternum also moves anteriorly by the spreading of the upper ribs, a pump handle motion. The sternocleidomastoid and scalenes facilitate the lifting and microrotation of the clavicles on the inhalation. The clavicles posteriorly rotate on the manubrium at the sternoclavicular joints as the sternum is elevated. The exhalation returns the clavicle by an anterior rotation motion as the sternum moves downward.

The mobility of the thorax is crucial for the amount of movement cascading down and up the ribs and spine. A stiff thorax inhibits this all-important movement. Side bending and rotations (spirals) of the spine are motions that maintain a more supple ribcage. The ribs approximate and expand with every breath and thoracic movement, especially side bending and rota-

> **Try it!**
>
> Sit upright on a chair. Start at the top of the head and side bend the head to the right as if pouring sand out of the crown of the head. Reach the right arm toward the floor and other arm up and over the head as if reaching for the ceiling. Inhale into the left side of the ribcage and expand the ribs as an accordion stretching its bellows open. Exhale slowly bringing the trunk back to center beginning at the lower ribs, shoulders and the head is last. Repeat on the other side (Fig. 5.7).

tion.

In Pilates, the "Mermaid" side bending movements are wonderful movements to include in a program. Try "Mermaid" on the Reformer or Cadillac with a straight arm on the bar for facilitating specific rib motion (Fig. 5.8).

Flared ribs

The lowest part of the front of the ribcage, along the border, is shaped like an inverted V. The width of this V-shaped border has a normal range of 75–90°. When the abdominal muscles are very tense (hypertonic) –

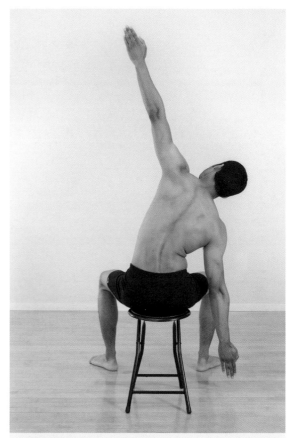

Figure 5.7
Rib mobility in side bending

especially common in people who overwork their oblique abdominal muscles by training the "abs" or who have respiratory issues – the width is decreased, reaching an angle as narrow as 38° (Bradley, 2014) (Fig. 5.9). The ribcage is braced and so unable to expand and relax with the breath. Without the expansion of the ribcage, the diaphragm is not able to move through its natural range, diminishing its strength and movement for its own blood supply (Clifton-Smith, 2014). Restoring the mobility of the ribcage and increasing the angle to a normal range will relieve the tension and allow the diaphragm to function well.

In Pilates, it is common to see the lower ribs protrude when the person lies down. In this case, the flaring of the ribs may be a result of thoracic spine extension (a lifting of the spine off the mat) at segments between T8 and T12. The lowest ribs are not

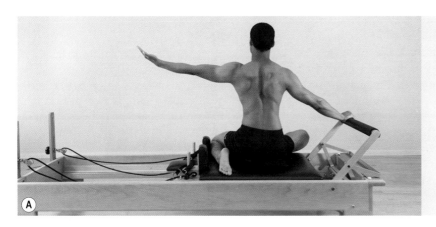

Figure 5.8 A
Start position with straight arm on the bar

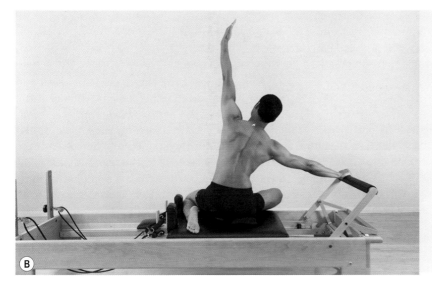

Figure 5.8 B
Side bending with length

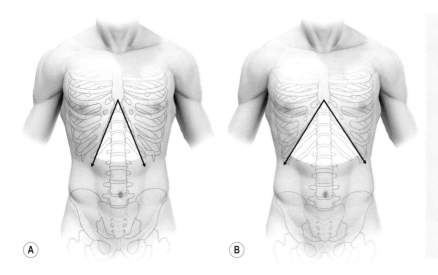

Figure 5.9
Inferior lateral angle of the ribcage

"anchored into the mat" because in an upright position, the upper thorax is flexed with a forward head. When the head meets the mat, the lower thorax has to lift to accommodate the lack of normal length of the thorax. Another contributor to the alignment of the spine while lying down is the position of the pelvis. When there is shortness along the psoas/iliacus/hip flexor line, lying with the knees bent and the feet flat on the floor removes the tension pulling on the front of the pelvis. The muscles and fascia rest in a shortened position, tilting the pelvis backward. The combination of a forward head, flexed upper thorax, and shortened anterior psoas line holds the ribs in a flared position. Releasing the area through breathing practices, release techniques of the trunk, specifically the psoas to hip flexor line, restoring abdominal length and working on the upper back/head alignment will all affect the angle and protrusion of the lowest ribs.

Stability and mobility

The diaphragm not only functions as part of the mechanism for breathing but also acts as a player for control of trunk stability (Kolár et al., 2012). Movement requires a grounding force (stability) to be present in contrast to a freely moving limb (mobility). As an example, when taking a step, the hip is moving the leg forward (hip flexion and

> **Practitioner note**
>
> A population of Pilates teachers are known to "correct" the flared ribs by compressing and closing the V angle. This is a dysfunctional cue to give and a disservice to the health capacity of the client. Improving the breathing and reorganizing the neuromuscular education of the abdominal muscles and upper back/head alignment will change the lower ribcage so that it does not protrude. The release and breathing techniques given below are recommended for restoring the ribcage. Also note: the "MET Release for the Lat-Pectorals and Abdominals" in Chapter 4 is excellent for facilitating new length of the trunk, especially the abdominals. Adding the "Lunge with Hip Drop" on the Reformer or physioball from Chapter 3 increases the length of the line into the hip.

leg swing) while, at the same time, the pelvis and spine are stabilizing the hip flexion tendons at the origin, allowing the leg to swing. And the standing side provides the stable ground from which to move. Without the stability of the pelvis, there would be no movement of the leg. The linking of the muscles and fascia signals a sequence of muscles beyond the hip joint through the spine working synergistically, alternating from a moment of stability and a moment of mobility.

CLIENT STORY

A Capoeira dancer and Pilates teacher came in for sessions, looking to alleviate repeated back pain after long dance sessions with her group. The dancer's trunk patterning was to shorten and compress her mid-section when moving into flexion or flexion with rotation. The abdominal muscles would bulge, creating a mound-like shape in the front with tightness in the inverted V of the lower rib angle. Her thorax was stiff and the range of extension was coming solely from her lower spine. The hip flexors were also tight, inhibiting her ability to extend from the hips with the back bends. Her breathing was contained, with little expansion movement of the ribcage. She was very strong but in a shortened compressed way that did not allow for her spine to move in the ranges

that spread the work from the hips through the neck. Retraining her trunk stabilizers was the key to improving the spinal motion she required for Capoeira and to her being pain-free the next day. The most influential work done was the "MET Lat-Pectorals Release" on the Small Barrel, "MET Intercostal Resistance Release," the "Breathing Sling," "Magic Circle Breathing" and psoas work such as "Lunge with Hip Drop" techniques. This was followed by reorganizing the trunk through Pilates apparatus work with a new sense of recruiting using breath in a balanced way. Her abdominal wall changed its contour; her pain lessened to fewer incidents; and her range of spinal motion for the dance was improved overall.

The central nervous system (CNS) is constantly monitoring the forces on the spine. It receives input from nerve sensors in the spinal tissues, including fascia, discs, joints, muscles and ligaments. In a fine-tuned body, the CNS is directing the amount of stiffness necessary for the movement being performed and anticipating the need for more stability or mobility. It is responsible for the appropriate activation and quality of the coordinated muscle activity. One doorway into the nervous system is the breath. The inhalation tends to stimulate the nervous system, bring energy up, and trigger the extensor group. Exhalation tends to relax the nervous system and stimulate the flexors of the body.

> **Note**
>
> Definition of all three types of muscle contractions:
>
> - isometric: tensing a muscle without changing its length
> - concentric: tensing with a shortening of the muscle
> - eccentric: tensing with a lengthening of the muscle.
>
> Coordinated muscle activity requires all three muscle contraction types for movement: concentric, eccentric, and isometric. When breathing, the diaphragm movement synchronizes the activity of the trunk musculature. On the inhalation the contraction types are:
>
> - Eccentrically for expansion:
>   - o abdominals
>   - o hip external rotators
>   - o rib intercostals
>   - o shoulders and neck (cervicothroacic diaphragm).
> - Concentric contraction:
>   - o diaphragm
>   - o pelvic diaphragm.
>
> The downward flattening of the diaphragm and the pelvic diaphragm resistance increases the intra-abdominal pressure (Fig. 5.10).
>
> - Isometrically to hold the shape, increasing the intra-abdominal pressure that stabilizes the spine:
>   - o muscles of the chest
>   - o abdominal wall.

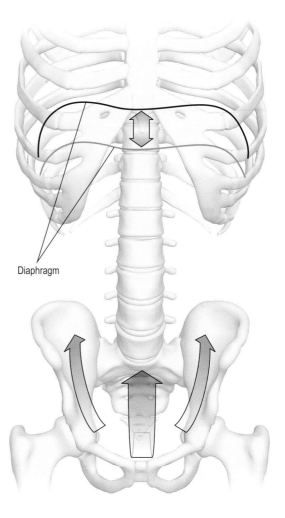

Diaphragm

Arrows indicate increase of abdominal pressure in pelvis area

Figure 5.10
Intra-abdominal pressure

Breath is present in every movement, therefore it plays a significant role in stability. The increased activation of the diaphragm has been documented when moving the arms repetitively (Hodges and Gandevia, 2000) and when lifting objects (Hemborg et al., 1985). One mechanism for stabilizing the spine is the co-activation of the diaphragms (thoracic and pelvic) and the wall of the abdominal cylinder, which increases intra-abdominal pressure (IAP). The fascia of the trunk, thoracolumbar, endopelvic and anterior abdominal is linked to the stability and synergistic work of the related muscles, the diaphragm with the transversus abdominis, pelvic floor, and multifidus (deep spinal muscle) (Lee, 2011).

According to Dr. Stuart McGill, this theory needs more evidence to describe the principles of IAP. In 2007, Grenier and McGill tested the strategies of abdominal hollowing, a transversus abdominis and internal oblique action, versus abdominal bracing, a complete abdominal girdle engagement. The discussion led to an examination of the role of the transversus abdominis (TrA) in stability of the spine. McGill defines stability as "the ability of the spinal column to survive an applied perturbation." His study concludes that the TrA has a limited role in lumbar stability and bracing is more effective. The load condition of this study determined that bracing produced a greater ability for spinal stability. As in most studies, the question being asked is very specific and the test is designed around a predicted result. This study tested the control of rotational buckling, trunk flexion, and lateral bending of the spine, limiting the investigation to one part of the TrA's role. Other studies have shown that TrA presets the torso preparedness prior to the torque movements of the column (Willard et al., 2012), and increasing the load challenge of the spine, the TrA co-contracted with the internal oblique. Some studies have shown that the TrA is linked to increasing intra-abdominal pressure (Hodges, 2008), thus contributing to spinal control and fascial tension of the lower back. The TrA has multiple roles, such as activation during gait, assisting exhalation, and at heel strike in time for change of trunk rotation (Hodges, 2008). The investigations continue, as do discoveries concerning the complex system of stability and the role the fascia (especially the thoracolumbar fascial layers) plays in stability or mobility for a pain-free and strong trunk.

Training the trunk is a whole system approach to challenging the body (not just a single muscle or a small group of muscles) spatially with varying loads for improved stability. In carrying out these exercises it is imperative to use the breath for the best possible coordination of the trunk muscles. A dysfunctional and uncoordinated trunk is one in which the musculature of the neck and shoulders is overworking and the spinal alignment inhibits the breath and

core activation. If this occurs, the training effect will be minimized and postural improvement will not be achieved. In addition, the dysfunctional breathing impacts the diaphragm, altering its synergy with the pelvic diaphragm. Training the abdominal group to brace restricts the movement of the thorax and stiffens the spine. If the thoracic segmental movement is not present or becomes stiffer, then inevitably motion will increase in the lower spine and neck. A well coordinated trunk with appropriate breath and a whole spine balance between stability and mobility is optimal.

Rhythms of breathing

> **Note**
>
> In medicine, diaphragm is derived from the Greek word "*phren*," meaning mind. The ancient Greek thinkers and philosophers saw the mind as being in the heart not the physical brain. The meaning of "phren" was extended to include the heart and diaphragm. The phrenic nerve innervates the diaphragm.

"Breath control is self control" (Paramahansa Harihananda, 1907–2002).

Breathing is both an unconscious and conscious activity. It is controlled by the conscious mind in activities such as singing or counting movement steps and in meditation with the focus on the breath. When we are at rest, the breath is controlled by the autonomic (automatic) part of the nervous system. One cannot just hold the breath and suffocate. Increasing physical activity increases the rate of the breath (anaerobic response) until a homeostasis of effort and breath (aerobic response) is met. Psychological factors can affect the pace of the breath too. A jaw-dropping surprise will stimulate a quick inhalation and holding of the breath. All of these scenarios are a physical response to an internal biochemical activity, which sends a signal to the nervous system to change the rate and depth of breathing.

Pilates, yoga, and Gyrotonic® exercise methods, as well as meditation practices, consciously choose specific breathing patterns, for example nasal versus mouth breathing, pumping the abdominals, and producing sounds. The purpose of these methods of breathing is to achieve specific training effects and to build capacity of mind and body. The conscious awareness of the breath is useful for distracting the "monkey mind," training the mind to focus, challenging the body physically (faster tempo with movement), and monitoring the effort of moving while hearing the breath's steady pace. The breath can be directed to facilitate enhancing movement of the trunk where there is restriction in the structure (recall Eve Gentry's one lung breathing technique in Ch. 4, "Rotation and Side Bending Cues"). Overall, the movement practices that incorporate conscious breathing improve the body's function and structure. Improved breathing also enhances overall energy within the body by balancing the chemical processes of the body's continuous exchange of oxygen and carbon dioxide.

The oxygen myth: fast versus slow

The normal rate of breathing when at rest is between 10 and 14 breaths per minute. The body takes in oxygen, exchanges it in the lungs, and expels carbon dioxide. The body has a high concentration of oxygen in the bloodstream under normal circumstances: at sea level there is 97–98% and above sea level 95% saturation. Approximately 75% of the oxygen breathed in is returned to the atmosphere without being consumed. During maximal effort, about 25% of the inhaled air is unused (Chaitow et al., 2014). The reserve of oxygen does not change readily for good reason, since oxygen in balance with CO_2 maintains the health of the body, especially the brain and heart.

The body's consumption of oxygen varies, increasing or decreasing in response to muscular activity, metabolism, and heart rate. The match between the rate and need (blood gases and pH balance) is controlled so as to sustain a steady supply of oxygen to the brain and heart. It is the amount of carbon dioxide in the blood that is the regulator of breathing, not the level of oxygen. Increased activity produces high levels of carbon dioxide and increases the need for oxygen, stimulating a faster breathing rate. Conversely, breathing becomes slower when the activity level is reduced, lowering the body's store of carbon dioxide and reducing oxygen need. Breathing with the intention of pulling more oxygen in or blowing CO_2 out is a myth about the process of oxygen being delivered to the tissues, especially the brain and heart.

The fast, rhythmic breathing taught in the Pilates "Hundred" exercise or in fast-paced breathing in yoga is said by some teachers to increase oxygen levels in the blood. This is not the case. Breathing fast rushes air into the lungs, lowering the level of carbon dioxide within the lungs. The body therefore draws more carbon dioxide out of the bloodstream into the lungs. A low level of CO_2 can be dangerous, however, affecting the delivery of oxygen to the tissues by changing the normal pH. The cells do not release the oxygen. The body has a protective mechanism when the smooth muscles of the cerebral vessels are constricting the blood flow to the brain; this results in the physical symptoms of light-headedness, tingling in the peripheral body areas, fainting, and more. Fast breathing actually lowers the amount of oxygen to the brain. It also excites the nerves, increasing the feeling of exhilaration, especially when focusing on the exhalation rather than the inhalation. The sensations experienced from fast breathing, of whatever type they may be, do not result from an increase in oxygen but from a decrease in CO_2 and from stimulation of the nerves.

Slower breathing has the opposite effect to fast breathing and is found to be therapeutic for mental stability. In yoga, ujjayi breathing involves a steady inhale and exhale with a ratio of 1:2. The rise in carbon dioxide in the bloodstream prompts the dilation of the cerebral blood vessels for increased oxygen supply to the brain. The mental benefits are a sense of calm, heightened alertness, and raw awareness. It gives an overall enhanced sense of well-being. Singing, chanting, and using sound reinforces the regulation and practice of slow breathing. Slow breathing is used for calming the nervous system and maintains better blood oxygenation (Bernardi et al., 2001).

It is important to remember (when not challenging the cardiovascular system) that fast breathing *decreases* blood flow to the brain whereas slow breathing *increases* blood flow. In his book "Return to Life through Contrology" (1945), Joseph Pilates' description of the "Hundred" exercise suggests breathing slowly, not fast as it is performed today. In his writing he emphasizes that you should "squeeze every atom of air from your lungs until they are almost as free of air as a vacuum." He also warns you that the impact of increased oxygen may cause light-headedness, though it is not the influx of oxygen per se but the decrease of CO_2 causing the constriction of blood to the brain. With the practice of slow breathing, fully emptying and filling the lungs without over-breathing (squeezing) will improve the balance of the blood flow to the brain, enhancing clarity and a feeling of well-being.

Nose or mouth breathing?

There is some variation in how breathing is taught in Pilates and other movement systems. When breathing is in through the nose and out of the mouth, usually fast paced movements are being performed, such as "Swimming"; in "Rolling Like A Ball," the four count breath is described as sniff, blow, sniff, blow. The exhale is synchronized with the flexion motion in both directions to facilitate a strong engagement of the abdominals. Exhalation with movement fosters the abdominal work while inhalation supports movement of extension and rotation. The breathing pattern may need to change to match the needs of the client, however. In rotation, for instance, the client may need to find the oblique cross of the abdominals. In this example, exhale is appropriate to cue. There is no one way to breathe in the system of Pilates. The important choice is focusing on the function of the breath in relation to the client's structure to facilitate movement.

Nose breathing has more resistance to the airflow (Bartley, 2014). This resistance benefits the perfusion rate into the body and it is thought to improve the elasticity of the lungs, which maintains optimal oxygen levels necessary for good heart function. Mouth breathing, which requires less exertion, usually occurs when there is difficulty in breathing. The lungs are filled more quickly with less effort, resulting in poor ventilation in the deeper spaces of the lungs. Healthy breathing is best served by nose breathing.

Breathing techniques

Specific breathing techniques can be useful tools for training the body's structure as well as improving its function for breathing. The following can be used in any movement form being practiced.

Joseph Pilates Breathing Wheel (Pinwheel Breathing)

- Sit or stand in an optimal alignment with the diaphragms aligned and wheels balanced (see Fig. 4.14)

- Inhale slowly through the nose to capacity but without over-breathing on the inhale.

- Purse the lips to blow the wheel, making it spin for the duration of the exhale without over-exhaling (Fig. 5.11).

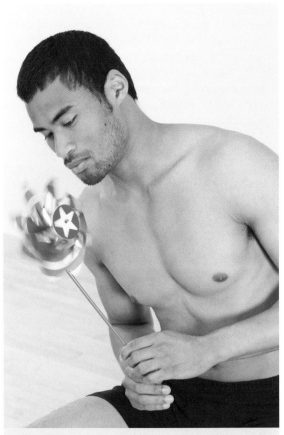

Figure 5.11
Pinwheel Breathing

- Be mindful not to change the body's alignment while inhaling or exhaling.

- Practice 5–10 times.

- Add any movement holding the breathing wheel to challenge the coordination of the breath with movement.

The pursed lips provide a resistance and help to keep the airway open for the exhalation. Ideally, try to have the 1:2 ratio of inhalation to exhalation.

Fogging the Mirror

- Can be done seated or moving in any form.

- Inhale through the nose to capacity without over-inhaling.

- Exhale slowly with the jaw relaxed and mouth wide open.

- Make a sound as if you are fogging a mirror.

- Close the mouth and inhale again.

- Repeat 10 times.

- Add this breathing pattern into any movement.

Focus in "Fogging the Mirror" is on the exhalation, which helps minimize any tension in the accessory muscles of breathing. The relaxed jaw also inhibits the accessory muscles and stimulates the abdominal work.

Walking Breathing

- Stand in good alignment, feeling the diaphragms and wheels aligned.

- Start to walk in an even rhythm of twos, as in marching, but walk with ease.

- Let the arms swing freely, as if you are pleased with yourself (fake it at first if you have to, then, over time, you will begin to really feel pleased).

- Breathe in for two steps.

- Breathe out for two steps.

- Choose to breath either way:

  - though the nose

  - in through the nose and out through the mouth with pursed lips

- Walk for 5–10 minutes in this way or as far as is possible for the capacity of the person.

Hissing Breath

- Sit at the edge of a chair, arms hanging down, palms facing out.

- Place the feet aligned under the knees; open the legs slightly wider and rotated out.

- Elongate the spine and stack the diaphragms.

- Inhale slowly through the nose but do not over-inhale.

- Exhale, making a hissing sound, with the lips slightly opened; the tongue is close to the back of the upper teeth and the hissing sound is like a balloon with a slow leak.

- Do not force the end of the exhale.

- Inhale and repeat 10 times.

Note: Many chair seats are at an incline from front to back. If this is the case, sit facing the corner of the chair.

Imagery for breathing practice

The mental practice of visualizing images while breathing improves the efficiency of breathing patterns through mindful control of the breath.

Double cylinders

Describing an image that mimics the motion is effective for better movement and capacity of breath. The double cylinder image (see Fig. 5.1) was used to describe how the diaphragm moves. Breathing in, the domed shaped piston is moving down, creating more space in the upper chamber and less in the lower. Feel the piston slowly moving down. On the exhale, relax the abdominal wall and allow the piston to reposition automatically.

Find the central axis

Aligning the trunk in a vertical axis is efficient for the excursion of the diaphragm and the coordination of all the muscles of breathing. If the pelvis is tipped forward (anterior tilt), the vertical axis of the crura is not in a position to assist the central tendon to move downward. The anterior fibers of the diaphragm will work more than the back half (Sweigard, 1974).

- Sit at the edge of a chair, arms hanging down, palms facing out.
- Place the feet aligned under the knees; open the legs slightly wider and rotated out.
- Align the diaphragms stacked over one another.
- Exhale and imagine the inner surfaces of the trunk are shrinking toward the center.
- The shrinking insides come toward the center to form a long pole in front of the spine.
- Inhale slowly and expand the inside to its original form.

The toothpaste imagery from Chapter 4 activates a whole body engagement to elongate the torso. The imagery above is for following the breath and internal expansion and contraction in alignment. It is good practice to find the central vertical axis in sitting, standing, lying on the back (supine), on the front (prone), and in quadruped. See the breathing positions described below.

Glass of water

Imagine the trunk as a drinking glass. Start with the glass empty and abdominals relaxed. Inhale slowly through the nose and fill the glass with water from the bottom to the top. Exhale slowly emptying the glass from the top to the bottom. This imagery focuses on relaxing the abdominals for better diaphragm movement, and the initial action of the pelvic floor. In response to the diaphragm movement downward, the pelvic floor supports the pressure downward caused by the increase of abdominal pressure. This imagery helps the chest breather to place their attention on the abdominal chamber rather then the shoulders and neck.

Positions to practice breathing

Constructive Rest Position

The Constructive Rest Position (CRP) is a position that requires no muscular effort, reducing the strain generally used for balancing the body. It was originally offered by Dr. Lulu Sweigard in her book *Human Movement Potential* (1974). The purpose of this position is to release any tension in the body. According to Dr. Swiegard, the ability when awake to rest the body without tension is as important as understanding good body mechanics (Sweigard, 1974). Practicing being in the CRP will release any unwanted held tension in the body that is restricting breathing.

> **Note**
>
> Dr. Sweigard began her research on what she would later call Ideokinesis at Teachers College, Columbia University, and completed her research at New York University where she received her PhD for this work.

- Lie supine on a firm surface with the knees bent, and feet in alignment with the hip joint.
- Tie a belt around the mid thigh so that the legs may completely let go without falling open.
- Reach the arms up toward the ceiling and then cross the arms, resting them on the chest (Fig. 5.12).

The shoulders may be tight and may slide off the chest or discomfort is experienced. The assessment here is that the shoulder area and upper ribcage need to be more flexible and supple. The head position may also cause tension in the neck and shoulders. If there is neck and shoulder tension in this position, place a folded towel under the head to support the head position.

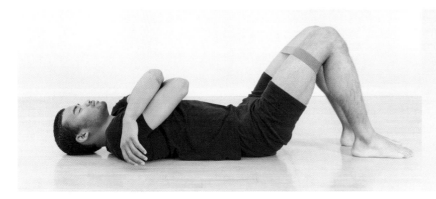

Figure 5.12
Constructive Rest Position

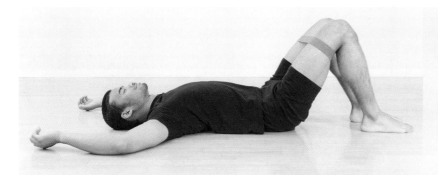

Figure 5.13
Constructive Rest Position:
arms overhead

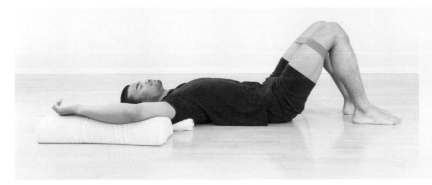

Figure 5.14
Constructive Rest Position
for tight shoulders

For the shoulders and crossed arms position try this:

- Relax the arms and reach them overhead with the elbows bent and resting on the floor (Fig. 5.13).

- If this position is difficult, then prop the arms into an angle that is comfortable (Fig. 5.14).

- Practice the hissing breath three times.

- During the hissing, imagine the tension melting away and dissolving.

- Return the arms to the crossed position.

- Notice if the body is less tense; if so, rest in this position and practice the breathing techniques.

- If still tense, repeat the arms overhead with hissing breath.

Most people's legs would fall open without a small amount of activation of the hip muscles. Tying a belt around the mid thigh or placing the legs up on to a chair for rest will alleviate the tendency for them to fall open.

Lying supine with props

If the CRP is too uncomfortable, rest in supine using props (Fig. 5.15). While lying with props, practice the breathing techniques.

Lying prone

Lying on your stomach is a challenge for chest breathers. The floor will be a resistance to the breath expanding the chest forward. Avoid the chest moving into the floor and imagine the breath moving into the lower back (Fig. 5.16).

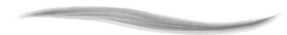

- Inhale wide into the lowest ribs and lower spine.

- Exhale and melt the shoulder blades down the back.
- Practice for a comfortable length of time and gradually increase the time spent on the front (prone).

Quadruped Breathing

The quadruped position is excellent for practicing breathing into the abdominal area. Imagine the breath moving into the lower ribs and back, and feel the recoil of the abdominal wall on the exhale against gravity. Use this breathing to coach the sensation of the TrA contraction.

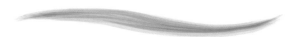

- Kneel in the quadruped position, wrists under the shoulders, knees under the hip joints.
- Find the central vertical axis in this position.
- Inhale feeling the lowest ribs expanding wide; allow the abdominals to relax without changing the position of the spine or pelvis (Fig. 5.17 A).

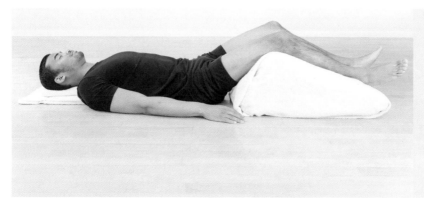

Figure 5.15
Lying with props

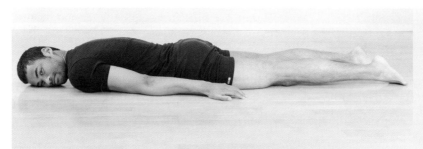

Figure 5.16
Lying prone

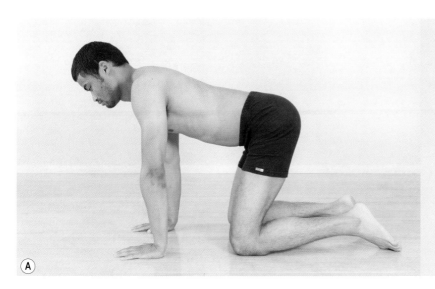

Figure 5.17 A
Quadruped Breathing:
abdominals relaxed

A

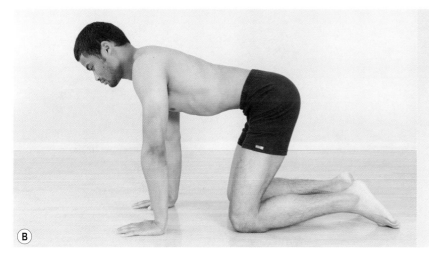

Figure 5.17 B
TrA contracting

B

- Exhale and feel a drawing in of the abdominals as a recoil action; try not to over-exhale; the spine and pelvis maintain their position (Fig. 5.17 B).

Breath movement re-education

Directed Breathing

To re-educate a faulty breathing practice, it is useful to use the hands to direct the breath and thereby redirect the pattern.

- Sit at the edge of a chair, arms hanging down, palms facing out.

- Place the feet aligned under the knees; open the legs slightly wider and rotated out.

- Align the diaphragms stacked over one another.

- Place one hand on the sternum and other hand at the mid belly (Fig. 5.18).

- Slowly breathe in and out.

- Feel which hand moved first.

- Inhale and feel the breath moving into the lower hand first, followed by the upper hand.

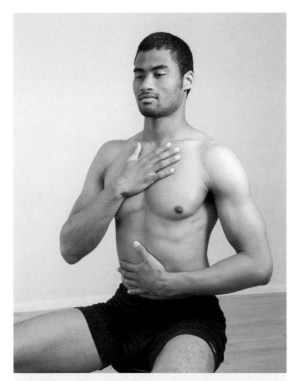

Figure 5.18
Directed Breathing

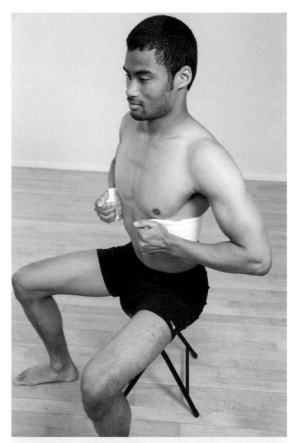

Figure 5.19
Towel Breathing

- Exhale and relax.

- Practice until the breathing becomes more natural, moving the lower hand first.

Towel Breathing

Eve Gentry (see Ch. 4) used this technique to teach how the breath expands in the back and sides of the lowest ribs.

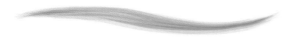

- Sit again in the position for practicing breathing.

- Wrap a hand towel or larger towel around the lowest ribs with the ends of the towel held at the front (Fig. 5.19).

- Inhale into the towel with the intention of stretching the towel; the towel becomes taut.

- Exhale and relax the ribs so that the towel becomes less taut.

Seated Breathing with arm movements

Minimizing the automatic tension of the pectorals when moving the arms sideways and up allows the upper ribcage to expand and lift. The tension in the pectorals tightens the chest and compresses resisting expansion. Performing release movements prior to the arm movements may be necessary.

- Sit again in the position for practicing breathing.

- Place your left hand on the right pectoral muscle, with the intention of feeling if and when the tension occurs.

- The right arm is hanging down and relaxed.

- Breathe in and notice the relaxed pectorals.

- Imagine the pectoral sliding away from the midline, elongating downward and under the armpit before the shoulder blade tip moves.

- Imagine the shoulder blade tip moving forward away from the spine.

- Slowly move the arm out to the side and up on inhalation; the thumb will face up.

- As the arm rises, imagine the shoulder blade moving under the armpit.

- Add the hissing breath on the movement of the arm.

Practitioner note
Hands-on

Gently place one hand on the front of the pectorals and one on the shoulder blade (scapula) (Fig. 5.20). As the client breathes and moves the arm, encourage, through a guiding touch, the lengthening and motion of the scapular rotation. Verbalize the intention and direction of the tissue.

Magic Circle Breathing

Magic Circle Breathing
VIDEO LINK V 5.1

The Magic Circle provides a resistance and feedback to the body as to the rib and thoracic spine movement while breathing. It is also a great tool to work with excessive kyphosis and a flat or reverse curved upper back. Whatever the shape of one's thoracic spine, it needs to be flexible and move while breathing.

- Set-up: Pilates box in the short position and a softer Magic Circle.

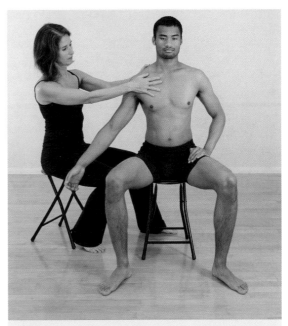

Figure 5.20
Hands-on breathing

- Kneel on the mat or table with the elbows placed on a box.

- Place the ring so that the sternum is resting on the Magic Circle without compressing it; use a soft pad on the end of the ring.

- The spine is in neutral position, head in alignment (Fig. 5.21 A).

- Specifically for the mid to lower thorax, cue the client to inhale as the sternum presses into the circle and the circumference of the mid thorax expands (Fig. 5.21 B).

- Exhale and allow the circle to recoil into the sternum, letting the sternum return to the starting position, with the spine neutral (Fig. 5.21 C).

- Repeat several times until the patterning is coordinated.

Practitioner note
Hands-on

Emphasize the direction of movement that is restricted and minimize the direction of ease. For example, if the client has difficulty moving the

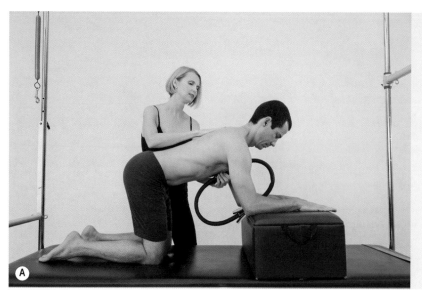

Figure 5.21 A
Magic Circle Breathing: start position

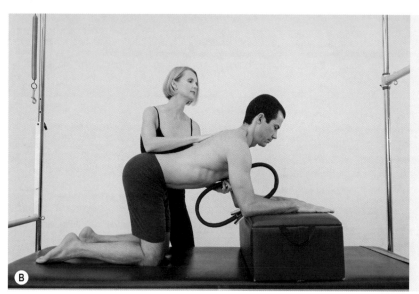

Figure 5.21 B
Inhalation

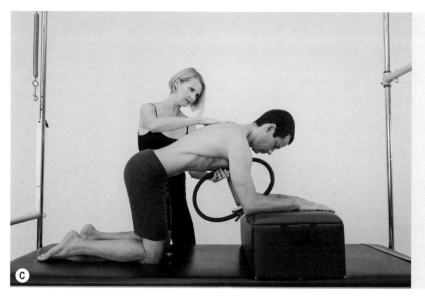

Figure 5.21 C
Exhalation

sternum into the circle with the mid thorax expanding, place one hand on the posterior lateral ribs on the back, and the other hand touching the ring in the front. Cue "Breathe into my hand, give a sense of weight of the hand on the body without pressing, and press into the ring." Tapping gently on the ring brings the attention to the ring. Watch for specific spinal motion. Be sure the shoulders remain in a good position on the ribcage without tension or elevation. The head follows the natural curve of the spine.

Breathing sling on Cadillac

 Breathing using the sling
VIDEO LINK V 5.2

The Pilates Cadillac has a bar that is suspended by springs, called a trapeze. In a non-traditional use of the trapeze, a special strap, a sling, is attached underneath the trapeze bar. Choose two long heavier springs (purple for a Balanced Body Cadillac) and replace the heavy short springs that are traditionally used. The sling is attached with two carabiners on the eyelets underneath the bar where a strap is hanging.

- Lie supine, the knees bent, with the feet flat on the table.

- Lift both legs so that the feet go through the sling.

- Slide the sling underneath the pelvis, moving into a bridge, and place the sling around the lowest ribs; lower the pelvis down (Fig. 5.22 A).

- Adjust the bar so that it is level.

- The springs will lift the lower thorax up a small amount (change to long yellow spring if the tension is too great) (Fig. 5.22 B).

- The objective is to breathe into the sling, moving the bar down a small amount.

- Practice inhaling and moving the bar down (Fig. 5.22 C).

- Watching the bar helps the action of the inhalation into the back.

- On the exhale, stabilize the bar, not allowing it to return to the lifted position.

- The work is to inhale, moving the bar down, and stabilize the bar on the exhale.

Once the coordination of the breathing and stabilizing the bar is achieved, add movements such as "Knee Folds" and "Leg Slides" (Figs 5.23 and 5.24).

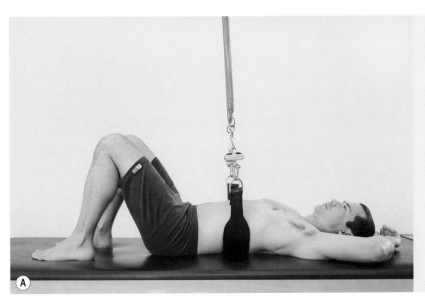

Figure 5.22 A
Breathing sling: start position

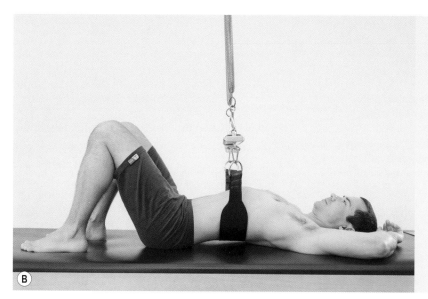

Figure 5.22 B
Relaxed trunk sling lifts spine off the table

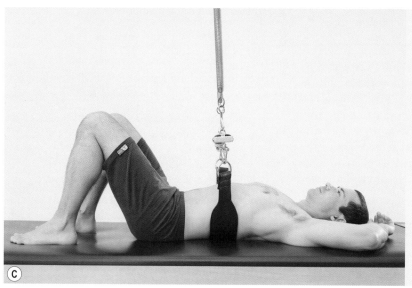

Figure 5.22 C
Inhalation into the sling moves spine into the table and lowers bar

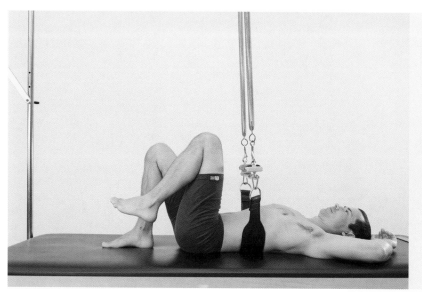

Figure 5.23
Sling with Knee Fold

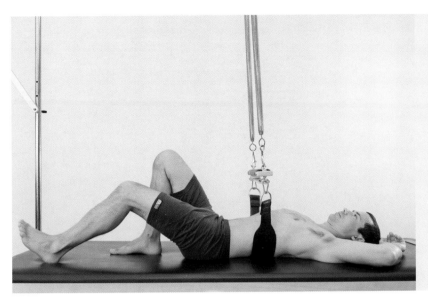

Figure 5.24
Sling with Leg Slide

Movement release techniques

Intercostal resistance release

 Intercostal/rib MET
VIDEO LINK V 5.3

The effort of breathing against a resistance followed by a relaxation facilitates a reorganization of the third and fourth regions of the thorax. Imagine the ribs as an accordion. In a relaxed state the accordion has little space between the folds and is not in tension. Visualize gathering up the folds using the hands; as air enters the accordion to spread the folds, resist the spreading of the folds.

- Lie supine, knees bent, feet flat on the mat, and arms by the sides.
- The practitioner places the palms of the hands on the posterior/lateral side of ribs 8–10; the finger pads are on the posterior side (Fig. 5.25).
- Place each finger as if it were a rib.
- The client exhales to begin to relax the ribs as best as possible; near the end of the exhale gather up the ribs.

- On the next inhale, give a gentle resistance by gently compressing the ribcage with the intention of preventing the ribs from expanding.
- On the exhale, release the resistance; near the end gather up the ribs again.
- Encourage a relaxation of the back, softening into the table.
- Cue the client to inhale and expand the posterior lateral ribcage without letting the abdomen rise.
- Keep the neck and shoulders relaxed.
- The centered vertical axis is undisturbed, the spine and pelvis are in neutral.
- Repeat several times.

Notice the change in the V angle of the lower front of the ribcage. The corresponding thoracic vertebrae T10–T12 are in better contact with the mat. This is an excellent technique for changing the unconscious holding of this area, which is usually seen as flared ribs.

Side lying positional release

This indirect approach works with releasing tension in the diaphragm area, internally and externally. Lying in a passive position of the body, into its ease rather

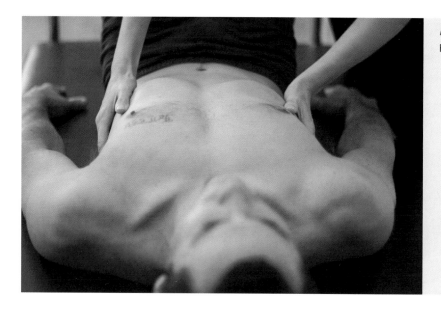

Figure 5.25
Hands-on ribs for MET

than resistance, reduces the sustained unconscious or involuntary contraction of the muscles in the targeted area. When the tension is taken away, the body and brain signal a shift, allowing for the release. The nervous system is no longer receiving excessive feedback from the muscles and fascia in the area, restoring the tone from spasm to resting. The resting tone is the release of tension, allowing for ease of movement and breath.

The position may be practiced on both sides or on the side of greater tension, such as the concave side of a curve.

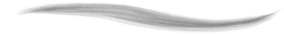

- Lie on the side of the concavity in the thorax.

- Hips are flexed to 70°; knees are fully flexed.

- Prop the head and upper torso, placing the thoracic spine in a side bending position without overpressure.

- The practitioner stands behind the client, placing one hand on the lateral ribs at the location of the diaphragm.

- The other hand is on the lower spine (Fig. 5.26).

- Gently place 5 grams of pressure medially, toward the mat.

- Hold the position for 1 minute.

Release work of the shoulder and neck (Chs 6 and 8) will benefit the ease of the breath. Follow the release with the "Intercostal Resistance Technique" (p. 191) and "Breathing Sling" (p. 189) on the Cadillac.

Stability with breath patterning

 Breathing using the sling
VIDEO LINK V 5.2

Leg Slide variations

Stability and alignment of the pelvis is crucial for the recruitment of the diaphragm in concert with the abdominals. Postural stability is the coordination of the diaphragm with the core muscles. It is common to find imbalances in strength and resilience between the deeper layers, transversus abdominis (TrA), pelvic floor (PF), and deeper spinal muscles, such as multifidus. The "Leg Slide Variations" focus on different recruitment patterns of the trunk with breathing.

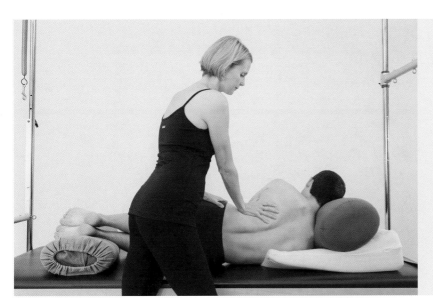

Figure 5.26
Positional release
of diaphragm

Practitioner note

Use two different hands-on positions to facilitate different effects of engaging for stability. One is to place the hands on the lateral sides of the ilium. The hands give a guiding touch to draw the right and left sides closer together, causing a narrowing of the pelvis. The intention is assist the TrA engagement at the pelvis. The second is at the greater trochanters using the same intention of drawing the hip joints closer together, bringing about a narrowing of the pelvic floor.

- Lie supine with the knees bent and the feet on the mat.

- The simple movement is to slide one foot along the mat until leg is straight in contact with the mat.

- Slide the foot along the mat, bending the knee to return to starting position.

- Observe the pelvis and lower spine for stability, tissue tension and muscular recruitment during both directions of the slide.

- Prepare the mind to move on inhalation.

- On exhalation slide the leg along the mat without changing the pelvis or spine.

- The practitioner introduces the narrowing hands-on as the leg slides, either at the top of the pelvis or greater trochanter.

- Pause at the point just before the pelvis loses its stability.

- Take a small inhale to renew the breath so the exhale lasts for the slide back.

- Once the coordination is achieved, eliminate the pause, then slide the leg out and back for the duration of the exhale.

- Repeat the slide with the narrowing hands-on at the pelvis and at the greater trochanter.

Breath sequences for leg slides with coactivation of core muscles

Breath 1: Expansion of the ribcage during leg slide movements:

- On inhalation, widen the lower ribs, imaging the expansion of the diaphragm.

- Compress the ilium at the upper rim toward the midline, cueing the transversus abdominis action,

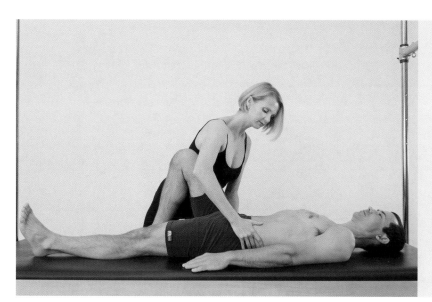

Figure 5.27
Stability with breath hands-on: compression of ilia

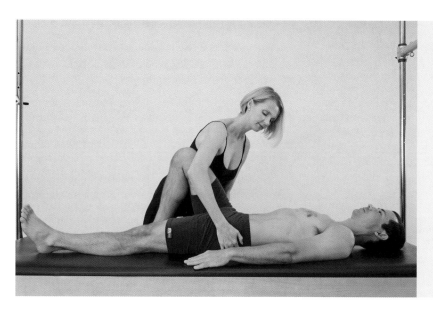

Figure 5.28
Stability with breath hands-on: compression of greater trochanters

or at the greater trochanter, cueing increased pelvic floor action (Figs 5.27 and 5.28).

• Exhale while sliding the leg out and back, maintaining the expansion of the ribcage.

• Repeat 5 times for each side.

Breath 2: Expansion on the inhalation and funneling inward of the ribcage on exhalation:

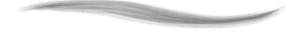

• On inhalation widen the diaphragm as above.

• Compress the ilium at the upper rim toward midline or at the greater trochanter.

• On the exhalation allow the lower ribs to relax the expansion and draw downward in a posterior and inferior direction, allowing for intercostal and oblique synergistic work with the recoil of the diaphragm.

- NOTE: the V shape at the inferior lateral angles of the ribcage does not close inward; the lower ribs are sinking into the mat and the ribcage is deflating from the active expansion part of the exercise.

The first breath exercise above is designed to focus on the activation of the TrA in conjunction with diaphragmatic movement and pelvic stability. The second breath exercise is layering the TrA and diaphragm action with the ribcage exhalation movement, specifically utilizing the intercostals and oblique systems. It is an excellent exercise for re-education of a ribcage that has flared or ski jumps for lower ribs.

Use these breathing sequencing exercises with the compression hands-on interchangeably with movement to challenge the breath and core work. In leg slide variations, one may slide the leg along the mat and add a small lift in the form of a straight leg raise to increase the challenge for stability (Fig. 5.29). A second challenge is to abduct the hip with pelvic stability, slide the leg down in external rotation, roll the leg into neutral and slide the leg back to the starting position. For a person to master the concentration of the breathing pattern, the movement task and monitoring the stability of the pelvis demands the whole nervous system become coordinated and in synchronization.

Upper thoracic Sphinx with belt

The upper thorax is an area where the segmental movement tends to be restricted, especially in extension. It inhibits breathing by not allowing the sternum to lift or the neck muscles to lengthen. The belt is a tool to bring awareness and to guide the movement of the upper thorax.

- The client lies prone (on stomach) with arms straight over the head, resting on the floor. If bare arms are resting on a wooden floor, use a towel underneath the arms for sliding if necessary.

- Place a yoga belt around the upper back just below the lower tips of the scapulae, the two ends under the armpits.

- The teacher sits in front of the client holding the ends of the belt (Fig. 5.30 A).

- Cue the client to move into a "Small Swan" (lying prone cues, Ch. 4) movement.

- When the head and chest are lifted, slide the arms, bending the elbows into a sphinx shape, resting on the elbows (Fig. 5.30 B).

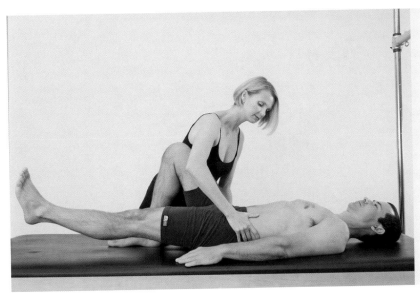

Figure 5.29
Adding a straight leg raise

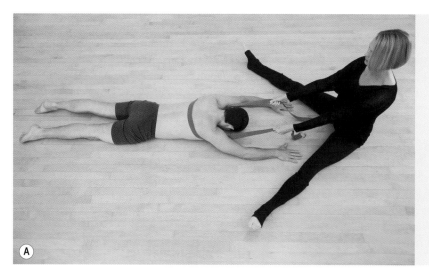

Figure 5.30 A
Upper thoracic Sphinx
with belt: start position

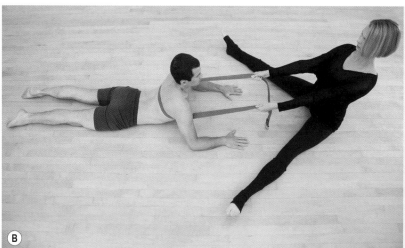

Figure 5.30 B
Sphinx on elbows

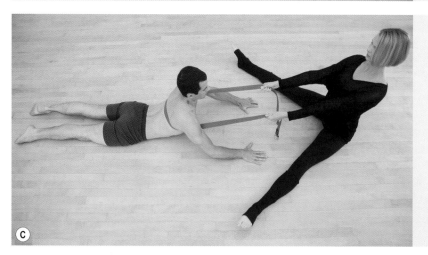

Figure 5.30 C
Sphinx with arms straight

- Cue the client to lift the chest a small amount, beginning to straighten the arms (Fig. 5.30 C).

- At this point prepare to lean back, creating a light pulling of the upper thorax and sternum forward.

- Cue to segmentally lower the chest, finishing with the head down and arms extended again (if using towel, slide the towel away).

- Repeat 3–5 times, gradually straightening the arms a small amount more.

- The intention is to keep the work in the thorax and not the lumbar spine.

Bridging to Chapter 6

Moving with integrity means learning and sensing one's own unique body and its development over time of habits, postures, and nervous system responses. Movement is a language in motion where life history and expressions of being human are seen. If feeling pain or a health issue arises, the body adapts its function and structure. Through mindful movement choices that specifically address the issue, or provide relief from symptoms, healing is made possible. Joseph Pilates believed that complete understanding of human movement, muscle coordination, principles of equilibrium applied to the body in motion and rest are the keys to attaining health and happiness. Studying the body's mechanisms helps bring a deeper sense of one's body for self-evaluation and intelligent movement choices.

Part 3

Resilient shoulders to head

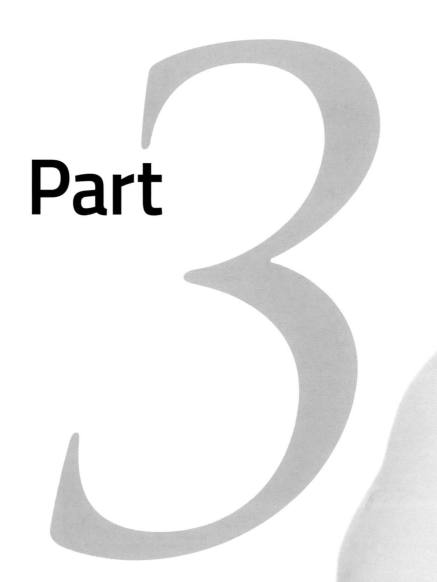

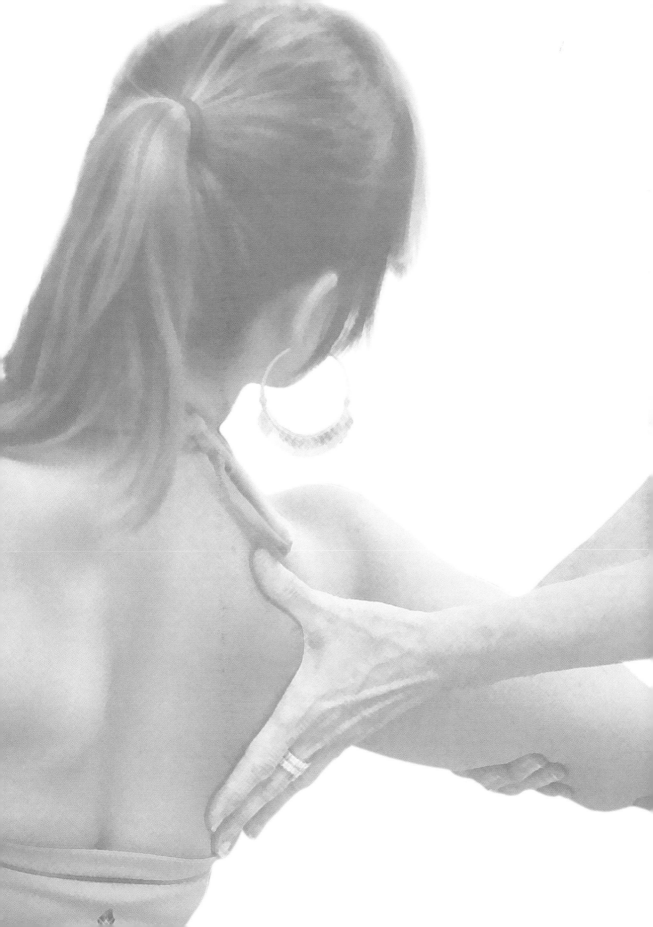

Resilient shoulders

"I opened my arms and love embraced me as a Lover"

Rumi

Contemplative awareness: towards and away

Touching, reaching, grabbing, pushing, and holding are human contact actions of the upper limbs. The arms are rooted in the body's core but extend beyond the body into the environment. The upper limbs, including upper thoracic spine, ribs, manubrium, clavicles, scapula, and the whole arm to hand complex, expand from the heart. This is a powerful center of exchange, of human emotion and expression, but consequently can be an area of great sadness and dysfunction.

The stages of movement development are well documented and begin very early, with the head. At first, an infant responds through reflexes, sucking being the primary one. By 3 months, there is more control of the head. The practice of lifting the head strengthens the neural pathways to move the upper back and arms. Lifting the head up gives the baby a limited view of the world but soon the chest and arms participate to widen it. In a prone position the infant learns to push up with the arms to extend the spine, giving an expanded field of view. Active hands pincer grip, shake objects, open and close, grasp the feet. The feet start to push away when they come into contact with a firm surface. All this activity is integrating both sensory and motor functions. By 7 months, the infant can roll the body, sit up, first with the help of the hands and then without help, reach with one hand, transfer objects from hand to hand, and use a raking grasp. Development progresses to more complex skills such as crawling, pulling the body up to standing, standing without holding momentarily, and eventually walking. The bipedal stance and the contralateral motion, the pattern of gait, help the upper body learn how to connect with the pelvis and legs.

There is naturalness to this organization, which, when referenced, provides a wonderful template of balanced, healthy movement patterning. Over the course of time, adults acquire postures that are less functional; they guard emotions, carrying everyday stress in their shoulders, joints, forearms, and wrists, and losing the fundamental and natural human movement patterning they had as infants. The lost ability to move in the most basic way causes physical issues and, in addition, portrays a person in a particular light, for posture and movement create a presence, a personality of the body. Feeling the chest open and lifted, the shoulders released, and the ribcage suspended projects positive self-esteem, confidence, and receptivity into the world.

Function and form

The development of function and form of the upper body is valuable for understanding movement patterns. Patterning is a neuromuscular action that is embedded in our cells during human embryogenesis. The upper limb cells begin their migration from the level of C5 to T1 from a ridge (the Wolffian ridge) where other sense organs, such as the nose, eyes, ears, nipples, and genitals, also develop (Schoenwolf et al., 2009). The hands and feet have far richer sensory receptors and proprioception than other parts of the body.

Sensory receptors in the body are distributed unevenly, with a higher concentration of sensory receptors in the body parts that need high acuity and dexterity. In the brain, the "map" of the sensory and motor connections looks disproportionate because the higher sensory receptor body parts (such as the fingers and lips) use more of the brain's cells or "real estate" (Blakeslee and Blakeslee, 2007) (Fig 6.1). The highly somatic receptors of the hands, lips, and tongue are directly connected to a response system affecting motor control, but differ from the trunk, knees or hips. The hands and feet link directly through the limbs to the brain.

Practitioner note

In the 1930s, Dr. Wilder Penfield, a surgeon, pioneered an operation in which he collected data from the surface of the brain that mapped the primary touch areas (the somatosensory cortex). He also mapped the motor cortex and found a similar map. Dr. Penfield called the map a "homunculus" ("little man" in Latin). The term is still used in modern neuroscience; however, there are now many maps (homunculi) interacting with one another. The web of information and responses shown by the maps is a reciprocal system creating a unique processing of the mind and body (Blakeslee and Blakeslee, 2007; Doidge, 2007).

As Phillip Beach (2010) observed, "The genesis of one's basic shape is derived from these processes that take place within the first 6 weeks post-conception, but shape continues to change over a course of a life time." To fully understand the function of the limbs is to follow the deep cellular processes of development. In embryogenesis, the upper limbs grow in a different way to the lower limbs (described briefly in Ch. 2). The growth pattern of the upper limb bud is a lateral rotation away from the body (Schoenwolf et al., 2009). The growth is on a proximodistal axis, meaning the path from the trunk toward the hand (see Fig. 2.1). As the bones, ligaments, and blood vessels develop, the growth pattern turns into a spiral in which the muscle mass separates into front (anterior) and back (posterior) components (Moore et al., 2011). The elbow is formed as the bones migrate to the final destination, the hand away from the elbow and the scapula and humerus toward the trunk. The upper limb progresses into forming the arms, which are held in a flute-player position, a pronation of the forearms. The limbs magnify the spiral motions produced from the body into the limbs. Using the analogy of the early growth process for movement provides a template we can use for changing dysfunction to function.

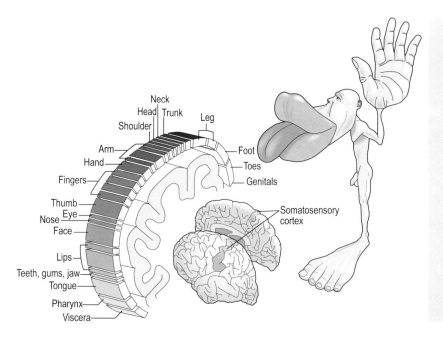

Figure 6.1

Map of sensory and motor connections

Neck
Head | Trunk
Shoulder | Leg
Arm — Foot
Hand — Toes
Fingers — Genitals
Thumb
Nose — Eye
Face — Somatosensory cortex
Lips
Teeth, gums, jaw
Tongue
Pharynx
Viscera

The spiral of the arm allows for the normal actions of the whole arm. The arms are not structured to bear weight as the legs are. The arms have a spring-like quality to them: imagine the motion of the forearms crossing and uncrossing. The function of the arm can be seen as the spring coiling around from the upper back and scapula to the hands, creating stability and strength. In addition, a fluid, soft quality of the arms is necessary for expression, touch, and sensitivity. Through life events, sports, and day-to-day habits, however, we can lose the functional spiral movement of the limb and trunk connection, which may cause undesirable structural changes. The dysfunction will be evident in the restriction of movement anywhere along the pathway from body to limb.

Root of the arms

The three dimensional trunk (described in Ch. 4, "Superficial and Deep," and Ch. 5, "Fascial Continuum") is continuous with the outreaching of the arms. Truly the root of the arms is a spiral continuum of the myofascial system, linking one side of the skull to the opposite shoulder, across to the front obliquely, to the opposite hip, knee, and foot (Myers, 2001). In a throwing action, the torso twists and spirals through the arm to release the object. The arms emphasize the trunk rotation from the head to the waist. The legs are the power for the twist of the torso from the pelvis to the waist. In gait, one can see the contralateral trunk motion amplified by the arms and legs (Fig. 6.2).

Shoulder and arm continuations

The muscles of the shoulder girdle travel in an oblique path from the trunk, continuing from the quadratus lumborum (laterally), which courses medially toward the spine where it crosses to the opposite side, to serratus posterior inferior, and following upward to the internal oblique, internal intercostals, crossing again to the opposite side external intercostals and on up to the pectoralis major (see Fig. 4.2), to the flexor side (anterior) of the arm, the forearm, and the palm of the hand (Beach, 2010).

The flexor reflex side of the arm is directly connected to pectoralis major with its attachment on the humerus. The pectoral fascia originates at the clavicle, with a superficial layer upward into the deep cervical fascia. Its deeper layer adheres to the clavicular

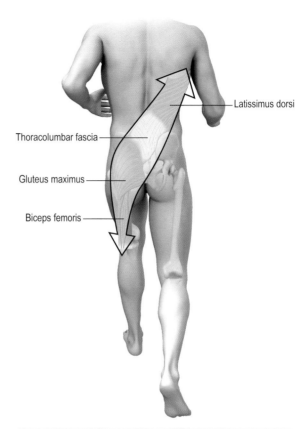

Labels: Latissimus dorsi, Thoracolumbar fascia, Gluteus maximus, Biceps femoris

Figure 6.2
Root of the arms into the myofascial system of the trunk

bone (periosteum). The lowest fibers of pectoralis major's origin, at the fifth and sixth ribs, are continuous through a fascial link of the abdominal aponeurosis, rectus abdominis and the contralateral (opposite) external oblique. The journey then continues into the pelvis, from pubic bone to adductors of the legs and down. A deeper layer, the clavipectoral fascia, underlies the pectoral fascia but has a distinct individuation, allowing the layers to glide over one another. The clavipectoral fascia is a strong layer arising from the clavicle, toward the subclavian and pectoralis minor. The fascia of the pectoralis major, the latissimus dorsi and deltoid muscles merge into the brachial fascia (Stecco and Stecco, 2012) (Figs 6.3 A & B). These connections of the arm into the trunk will participate in creating the movement in a variety of arm movements.

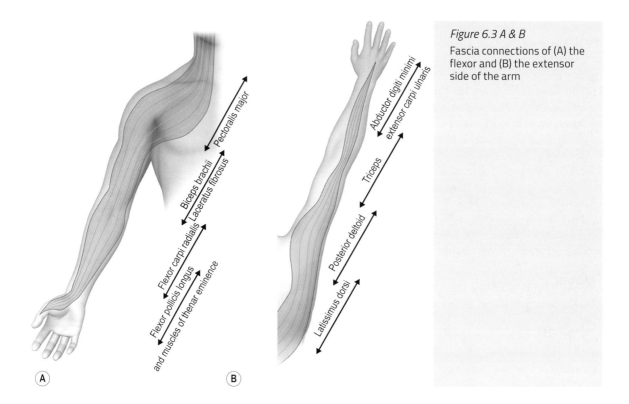

Figure 6.3 A & B

Fascia connections of (A) the flexor and (B) the extensor side of the arm

Try it!

Hang with one arm from an overhead bar, and try to pull the body up – a one arm pull-up. Or simply keep the arm straight and pull up. It is possible to feel this with both feet on the ground, with only a little weight being pulled up by the arm. Or imagine it. Feel how the arm flexors contract and feel it into the pectoralis major, and into the abdominals (Fig. 6.4).

The continuous path of the extensors of the arm stems from the internal oblique on one side, to the external oblique on the opposite side, up to the same side external intercostals, traveling back to the opposite side trapezius, latissimus dorsi, rhomboids, infraspinatus, teres major and minor, down the back (posterior) of the arm, the forearm and the back of the hand (Beach, 2010). The fascial trail is continuous from the latissimus dorsi in both a superior and an inferior way. The latissimus dorsi emerges from the thoracolumbar fascia and joins into the superficial lamina of the lateral raphe and sacrolumbar fascia. The fascia of the

gluteus maximus also attaches at the sacral crest (Vleeming, 2012). Superiorly affecting the shoulder, the thoracolumbar fascia runs up to the posterior deltoid where it merges into the brachial fascia (Stecco and Stecco, 2012) (see Figs 4.3 and 6.3).

The strength and support for the upper limbs come from the relationship of the front of the shoulder with the back of the shoulder and its trunk connections. And this relationship of the front to the back will also determine the position and movement ability of the humerus and scapula. When the humeral head is forward, the pectoralis major is shortened, pulling the shoulder down and forward (Fig. 6.5). The latissimus dorsi, when restricted, pulls down and internally rotates the head of the humerus, holding the humeral head forward. The attachments in the deep layer, clavipectoral fascia on the pectoralis minor and subclavian, will inhibit the motions of the clavicle and scapula. The co-tightening of these muscles and lack of independent glide of the fascial layers restricts the ability of the humeral head to move in relation to the other bones around it, causing dysfunctional movement.

tightness is in the thoracolumbar fascia side of the body, the spine will arch while hanging. If the front of the chest is curled in, then the abdominal/pectoral fascia is tighter. One can also observe how the scapulae sit on the ribs in relation to the spine.

- The client is kneeling on Cadillac, holding the upper bars or a chin-up bar, with the legs supported by the table; if the knees do not reach the table, place a small box underneath the knees; move the knees forward, assisting the spine to hang long (Fig. 6.6 A).

- The practitioner observes the side plumb line.

- The hanging client feels the lengthening.

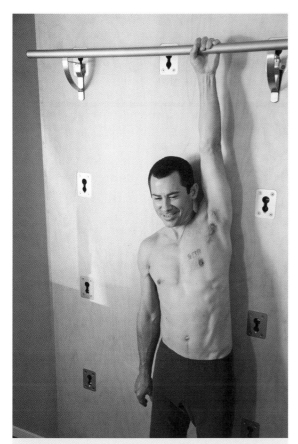

Figure 6.4
Hanging from one arm feeling the arm flexor

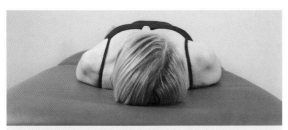

Figure 6.5
Pectoralis area shortness on the right side

Latissimus stretch and activation of shoulder girdle

Using the overhead bars of the Pilates Cadillac or another high bar as a chin-up bar, hanging with both arms clearly shows where the imbalance lies. If the

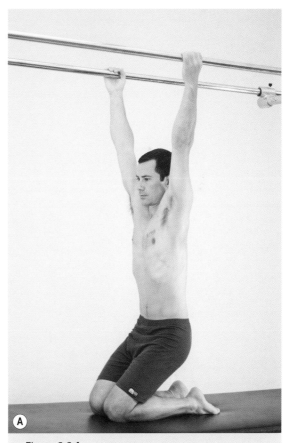

Ⓐ

Figure 6.6 A
Latissimus dorsi activation and stretch on Cadillac

- Cue the client to keep the arms straight and lift the trunk or crown of the head up toward the sky, then exhale (Fig. 6.6 B).

- Observe the path and shape the body takes; it is common to see the spine extend, which is a sign of the latissimus dorsi overworking while the serratus anterior is inhibited and lacking its connection to the external obliques.

- Cue the client to feel scapula glide down as the body moves vertically up.

Practitioner note

Be aware of possible overuse of the flexors of the arm and extensors of the back. Cue manually where the client needs to draw their attention to connect into the balanced lines of pull.

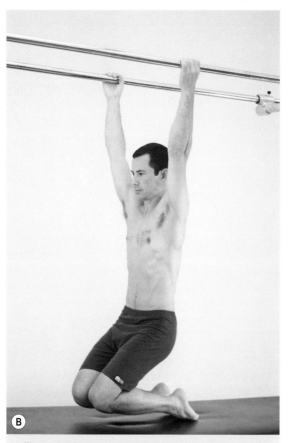

B

Figure 6.6 B
Lifting the trunk

The balance of the trunk in movement will allow the arms to move more freely. Shoulder movement requires the scapula to be mobile in order to move the shoulder (glenohumeral) joint for the many shifting positions of the arm. Stability of the scapula is also required so that the arm is supported, to avoid impingements of the shoulder joint at certain ranges and weight bearing on the arms. Finding the best position of the scapula on the ribcage will give it the best opportunity to move without effort or strain. A balance of the muscles that surround the scapula and motor control of the rhythm of the bone movements are the key elements to work with the shoulder.

Shoulder network

The shoulder network is a perfect example of balanced tension required for optimal movement. The arms move as part of a kinematic chain, movement of one segment producing movement in other linked segments.

The bones of the functional shoulder are (Fig. 6.7):

- upper thorax

- first and second ribs

- manubrium

- scapulae

- clavicles

- humeri.

Figure 6.7
Bones of the functional shoulder

Practitioner note

When weight bearing on the arms, the radius, ulna, carpal and metacarpal bones play a role in the dynamic movement of the shoulder (see Ch. 7, "Weight Bearing on the Hands").

The shoulder (glenohumeral) joint is a ball and socket joint made up from the head of the humerus and the scapula glenoid fossa. The glenohumeral joint is the most mobile joint in the body. Its neighbors, the other structures related by attachments and location, move in a sequence that is responsible for its great range of motion. The relative relationship of the bones of the functional shoulder and their timely dance create happy shoulders.

The scapula's normal position is resting on a rounded shape of the ribcage between ribs two and seven. The angle of the scapula runs obliquely at about 30° and is often called "scaption" (a shortened form of "scapular plane elevation") or the scapular plane. Its superior and medial angle lines up with the first thoracic vertebra. The spine of the scapula corresponds to the third thoracic vertebra and the inferior medial angle is at the seventh or eighth thoracic vertebra. The distance from the spinal border of the scapula to the thoracic spine is 3 inches (5–6 cm) just below the spine of the scapula. At the inferior angle, it lies about 7–8 inches (18–20 cm) from the spine.

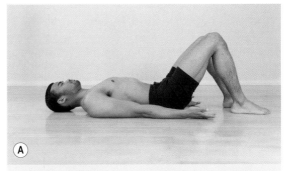

Figure 6.8 A
Finding scaption angle: start position, setting scapulae

Try it!

Find the scaption angle that is optimal. Lie down, knees bent and feet flat on the floor. Place the arms at the side of the body with the thumbs facing outward. Feel the contact of the upper back with the floor. Gently press the feet into the mat and slightly away to slide the scapula downward and in contact with the ribs (Fig. 6.8 A). Check in with the lower ribs; be sure there is contact with the mat. Look straight ahead; turn the hands so the thumbs are facing forward, palms facing each other. Slowly lift the arms up between 60° and 90° (Fig. 6.8 B). Slowly move the arms away from each other, opening the arms wide (Fig. 6.8 C). Notice and feel only the arms moving. Try to feel if the shoulder blades begin to move. Keep the arms straight. Pause the movement at the point where the lower ribs lose contact with the floor and/or the scapulae move. Look at the angle of the arms. This is the scaption angle.

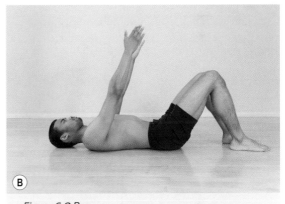

Figure 6.8 B
Arms raised

Practitioner note
Hands-on

To set the shoulder girdle, the client lies in the supine position. Stand on the left side of the client facing the head (superiorly), and place the left hand underneath the trunk, with the fingertips at the medial border of the scapula. Place the right hand on the superior part of the spine of the scapula. In one smooth and synchronized movement, glide the scapula inferior

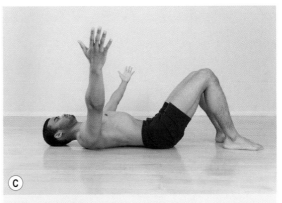

Figure 6.8 C
Moving into scaption angle

and lateral (Fig. 6.9 A). Use the hand on the spine of the scapula, moving it inferior, and the hand on the medial border laterally in a combined movement (Fig. 6.9 B). If the client's scapula is too medial to begin with then do not emphasize the medial direction, but focus instead on the superior hand motion, moving it inferior with both hands.

Scapulohumeral rhythm

"Scapulohumeral rhythm" is a term used to describe the combined motion of the scapula and humerus. The motion, however, is not isolated to these bones but includes a whole torso involvement, especially the upper thorax, clavicle, and manubrium. Watching the timing of the bones as the arm is moving is helpful in coaching healthy shoulder movement and identifying which lines of tissue are restricting the motion.

Since the arm (humerus) is attached to the scapula (glenoid fossa), the combined motions of the ball and socket joint fully elevate the arm to 180° of

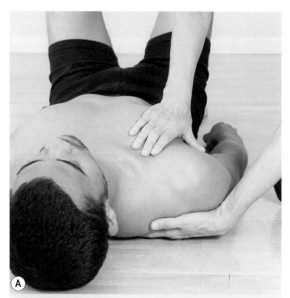

Figure 6.9 A
Practitioner's hands-on: setting the scapula hand placement

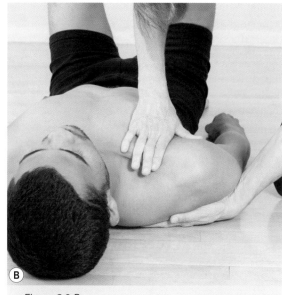

Figure 6.9 B
Glide of the scapula into place

humeral extension. Any movement of the scapula affects the glenohumeral joint. The socket part of the joint, the glenoid fossa of the scapula, is maintaining an optimal position to receive the humeral head for a harmonious joint. The shape of this joint is incongruent for stability compared to the ball and socket joint at the hip. The shoulder joint sacrifices stability in exchange for the mobility needs of the arm and hand.

Sternum to clavicle to scapula

Three other joints are important to the elevation of the arm, whether to the side (abduction) or front (flexion) of the body. The sternoclavicular (SC; sternum and clavicle) and acromioclavicular (AC; acromion, which is part of the scapula, and clavicle) joints are part of the kinematic linkage of the arm. Another non-bony joint is the scapulothoracic joint, which is a functional articulation where the scapula slides along the ribcage. The movements of the scapula along the ribcage are associated with the SC and AC joints. The AC joint is the acromion of the scapula articulating with the lateral edge of the clavicle; the medial edge of the clavicle attaches to the manubrium at the SC joint. Looking at the structures and the chain of movements, it is clear that any movement of the scapula will facilitate motion of the clavicle.

The only axial skeletal attachment of the shoulder complex is at the SC joint (see Fig. 6.7). The scapula relies on the suppleness and resilience of the tissue in which it is embedded. The motions of the scapula are classically described in the three planes and are translatory motions:

- superior to inferior (elevation and depression)
- coronal (abduction and adduction or protraction retraction)
- rotational (upward and downward rotation).

Winging, tipping, and spinning

There are two other less frequently described motions, namely the winging and tipping of the scapula that maintain the contact of the scapula with the ribcage as it navigates the contour of the ribcage. The term "winging" is usually associated with a dysfunction of the coupled muscular movements of the scapula and loss of scapula contact on the ribs. There is normal winging necessary during rotation of the scapula. If the scapula did not move around the sides of the ribcage as the arm elevates, then only the spine edge or medial side of the scapula would remain on the ribcage. Because of the ribcage contour and the scapula linkage at the AC and SC joints, pure movement is prevented. Tipping motions occur during arm elevation and depression to maintain contact to the ribcage. As the scapula glides up, the lowest end (inferior angle) moves back (posterior), conforming to the increased curvature of the ribcage. Tipping occurs at the AC joint and is linked with clavicle rotation since the two are the joints of the clavicle.

The clavicle mirrors the action of the scapula with the attachment of the scapula to the distal end of the clavicle. Rotation of the clavicle is a spin at the manubrium. From its resting position, the clavicle only rotates in one direction, that is, posterior.

As the arm is elevating, the inferior surface of the clavicle is now facing front (anterior). The clavicle is rotating backward around its long axis producing further elevation of the acromial end (AC joint), which increases scapular upward rotation for another 30°. Once the arm is at its height and begins to lower, then the clavicle rotates anterior back to its resting position.

> **Practitioner note**
>
> On the surface, it is often difficult to observe the movement of the clavicle. Focus on the lateral end of the bone in order to see or feel the motions.

Phases of bone rhythm

The scapulohumeral rhythm is the combined motions of all three planes of all the linkages. The first phase is a setting phase, where the scapula is providing stability for the humeral movement. In this phase, the motion is generally at the glenohumeral joint unless the arm is loaded. Adding a stress to the arm may activate the scapula. The axis of the motion is centered at medial end or base of the spine of the scapula, with a range of 60°.

Several important force couples act within the shoulder girdle to rotate about its axis of motion. The glenohumeral joint's shape is not congruent so the axis of motion is not pure spin but requires motions of rolling and gliding of the humeral head on the glenoid fossa. The head of the humerus moves in the opposite direction to the shaft of the humerus. The deltoid and rotator cuff act as a force couple. The rotator cuff muscles guide the head of the humerus within the glenoid fossa and provide the external rotatory force necessary to prevent impingement (the humeral head butting up against the acromion) while the deltoid, considered the prime mover for humeral abduction, pulls the humerus outward and upward. This motion of upward and outward is crucial to guide arm movement to create interarticular space through gliding and maintain apposition (close proximity) of the joint surfaces (Norkin and Levangie, 2011).

When the arm reaches 60–90°, the scapula begins upward rotation. Every 1° of scapula rotation is accompanied by 2° of humeral elevation (Norkin and Levangie, 2011). The force couple of the lower trapezius and serratus anterior produces the rotational motion of the scapula. The lower trapezius and lower serratus become more active as the scapula progresses through upward rotation above 90° (Fig. 6.10). The action of the lower trapezius is greater in abduction and must relax to allow forward flexion. The lower fibers of the serratus anterior become more active in forward flexion. The rhomboids and middle trapezius are synergists, eccentrically contracting to control the change of position of the scapula. The latissimus dorsi and pectoralis major give some resistance through being lengthened. It is common to find the inability to raise the arm due to the tightness of these muscles. Prior to strengthening the upward rotation movements, releasing the latissimus and pectorals is recommended (see Ch. 4, "MET Release for the Lat-Pectorals and Abdominals").

As the scapula continues upward rotation, it produces elevation of the acromial end of the clavicle. Ligaments become taut (costoclavicular at the SC, conoid and trapezoid at AC), preventing the continued upward rotation of the scapula. Winging and tipping is sustaining the contact with the contours of the ribcage. The action of the muscles rotating the scapula, the trapezius and serratus anterior, against the restriction of the clavicle elevation stimulates the posterior rotation of the clavicle. The elevation and

rotation of the clavicle moves the manubrium up and the first and second rib rings descend in the back, which extends the upper thorax.

> **Practitioner note**
>
> According to Kapandji (1982), abducting the arm is in three phases:
>
> - Phase one, from 0° to 60°, takes place only at the shoulder joint.
>
> - Phase two, from 60° to 120°, requires recruitment of the scapulothoracic "joint" (the space between the scapula and the serratus anterior).
>
> - Phase three, from 120° to 180°, involves movement at the shoulder joint and the scapulothoracic "joint," and the clavicular elevation/rotation with thorax spine side bending to the same side, a concavity toward the arm.

Scapulohumeral rhythm training with pole

 Scapulohumeral training with a pole
VIDEO LINK V 6.1

The movement will be elevation of the humerus in the scapular plane (flexion and abduction), beginning from low angle to as high an elevation as is possible while still maintaining good scapulohumeral mechanics.

- The client is seated, holding the pole at a low angle with the arm straight, the humerus in a neutral forearm, supinated with the thumb facing up.

- The practitioner stands behind the client, holding the top portion of the stick (Fig. 6.11 A).

- Pull or adjust the tension on the stick to place the scapula and humerus in an optimal position to start; use the other hand to adjust the scapula if necessary.

- Cue the client to gently pull down on the stick to feel the depression of the scapula; practitioner resists this motion lightly to prevent the stick from moving.

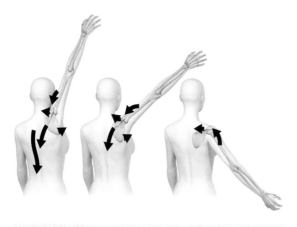

Figure 6.10
Scapulohumeral rhythm

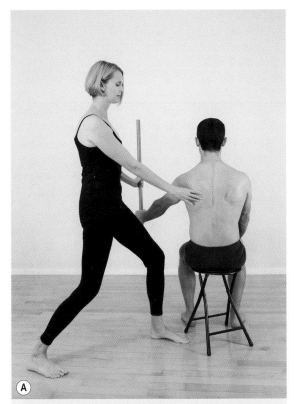

Figure 6.11 A
Scapulohumeral training with a pole: start position

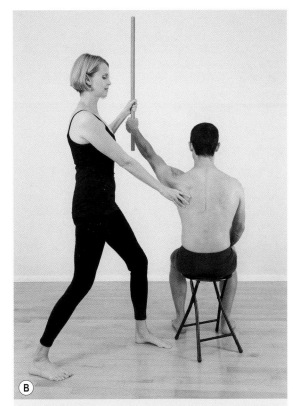

Figure 6.11 B
Guiding the scapulohumeral rhythm with the pole

- Instruct the client to maintain the resistance downward but allow the stick to be moved up matching the resistance (the amount of upward pull created by practitioner); cue "meet my resistance as I move the pole up" (Fig. 6.11 B).

- Use the free hand to feel and cue the serratus anterior.

- When the client begins to elevate the humerus instead of the scapula rotation, pause and ask them to pull down the pole to reinstate the muscle activation.

- On the descent of the humerus, the client may pull the pole down, activating assistance from the latissimus dorsi; do not offer too much resistance.

- The trainer can use the hand not pulling the pole to guide the scapula and tactile cueing for proper muscle pattern activation.

- Repeat 2–3 times; note that clients tend to become very sore in this action.

Downward movement

There is no consistent rhythm patterning for the downward movement or depression of the shoulder. The scapula tends to downwardly rotate and adduct as the arm is returning to the hanging position. Seeing the return of the scapula to its original optimal position on the ribcage is preferable, so that the tone of the area is balanced. A forceful downward movement of the humerus in relation to the trunk is a retraction and depression of the scapula produced by the lower trapezius and the rhomboids. The levator scapula retracts and rotates the glenoid fossa inferiorly (Kapandji, 1982). The latissimus dorsi and pectoralis major are prime movers in adduction with assistance from the pectoralis minor, which acts directly on the scapula.

Practitioner note

The upper fibers of serratus anterior are attached on the anterior side of the superior/medial border of the scapula, opposite the levator scapula (Fig. 6.12). Both muscles, when in held tension, cause an elevated scapula, inhibiting the downward movement and dysfunctional winging of the scapula. A scapula that is held high on the ribcage, with the inferior medial edge off the ribcage, minimizes the contact of the scapula gliding along the ribcage. Without this contact, movements thought to strengthen the shoulder girdle and shoulder will be limited, if not impossible. Release the upper serratus anterior prior to scapula stability work.

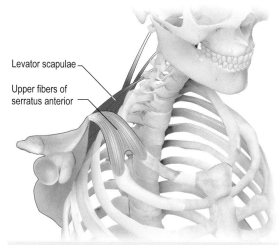

Levator scapulae

Upper fibers of serratus anterior

Figure 6.12
Relationship of the upper fibers of serratus anterior and levator scapula

Side lying release of the upper serratus anterior and levator scapula

Side lying upper serratus/levator release
VIDEO LINK V 6.2

It is easier to access this area using the push-through bar on the Pilates Cadillac apparatus. The bar gives the practitioner a third hand and a closed chain effect of the client's arm. This may be performed without the bar, though it seems to involve more work for the practitioner and not to be as effective.

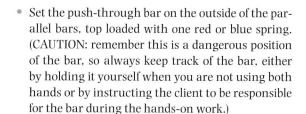

- Set the push-through bar on the outside of the parallel bars, top loaded with one red or blue spring. (CAUTION: remember this is a dangerous position of the bar, so always keep track of the bar, either by holding it yourself when you are not using both hands or by instructing the client to be responsible for the bar during the hands-on work.)

- The client is side lying with the head at the push through bar end with the arm to be released up).

- The client holds the push-through bar at an angle of approximately 130–150° abduction and flexion of the shoulder and with the elbow softened.

- Stand to the back and side of the client and place one hand on the inferior angle of the scapula and the other hand in front of the superior angle of the scapula.

- Cue the client to allow the bar to move away slightly and move the scapula into upward rotation manually, if needed (Fig. 6.13 A).

- Fix the inferior angle by using the inferior hand to block the movement of the scapula.

- Place the superior hand underneath the superior angle, lifting it to introduce a winging position of the upper scapula.

- The practitioner stands in a comfortable, grounded way in order to introduce resistance to the arm. First the practitioner fixes the inferior angle so no movement occurs and changes the superior hand position (to block the arm with the pull of the bar) (flexion of shoulder) (Fig. 6.13 B).

- Hold for 5 seconds.

- Cue the client to stop the engagement; change the hand back to the superior angle.

- As the client lengthens the bar slightly away, the practitioner attempts to create a superior winging, bringing the upper scapula away from the chest wall and thus creating a stretch.

- Repeat 2–3 times.

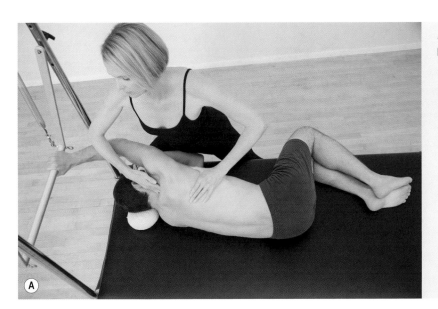

Figure 6.13 A
Moving bar away

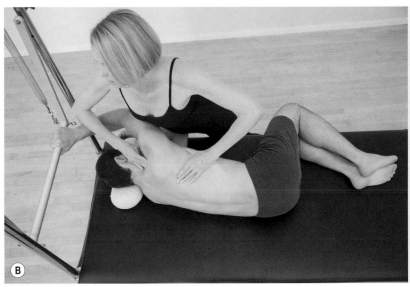

Figure 6.13 B
Pulling bar in and blocking
the movement of scapula

Practitioner note

A forceful movement of the trunk in relation to a fixed
arm, as in a push-up, is also a downward movement of
the scapula moving the thorax on the arm. When the
arm is bilaterally fixed, the latissimus dorsi will pull the
lower attachments on the pelvis toward its attachment
on the humerus. If the spine is in a neutral position, a
co-contraction of the pectoralis major and its fascial
connections into the abdominals will be called to work.
(See also Ch. 7, "Weight Bearing on the Hands".)

Thorax: nature and arm movement

The shape of the thorax is vital for the contact of the
scapula on the ribcage. When the normal kyphosis is
lost, it changes how the scapula functions. One possibility is a reversed curve where the spine and ribs
move away from scapula surface. This presents as a
hollowing in the upper thoracic spines and prominent
medial edges of the scapula – a dysfunctional winging (Fig. 6.14 A). Or there may be excessive kyphosis
where the scapulae are glued to the surface, unable

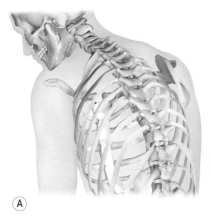

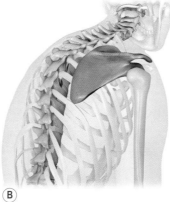

Figure 6.14

A Reversed thoracic curve with minimal contact of scapula on ribcage

B Excessive kyphosis with head forward

(A)

(B)

to glide and too abducted, placing the glenohumeral joint in an anterior and downward orientation (Fig. 6.14 B). Both scenarios set up the shoulder for poor movement, compression of the thoracic outlet, and impingement of rotator cuff muscles. The whole body posture is compromised, affecting the cervical spine and the ability to connect into core support. Breathing is certainly also compromised.

Practitioner note

The thoracic outlet (see Fig. 6.7) is the space where the brachial plexus and blood vessels travel from the neck through the scalenes and slip through a small space under the clavicle, in front of the coracoid process of the scapula and down the arm. When the space is narrowed through poor posture, the scapulohumeral rhythm becomes asynchronous. Then the tissues in the area become tight and densify, restricting the space and impinging on the supraspinatus muscle. The compression may cause symptoms such as tingling down the arm or into the neck, cold hands, and weakness of the hands.

The upper thorax responds to end range of lifting the arm by extending and side bending, a lateral movement (translation) away from the arm (Theodoridis and Ruston, 2002). Since the upper thoracic spines are continuous with the ribs' concentric ring attaching to the manubrium and sternum, the motion in the spine will be reflected in the front. The first and second ribs move as a whole ring. The ring moves up in the front as the back moves down for extension. As the left

arm lifts, the whole ring is also translating left (apex right) and rotating to the right (Fig. 6.15). The manubrium will face to the side of the rotation. Watching the manubrium while someone is moving the arms is a great indicator of how the thoracic spine is moving.

Practitioner note

Observing the manubrium in a static position will show how the upper T spines are situated. It is not uncommon to see a manubrium facing left. If the entire rings of the first and second ribs are rotated to the left, the myofascia attachments from above and below the ribs are at a slant, an oblique orientation. The lines are lengthened on one side and shortened on the other creating a length tension. Imagine a hot air balloon. The rib rings are the basket with a medallion on the front, the strings are the neck, and the balloon the head. As the right side of the ring (basket) rotates forward, the left side moves backward with a coupled movement of side bending. The strings of the balloon will be in tension, with one side shortened and the other lengthened. The long held strings represent the anterior and middle scalenes, and SCM (sternocleidomastoid) on the left. The shortened held strings on the right are the levator scapula, the upper fibers of serratus anterior, and rhomboid minor. The rotation of the manubrium follows the rotation of the pelvis and sacrum in most instances (refer to Ch. 3 for the transition of the spine; T1–T2 is such a place). Working to release the shortening and establishing normal length of these tissues will add to freeing up scapula and cervical movement. The releases will be described in Chapter 8.

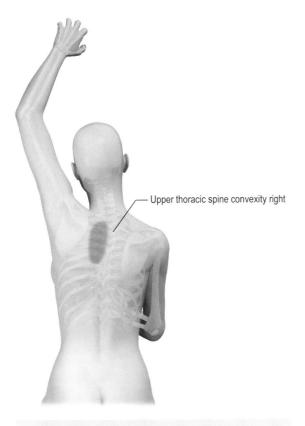

Upper thoracic spine convexity right

Figure 6.15
Thoracic spine movement (apex right) while arm raises

Movement release for rotation of vertebromanubrial region

This movement, especially with the added resistance, enhances the movement of rotation of the first and second rings. Observe the whole body while cueing the movement (the tendency is to rotate in the lower chains, at the T/L junction, pelvis and hip joints, rather than at the segment desired). This exercise is effective for upper thorax, arm elevation and neck restrictions. Some people find that sacral tension is released too.

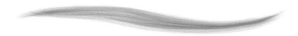

- Lie back on an incline, for example a Pilates Arc, with a support under the head; the upper spine is in slight extension with the lower ribs in contact with the Arc.

- Cross the arms, with hands holding the elbows slightly lifted off the trunk at about 45°.

- Hold the occiput to stabilize the skull by placing the metacarpal joint of the second finger on the mastoid and cup the occiput with the palm of the hand (Fig. 6.16 A).

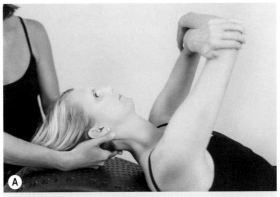

Figure 6.16 A
Movement release for vertebromanubrial rotation: start position

- Cue the client to slowly rotate the thorax to the right.

- At the point of tension under the hands, cue to pause and note the range of motion.

- Cue the client to rotate to the left; feel for range of motion.

- If the arms move in adduction/abduction rather than spinal rotation, cue to rotate from the ribs and not the arms. (Imagery: image the clavicles as a seesaw, with one side moving down as the other side rises.)

- Choose the more restricted range of motion.

- Add a resistance by rotating the trunk to the restricted side (left for example) and pause just prior to the end range, at the barrier.

- Introduce resistance by placing a hand on the outer edge of the left arm near the elbow (Fig. 6.16 B).

- Ask the client to press against the hand, thinking of rotating to the left, but the practitioner blocks it, creating an isometric contraction.

- Hold for 5 seconds.

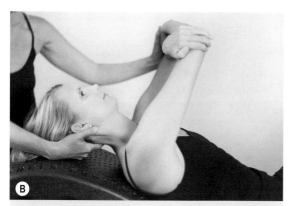

Figure 6.16 B
MET

- Stop the resistance and continue to move into the left rotation to the new barrier (moving past where your started), then add resistance again; repeat 3 times.

Restriction of scapula movement disrupts the patterning of the arm, the scapulohumeral rhythm as described above. If the entire shoulder girdle and the upper thorax are restricted, this alters the ability to stretch the arm out, as, for example, when reaching into a high cabinet. The shoulder girdle and arm move as one unit, displacing the humeral head and compressing the thoracic outlet. The humeral head is not congruent with the glenoid fossa. When it is not congruent, imbalances occur around the shoulder, as for example the anterior ligaments are restricted with the external rotators (infraspinatus and teres minor) tightening inhibiting internal rotation of the shoulder. And the deltoid muscle is shortened and has inadequate tension for the elevation of the humerus necessary for bypassing the thoracic outlet. Clearly, this is a situation to be changed through movement work for balance and re-education of the functional pattern.

Pectoral–deltoid fascia release

Pectoralis fascial stretch: hands-on

Pectoralis–deltoid fascia release
VIDEO LINK V 6.3

- The client lies supine on an incline such as the Pilates Arc with approximately T4 resting on the apex of the Arc; support the head in alignment and have knees bent and feet on the floor.

- Arms are at 90° flexion, with externally rotated shoulders and supinated forearms.

- First set the scapula in a neutral position on the thoracic cage (see Fig. 6.8 A) and assist placement of the humerus in an externally rotated position.

- The practitioner stands in front of the client.

- Guide the client through movement of the humerus from the starting position, 90° flexion, to 90°abduction (Fig. 6.17 A).

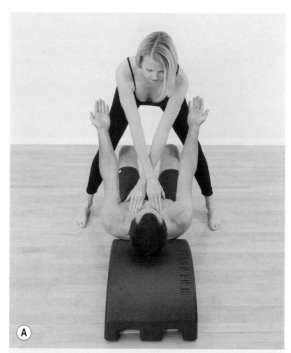

Figure 6.17 A
Pectoralis–deltoid fascia release: start position

- The scapulae remain in their position on the thoracic cage and the head of humerus does not displace anteriorly or superiorly.

- Practice the range of motion, maintaining integrity of the scapula and humeral head positions.

- Using a light coating of massage oil or cream on the finger pads, begin a fascial stroke from the center of the sternum, underneath the clavicles, along the length of the clavicles and on to the anterior surface of the humerus, following the movement of arm abduction (Fig. 6.17 B).

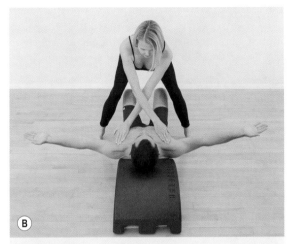

Figure 6.17 B
Fascial stroke

- Reaching the end range of the arm in abduction, simply cue to bring the arms straight in, back to the starting position, maintaining the external rotation of the humerus.
- Repeat the stroke 1 inch (2.5 cm) below the first line.
- Repeat a third stroke, 1 inch (2.5 cm) below second line.

MET in doorway

A self MET release of the pectoral–deltoid fascia which also enhances the range of external rotation by lengthening the tight internal rotators and activating the external rotators.

- Stand in a doorway so that one (or both) inner arm(s) and palmar side of the hand is placed on the frame of the door; the elbow begins at about

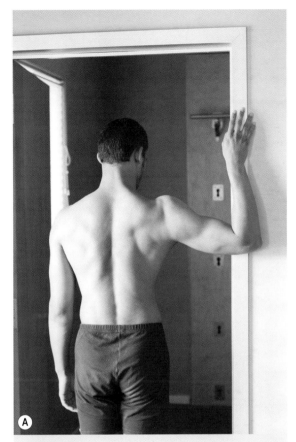

Figure 6.18 A
Doorway shoulder activation and stretch: start position

60° abduction and normal scaption of humerus to scapula (do not stand in the doorway at first, but find the proper angle of the arm which determines where the stance is in relation to the arm position) (Fig. 6.18 A).

- Take a small lunge step into (but not far into) the doorway.
- Press the whole inner forearm and hand into the frame and count to 5.
- Stop pressing and peel the forearm off the door frame, keeping the elbow planted on the frame (Fig. 6.18 B).
- Step or lean into the doorway further, generating an elongation of the front of the chest and shoulder.

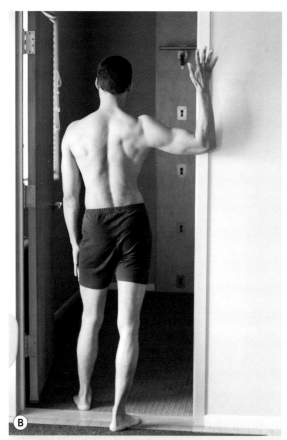

Figure 6.18 B
Activation and stretch

* Stay at the new stance position and press again.

* Stop, repeat the peel of forearm, and step further into the doorway.

* Repeat 3 times.

* Change the angle of the arm to 90°; repeat the above sequence 3 times.

* Change the angle to 110° and again repeat the sequence 3 times.

After releasing the pectoral–deltoid fascia and activating the posterior shoulder, integrate the new position through movement awareness such as the "Coronal Arm Circles" and other movements below.

Coronal Arm Circles

Generally, people shrug and circle the shoulders in a forward and backward direction. The forward and back circles promote forward humeral head motion, which for many people is too flexible in the front and tight in the back of the joint. It is not possible to reach the posterior part of the joint moving in this range. "Coronal Arm Circles" are sideways circles encouraging scapula range of motion of all the planes along with the distraction of the humeral head laterally and back.

* Stand facing a wall and place the hands on the wall at shoulder height.

* Elbows are bent, arms at ease.

* Move the scapulae in toward the midline (adduction or retraction) (Fig. 6.19 A).

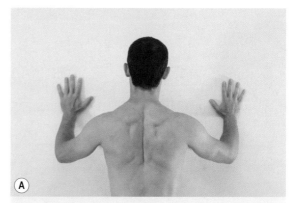

Figure 6.19 A
Coronal Arm Circles: adducting

* Elevate the scapulae (Fig. 6.19 B).

* Abduct the scapulae (Fig. 6.19 C).

* Depress the scapulae (Fig. 6.19 D).

* Repeat three times; smooth out the corners.

* This exercise can also be done sitting cross-legged or in a chair on top of sits bones with an elongated spine and diaphragms stacked.

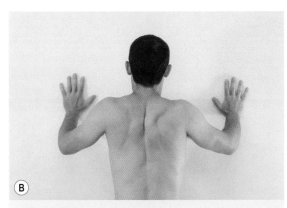

Figure 6.19 B
Elevating

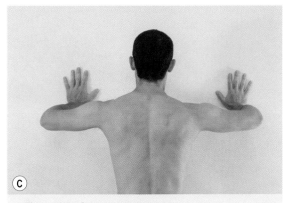

Figure 6.19 C
Abducting

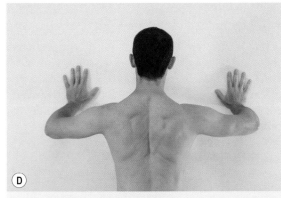

Figure 6.19 D
Neutral

Lead the movement with the scapulae, not with your elbows. If the client is having difficulty with the individuation of the scapulae, place their hands on a wall so that the hands are stable and making small circles reflective of the scapulae.

> **Tip**
> **Visual cue**
>
> "Wax on wax off"

> **Practitioner note**
>
> Guide the movement by placing the hands on the edges of the scapulae. Hold in the following manner: finger pads of fingers 2–5 on top of the spine of the scapulae and the thumb at the inferior angle. Guide the circling motion of the scapula.

Exercises for mobility and stability of the thorax and shoulder girdle

Scapula Reaches

This exercise brings awareness to the line of movement from the lower tip of the scapula through the little finger side of the hand. "Scapula Reaches" articulates the upper thoracic spine with small rotational motions of the spine, and glides the scapula and elongates the tissues along the line. Imagine lengthening from T2–T6 to the medial border of the scapula (rhomboids, upper trapezius), across the scapula to the latissimus dorsi/teres major merging into the humerus and along the outer edge of the arm (see Fig. 6.3).

- Lie on the back with knees bent and feet on the mat.

- Raise arms up toward the ceiling at 80° shoulder flexion with the fingertips reaching up to the ceiling, palms facing each other (Fig. 6.20 A).

- On an inhale, reach the right arm toward the ceiling, externally rotating the arm as if you were

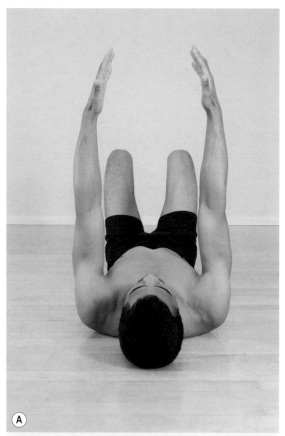

Figure 6.20 A
Scapula Reaches: start position

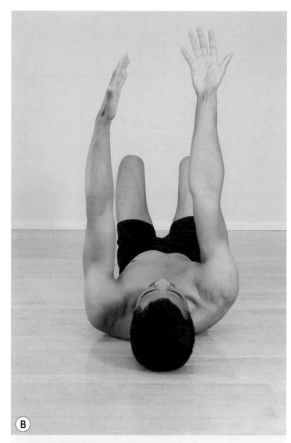

Figure 6.20 B
Externally rotate and reach

screwing in a light bulb; the pinky finger will rotate toward the midline (Fig. 6.20 B).

- On the exhale, internally rotate the right arm as if you were unscrewing the bulb, back to a neutral shoulder position, feeling the back of the shoulder resting on the floor.

- Repeat the movements with the left arm.

- Alternate sides.

- Pay attention to the opposite shoulder, maintaining contact/resting on the floor as the other arm moves.

- Reverse the movement, internally rotate and reach, externally rotate to return to neutral (Fig. 6.20 C).

Ribcage Arms

This exercise teaches and re-educates the connection of the shoulder girdle and arm complex connection to the trunk's core. It is necessary for the supine position to have anchor points of the lowest ribs to the mat with the pelvis in neutral (sacrum anchor point). A head support may be required to contact the mat properly.

- Lie supine as in "Scapula Reaches," with straight arms at 80° flexion in a neutral shoulder placement, palms facing each other (Fig. 6.21 A).

- Inhale and feel elongation of the body without moving.

- Slowly exhale, feeling the co-contraction of the core and rib anchor point into the mat; move the straight arms overhead to the point where the anchor point may lose contact (Fig. 6.21 B).

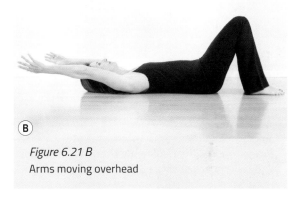

(B)

Figure 6.21 B
Arms moving overhead

- Inhale a small amount, holding the position.

- Slowly exhale, sliding the scapulae down the back, followed by the arms.

- Repeat 3–5 times.

Pay close attention to the coordination of the breath with the movement pattern. Notice that the length between the bottom of the sternum and pubic bone stays consistent. Add holding light weights or a pole with an ankle weight wrapped and secured on the pole. The pole provides feedback to the differences in right and left shoulder discrepancies.

Quadruped thorax and shoulder series

In quadruped, the arms are fixed and weight bearing, placing the work directly into the thorax and shoulder girdle. This requires a core connection and good breathing skills.

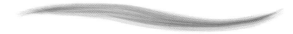

- Kneel in a quadruped position with the heel of the hands under the shoulders and the knees under the center of the hip joint, with a neutral pelvis and spine.

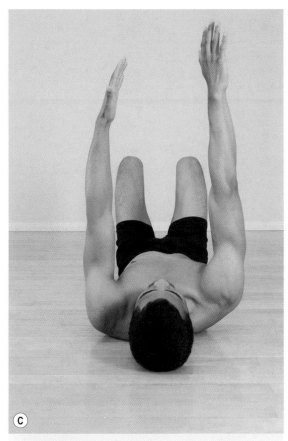

(C)

Figure 6.20 C
Internally rotate and reach

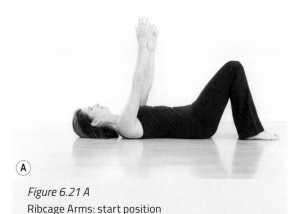

(A)

Figure 6.21 A
Ribcage Arms: start position

- If a quadruped position is not possible, all the movements may be performed standing facing a wall and placing the arms on the wall as if it were the floor.

Protraction/retraction (mobility)

- Place the attention on the sternum.

- On an inhale, move the sternum toward the floor, allowing the scapulae to adduct toward the spine (retraction); be clear that the retraction happens because of the movement of the sternum to the wall or floor (Fig. 6.22 A).

- On the exhale, soften the sternum into the body, away from the floor, allowing the scapula to move wide without excessively rounding the thorax (protraction) (Fig. 6.22 B).

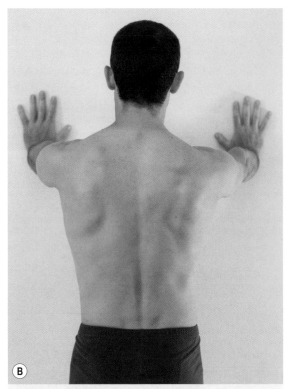

B

Figure 6.22 B
Sternum away from floor for protraction

- Direct the in breath into the upper chamber of the thorax to access the motion in the shoulder blades and upper T spines.

- Repeat 3 times, slowly.

Tip

Bring awareness to the stability of the lowest part of the ribcage and mid to lower thorax. The movement is to occur at the upper T spines and mainly sternal and scapula motion.

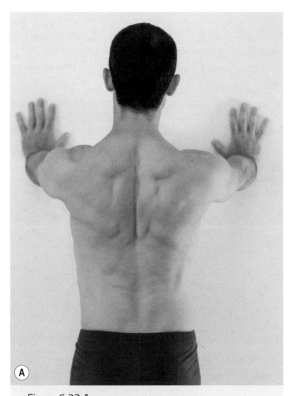

A

Figure 6.22 A
Quadruped shoulder retraction and protraction: sternum to floor for retraction

Practitioner note

Guide the client to move in their true range by bringing awareness to where in the body the movement is occurring and where the place of stability is located.

Thoracic extension/scapula rotation on large ball

The ball helps enhance the scapula motion coordinated with the thoracic movement. It can also be used to mobilize specific segments that are not responding to the upward movement of the humerus. Hands-on work is added to assist in thoracic spine motion.

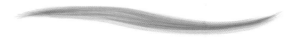

- Props needed: 65 cm (26 in) or 55 cm (22 in) physioball and a mat or padded surface.

- Kneel on a padded surface with the elbows and shoulders bent at 90° or less and forearms resting on the ball with the spine in a long neutral position.

- The practitioner stands to the side of the client.

- First find the position of stability and alignment (Fig. 6.23 A).

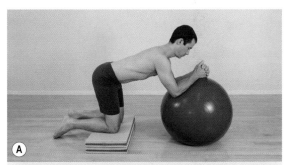

Figure 6.23 A
Thoracic extension on the ball: start position

- Inhale and move the ball away by lifting the hands and forearm off the ball and pressing the ball forward with the elbows creating upward rotation of the scapula, humeral flexion and upper thoracic extension (Fig. 6.23 B).

- On the exhale, press the elbows down into the ball and drag the ball back as the forearms return to touching the ball.

- The lower thoracic and pelvis remain in neutral and stable; knees stay under the hips.

- The head and neck respond to the posterior rotation of the clavicles and forward motion of the sternum.

- Repeat 3 times.

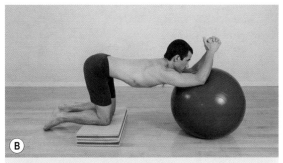

Figure 6.23 B
Rolling ball away for extension

Practitioner note
Hands-on

Hold the wrists of the client with one hand and place other hand at the area of the spine needing guidance. Softly fold the fingers and place them in the area on either side of the spine, not on the vertebrae (Fig. 6.24). The thumb is on one side and the knuckle of the index finger on the other. As the client rolls the ball away and moves into the area needing to move, pause momentarily. Cue to inhale and on the exhale, lift the wrists up slightly so the elbows unweight but stay in contact with the ball. The hand on the thorax will guide the movement of the area inferiorly and slightly anterior. The intention of the movement is to continue the forward motion of the ball. When completing the exhale, cue the client to drag the ball back, flexing the upper thorax slightly. The movement is a micromovement at the area, drawing the attention to moving the area. Remember while enhancing movement using hands-on skills, use the pleasure barometer, an emotional response of joy rather than suffering.

Scapula movement freedom on Pilates Cadillac

Side lying Ribcage Arms

The practitioner guides the client through a full range of arm and thorax motion with intuitive hands-on. It facilitates fascial gliding of the serratus/oblique/latissimus complex and improves mobility of the ribs and vertebrae of the vertebrosternal region. It enhances scapula motion if it has adhered to the fascia underneath the scapula. It retrains motor skills for moving the arm in various ranges of

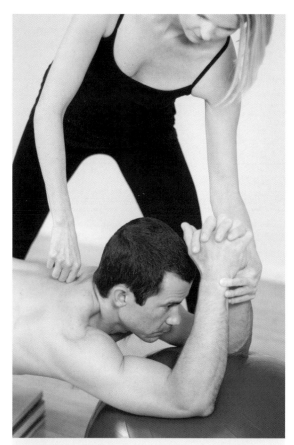

Figure 6.24
Practitioner hands-on

movement. Changing the angle of the hand on the bar will provide multiple possibilities for diagonal motion.

- The client is side lying on the Cadillac with the working arm side up facing the push-through bar; the legs are supported by the Wunda Chair pushed against the side of the Cadillac table.

- The side lying position is in proper alignment; support the head.

- The Cadillac should be top loaded with a blue or red spring on the reverse side.

Practitioner note

CAUTION: as in the "Upper Serratus Stretch" above, remember this is a dangerous position of the bar. Always keep track of the bar either by holding it yourself when you are not using both hands or by instructing the client to be responsible for the bar during the hands-on work. The red spring is stronger so it will pull the arm more than the blue spring. Use the red spring for very tight, larger people. The blue spring is for smaller and looser folks.

- Begin with the bar through the side poles, arm extended, body in proper alignment to start (for example the right arm) (Fig. 6.25 A).

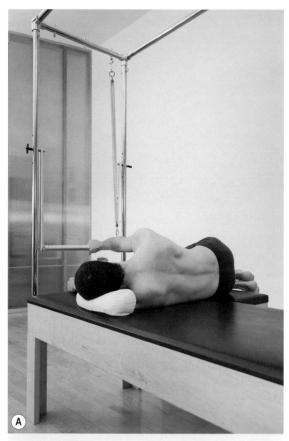

Ⓐ

Figure 6.25 A
Side lying Ribcage Arms: start position

- Cue the client to allow the bar to pull them further into a left rotation.

> **Practitioner note**
> **Hands-on**
>
> One possibility is to place one hand at the serrratus anterior, close to the pectorals, and the other hand on the posterior side, on the scapula; guide the rotation through the ribs, allowing for tissue gliding but not displacement of the relationship of the humeral head and torso; the posterior hand may provide an intention of scapula movement on the ribcage (scapulothoracic joint), with the front hand preventing a feel of too much pull and shortening of the pectorals.

- Cue the client to rotate back to the starting position; encouraging movement from the thorax posteriorly, with an intention of the thoracolumbar fascia from the pelvis to the arm gliding back with the ribcage connection.

- Cue to rotate to the right as the elbow bends, reaching the elbow wide, creating length in the pectorals while maintaining length of the posterior shoulder; this position of the arm remains as the thorax rotates (Fig. 6.25 B).

- If appropriate, continue the movement into the twist.

- The arm will follow the pull of the bar as it rises up by straightening and the trunk will de-rotate to side lying again with the arm in abduction and fully extended (Fig. 6.25 C).

- To reverse the movement path, the thorax begins a rotation to the right as the bar descends and the elbow bends.

- Follow the reverse path to the starting position.

The practitioner's hands-on and guiding is in the moment, and what is being seen in the body moving. The weave of trunk rotation from the pelvis through the head (as described in Ch. 4) and the shoulder continuum above is the gliding and sliding that should be observed. Pause the movement if the movement and integrity of the alignment are not apparent. Cue the breath into the areas that are stagnant or held.

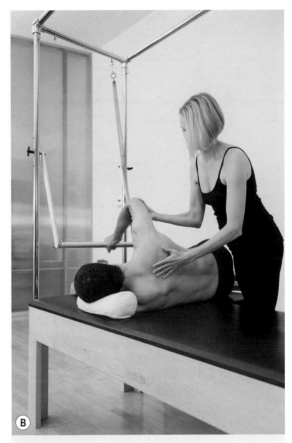

Figure 6.25 B
Rotating trunk back

Practice a smaller range or part of the whole movement until the quality is present. Allow the hands to touch and enhance the direction of the glide. Move slowly and mindfully.

Upper arms prone on Cadillac (unilateral)

Lying prone on the table gives the practitioner access to the posterior first rib and scapula. The table provides feedback to the client as to their alignment with an opening and lengthening of the front of the shoulder and inability to drop the chest downward. Use the pleasure barometer (see practitioner note above) as to the appropriateness of this position for the client.

The push-through bar is reverse loaded: place the bar on the outside of the table and top load it with one blue

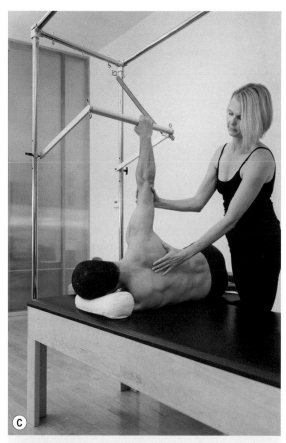

Figure 6.25 C
Fully extending arm

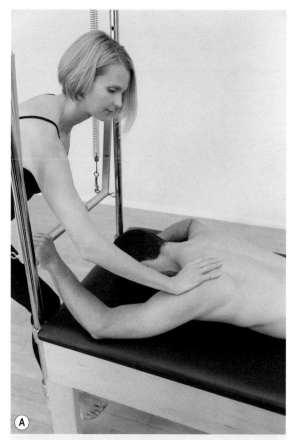

Figure 6.26 A
Upper arms prone on Cadillac: start position

or red spring. Note this is a risky bar placement, so keep one hand on the bar at all times.

- The client lies prone on the Cadillac under the push-through bar, holding the bar with one arm (Fig. 6.26 A).

- The position of the body on the table needs to be where the bar is pushing into the body rather than pulling the arm away.

- The practitioner places the thumb along the length of the first ribs and the palm of the hand

on the scapula with the fingers at the inferior edge (Fig. 6.26 B).

- As the arm bends, assist the rib and scapula to move inferiorly.

- Hold the position of the rib; as the arm begins to straighten, hold the rib in place and assist the scapula rotation.

- Press the bar away to the best straight arm position possible (Fig. 6.26 C).

- Slowly bend the elbow, externally rotating the humerus in the scapular plane (scaption).

- Slowly press the bar away, straightening the arm.

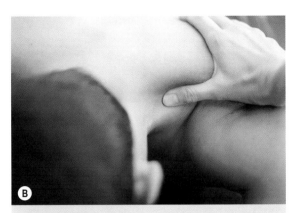

Figure 6.26 B
Hand position

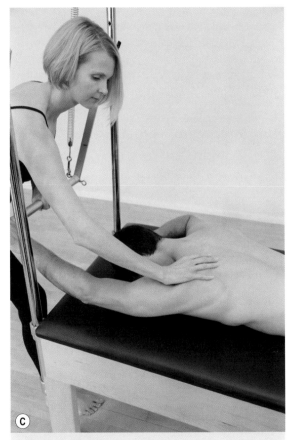

Figure 6.26 C
Arm extending

- Repeat the hands-on 2–3 times then allow client to move without the hands-on 3 times.

Scapula Glides

"Scapula Glides" are another option for accessing the first rib posteriorly with scapula movement. For people with extremely tight neck and upper shoulder muscles and fascia, gliding the scapula seated is a better choice for positioning the arm well. Scapula glides have access for assisting clavicular motion.

- The client is seated on a box placed on the floor at the push-through bar end of the Cadillac.

- The bar is top loaded on the outside of the table with one red or blue spring.

> **Practitioner note**
>
> CAUTION: remember this is a dangerous position of the bar, so always keep track of the bar either by holding it yourself when you are not using both hands or instructing the client to be responsible for the bar during the hands-on work.

- The client holds the bar with a straight arm and shoulder fully flexed; place the hand on the bar so that the arm is in scaption plane and supporting the arm (Fig. 6.27 A).

- Without bending the elbow, glide the scapula downward, lowering the bar (Fig. 6.27 B).

- The practitioner sits behind the client to guide the movement of the scapula.

- From the side or front, observe the clavicle rotation; when the arm is flexed (overhead) the scapula is upwardly rotated and the clavicle elevated and posteriorly rotated; it does not elevate without the rotation.

- As the scapula glides downward, the clavicle rotates anteriorly returning to its neutral position; add bending the elbow (Fig. 6.27 C).

- Observe the motion of the first rib when the arm is fully flexed; add hands-on if needed.

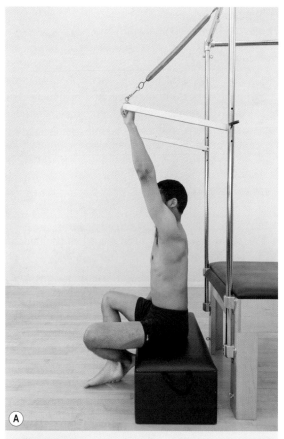

Figure 6.27 A
Scapula Glides: start position

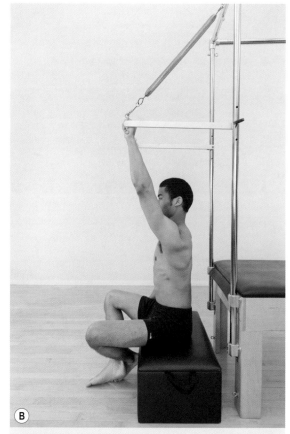

Figure 6.27 B
Straight arm pulldown

One arm lat pulldown

This simple movement is both a re-education tool and a way of strengthening a functional shoulder girdle by adding more resistance (spring load). Cue the client based on what you observe, how they move in relation to the scapulohumeral and rib notions described above.

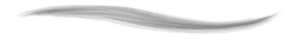

- The client sits sideways on the table with the side of the arm to be worked facing the bar; use 1–1.5 loaded springs.

- Set the body position by first having the client pull the bar down completely; check for a good angle of the elbow (scaption) so that the arm can easily extend without disrupting the trunk and shoulder (Fig. 6.28 A).

- Cue and assist the scapula into upward rotation and guide the humerus into scaption to maintain contact of the posterior humeral head with the glenoid fossa.

- Pull the bar down and the scapula moves into the downward position.

- When the scapula reaches its neutral position at about 40–60° humeral abduction, cue to stabilize

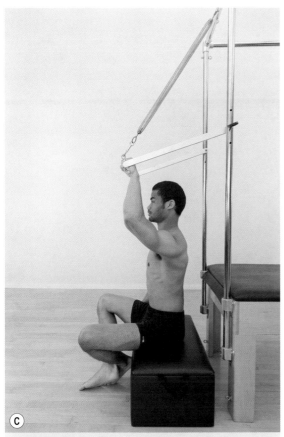

Figure 6.27 C
Adding bending elbow

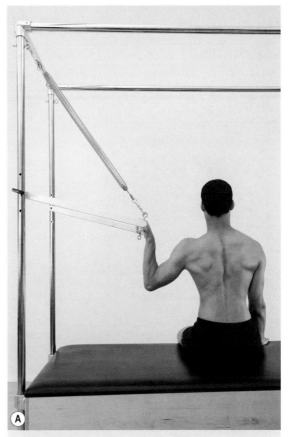

Figure 6.28 A
One arm lat pulldown: setting the arm with the elbow bent

the scapula and continue the movement with only the arm (Fig. 6.28 B).

Practitioner note
Hands-on

Guide the scapula into upward rotation with the thumb side of the hand on the inferior medial border of the scapula; the top hand is encouraging lift of clavicle; hold underneath the elbow, encouraging a spin of the humerus while staying in the scaption angle (Fig. 6.29).

- After a few repetitions of the single arm, a choice is to add a side bend of the thorax toward the bar; the

free arm reaches out to the side and upward as the spine side bends toward the bar (Fig. 6.30 A).

- The practitioner anchors the pelvis on the side of the free arm as the client leans, moving the push-through bar.

- Return to the upright seated position by reversing the movement sequentially from the pelvis through the ribs and the shoulder, then move the head to the center while resisting the bar pressure into the body (press away as it moves in) until the bar is unweighted.

- Feel the center then continue to extend the arm, holding the bar upward, pushing the bar up,

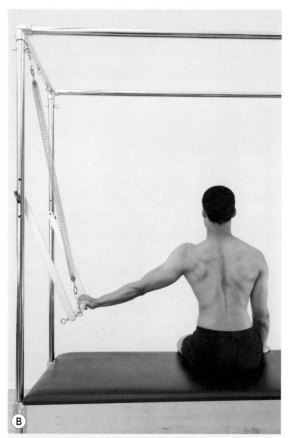

Figure 6.28 B
Arm extending

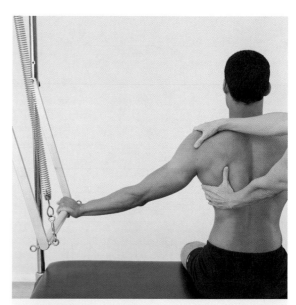

Figure 6.29
Hands-on one arm lat pulldown

elongating the side of the body and fully rotating the scapula of the bar arm.

• Leaning and breathing (inhale) into the elongation opens up the armpit and side ribs (Fig. 6.30 B).

• Repeat 2 times.

Humeral head

The anterior placement of the humeral head is a common and dysfunctional pattern. The ligaments around the humeral head become stiff, typically in the anterior area, and loose in the posterior area. Alternately to manual bodywork, which helps release the held position, these movements allow for changing the holding of the humeral head to restore it to an improved position.

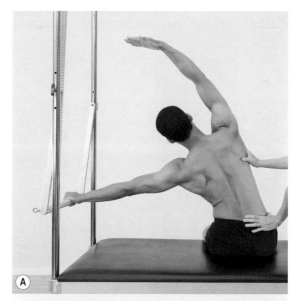

Figure 6.30 A
Adding side bending and hands-on to one arm lat pulldown

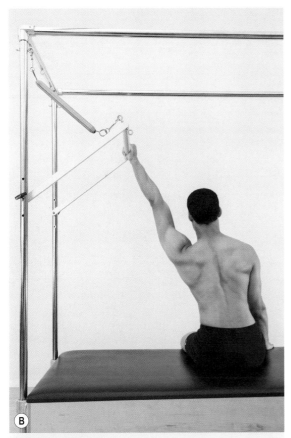

Figure 6.30 B
Lengthening side

Rotating Arms

- Lie supine with the arms stretched out to the side in a low T position with the palms facing up; the abduction of the arms matches the available range of the client so that the scapulae are set in the best position on the ribcage; the range may be from 90° to 75° (Fig. 6.31 A).

- Inhale, internally rotate the right arm, turning the palm toward the floor as the head turns to the left, looking toward the palm-up side; allow the arm to

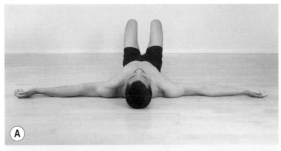

A

Figure 6.31 A
Rotating Arms: start position

spiral from the hand all the way to the clavicle and scapula; allow the humeral head to move off the floor; roll across the upper back to shift the weight onto the externally rotated shoulder; on the palmar side lift the little finger, emphasizing the external rotation of that arm. Both arms are actively rotating (Fig. 6.31 B).

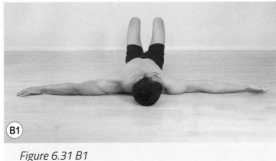

B1

Figure 6.31 B1
Rotation of arms

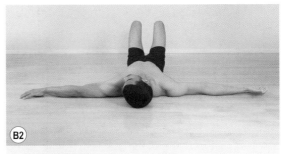

B2

Figure 6.31 B2
Rotation of arms

- Exhale, returning to the center with both palms up.

- Repeat on the other side.

- Repeat until the movement feels connected and easy.

- Reverse the head rotation and arm rotations.

- Look toward the internally rotated shoulder, emphasizing the rotations.

- Repeat until the movement feels connected and easy.

- Add a fluid motion:

  • begin the movement but do not pause in the center; move easily and continuously

  • inhale to look at the hand

  • exhale while transitioning through the center

  • inhale to look at the opposite hand.

- Continue alternating rotation of arms with each breath.

The cervical spine is rotating the head. It is common to see the head tilt to look at the hand rather than a cervical rotation. Cue the "eyes in the back of your head" looking at the opposite hand. If looking with the eyes to the right hand, the "eyes in the back of your head" are looking at the left hand.

Seated Screwdriver on the Cadillac

As the name suggests, the motion is a winding and unwinding of the shoulder complex and arm that connects to the pelvis. This may be performed with or without hands-on. The hands-on actions guide and enhance the movements the body on its own will not be able to access.

- The client is seated on the Cadillac facing away from the push-through bar and toward the left side.

- Working the side of the body, sit so that the right hip is externally rotated with the knee bent resting on the table; the left foot is on the floor, knee bent; both sits bones are on the table with the pelvis level (Fig. 6.32 A).

- Turn to the right and hold on to the top loaded bar with one blue spring, palm down.

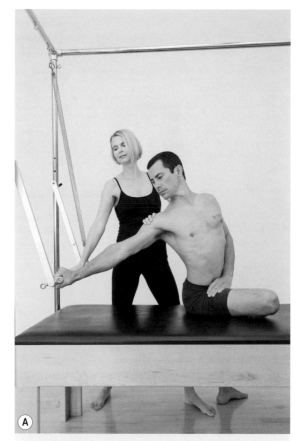

Ⓐ

Figure 6.32 A
Screwdriver: start position

- Inhale slowly and lean into the bar rotating to the right with small upper thoracic extension; the head is looking at the hand on the bar.

- As the humeral head is externally rotating with the thoracic extension the scapula is moving under the armpit in a small amount of upward rotation.

- Moving into flexion, there is left rotation and left side bending and internal rotation of the shoulder.

- Exhale slowly, beginning the movement by shifting the weight from the right sits bone to the left side, sequentially moving the spine rotating left with flexion and internal rotation of the shoulder; the head follows the path of the sternum, making a curved path to finish over the left ilium (Fig. 6.32 B).

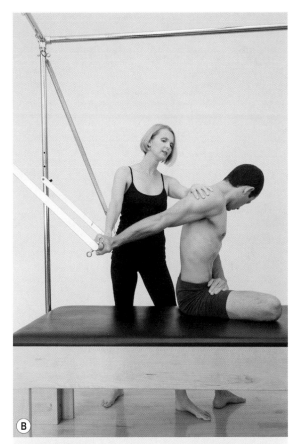

(B)

Figure 6.32 B
Rotation of the shoulder

- Repeat the movement, starting at the pelvis and shifting the weight toward the right sits bone, spiraling through the spine and sternum into the extension.

- Repeat until the movement feels connected and easy.

Practitioner note
Hands-on

As stated for the hands-on directions for the "Side Lying Ribcage Arms" exercise above, the guiding of the movement is in the moment, based on how the body is moving (or not moving). Do not be afraid to pause, or to slow down and limit the range of motion. The micromovements are a powerful way to allow the body to let go of holding.

Enhancing Screwdriver motion

 Enhancing Screwdriver
VIDEO LINK V 6.4

The practitioner stands behind the client's left side if working the right arm. The hands will be working with the bar, the humerus, the scapula–clavicle, and the left side of the pelvis and thigh. On the external rotation movements, encourage the external rotation of the humerus by using the bar for a light distraction as the other hand emphasizes humeral head rotation. Place the hand on the anterior side of the humerus under the biceps and spin it upward. Another area to assist is at the inferior angle of the scapula, moving it under the armpit, gently pressing it into the ribs. A third choice is to reach around to the front and lift the pectoralis up and back.

For the internal rotation motion, hold the bar and cue the client to continue to leave the bar behind them and not allow the bar to press into the body. With one hand, encourage the scapula to ride along the ribs. The ribs are flexing, creating a curved contour. A cue at the sternum may be necessary to soften and assist upper T spine flexion.

Side arm pull on the Reformer

This strengthening movement of the shoulder complex plus stability of the trunk is a perfect example of the whole body emphasis in the Pilates repertoire. Before being able to perform this advanced movement, it is vital for all of the motions of the shoulder components and attachments to the pelvis to be available, in order to receive all the potential benefits of this exercise.

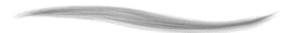

- The Reformer is set with the ropes of a length to match the arm expansion and the amount of tension desired; the lighter the better for optimal bone rhythms; use a light spring.

- The client is kneeling facing the side; the side of the knee can be braced against the shoulder rest for added stability or challenge with no bracing (Fig. 6.33 A).

- When working the left arm, the right side of the leg is toward the shoulder rests; reach across the body to hold the rope.

- The arm position is as if reaching over to the hip on the opposite side to draw a sword from its sheath; the movement is to pull the sword out across the body to a high angle at the opposite side, at the end of the *"en garde"* stance.

- More precisely, the arm is in internal rotation, adduction and flexion (hand reaching to opposite hip).

- The movement leads from the elbow toward abduction, to a range available to the client, potentially from the midline of the body or just past (humerus at about 30–35° abduction) (Fig. 6.33 B).

- At this point the humerus externally rotates, abducts and extends; the hand is in the upper right diagonal (130–150° abduction) in the scaption plane (Fig. 6.33 C).

- The path reverses from the abducted, externally rotated, extended arm down across the body, adducting, internally rotating, and flexing.

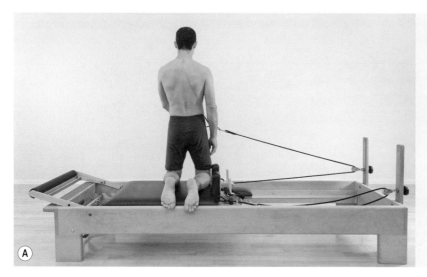

Figure 6.33 A
Side arm pull: start position

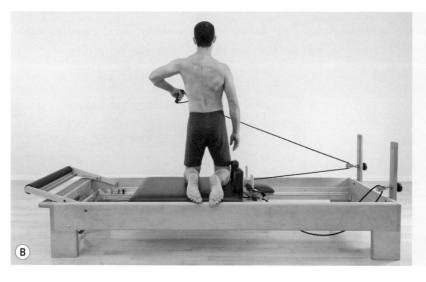

Figure 6.33 B
First motion of the arm pulling

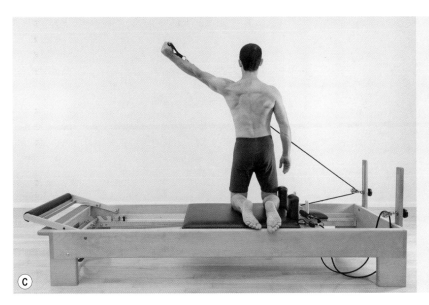

Figure 6.33 C
Final extension of the arm

- The torso maintains its good alignment and balance, creating a strong recruitment of the whole stability system of the body.

- Inhale as the arm moves through the extension path and exhale on the flexion path.

Again, the eagle eye observes the whole patterning of the movement of the bones and tissue tensions in the healthy patterning.

Thorax moving on the scapula

Forearm supported Knee Stretch on the Reformer

An effective training technique is to work the scapula relationship to the thorax by moving the thorax when the arms are fixed. This reverses which end is stabilizing and which mobilizing. When the scapulae glide on the rib cage, the origin of tissue (serratus anterior et al.) on the scapula is moving toward the stable ribs. Reversing this challenges the connections by moving the rib end while stabilizing the scapula side.

This description works on a Balanced Body® studio Reformer. Be creative with the style of Reformer being used. Set up the Reformer with the foot bar in the down position. Place the box in the long position between the foot bar and the carriage. It needs to be firmly placed on the top and against the foot bar for security. Choose one light to medium spring based on the client's size and strength. The right spring will enable the proper bone rhythms with resistance.

- Kneel on the Reformer in a quadruped position (as "Knee Stretch" position, below), placing the forearms on top of the box; the feet are crossed at the ankles and resting on the carriage (not on the shoulder rests as in "Knee Stretch").

- Establish a neutral starting position; check the knees are under the hips; press the carriage out with the legs to establish knees under hip joints (Fig. 6.34 A).

- The practitioner stands at the foot bar end, holding the box until sure that the client is moving from the spine and not pushing with the arms (an action which will dislodge the box off the foot bar).

- Inhale and move the carriage away from the box by moving the thorax away through the arms (Fig. 6.34 B).

- On the exhale return the carriage home.

- Repeat 5–8 times.

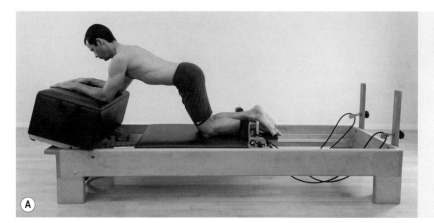

Figure 6.34 A
Forearm supported Knee
Stretch: start position

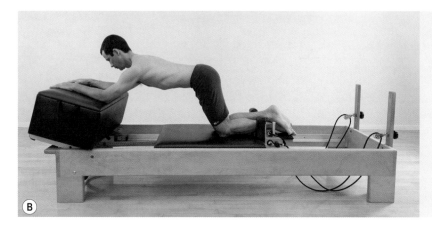

Figure 6.34 B
Movement pressing away

Tip

Observe for the small upper thoracic movement into extension at the end range of the scapula upward position; the head will lift slightly in response to the sternal motion. Be aware of the lower rib connection into the trunk. The stability of the thoracolumbar junction is important to the ability to extend the upper thoracic spine with the scapulohumeral motion.

Side forearm supported plank

Using the same set-up on the Reformer, the box provides a support for the arm, taking the stress out of the wrists when weight bearing during plank movements. Practice a side bridge on the forearm prior to doing it on a moving Reformer.

- The client is facing to the side, kneeling on the Reformer.

- Place the forearm on the box with a 90° elbow bend, elbow under the shoulder with the hand pointing to the front (a kickstand position of the arm); the body is at an angle and therefore the kneeling is not on both knees but on the knee closest to the box; the knees need to be level with one another so that the pelvis is level.

- Inhale while remaining in the position (Fig. 6.35 A).

- Exhale and move the carriage away from the box (Fig. 6.35 B).

- The trunk is moving on the scapula with a stable arm.

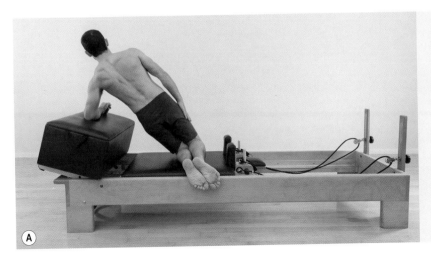

Figure 6.35 A
Forearm supported side body position

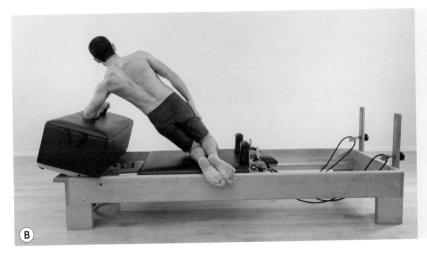

Figure 6.35 B
Movement pressing away

- Repeat 5–8 times on each side.

> **Tip**
>
> Side body alignment and lift of the spine throughout the movement are important. The tendency will be to sag the ribcage, presenting the shoulder joint elevated and impinging. The practice is to maintain the elongation and narrowing feel while moving.

Knee Stretch series on the Reformer

"Knee Stretch" is a central exercise in the Reformer repertory, and another example of the whole body coordination and strength training of Pilates. The movement and breath are the same as in the "Forearm Supported Knee Stretch" above. The full pose is without the box, with the bar in the high or low position, with the hands on the bar and the arms straight, and with an evenly rounded spine. The feet are placed with the plantar side of the foot and heel against the shoulder rests; the toes are curled up so that the metatarsals are on the carriage. This position is called the foot being "on the walk." The heel is pressed against the shoulder rest. The balls of the feet are a short distance away from the shoulder rest to match the shape of the arch of the foot (Fig. 6.36).

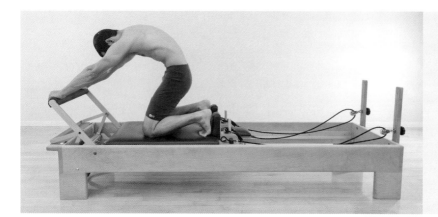

Figure 6.36
Knee Stretch

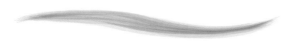

- Start at the home position of the Reformer using two springs (one light, one medium).

- Maintaining the body position, the body moves the carriage out (inhale) and pulls it in (exhale) in a rhythmical pace.

- The rhythm is not even; the press out is a half beat, the "and" before the 1 count, and pulling in is a full beat; going out is a quick motion (inhale) and the resistance of the carriage pulling in is sustaining the exhale.

- The shoulders are stable; the shoulder girdle does not move backward and forward with the rhythm of the body.

- The practitioner stands at the foot bar and places the hands on top of the client's shoulders for feedback to the client. Cue "there is no change of contact between my hands and your shoulders; the pressure stays the same."

- The motion of hip extension and flexion drives the movement, with stability in the thorax and shoulders and a balanced curved spine.

Thoracic stability with overhead arms

Lifting the arms overhead bilaterally requires the mid-thoracic local stabilizers to turn on as the glenohumeral joint flexes, and the scapula upwardly rotates and stabilizes. When challenging clients with overhead resistance work the thorax does not rotate, side bend, flex, or extend. Observing the client's ability prior to training in overhead resistance work is important information for program design.

Observe arm lift incline prone

Use an incline bench or create an arrangement using boxes at the end of a table. A sloped incline position for the trunk is necessary for this exercise. Using the Reformer, two boxes are needed. Place one box in the long position on top of the Reformer. Place a second box over the shoulder rests on a slope to rest on the floor. Have the client lie prone on the long box on top of the Reformer; the head and upper torso will lie on the inclined box with arms placed overhead. The whole body is resting on the boxes. The body's position is in flexion, allowing for a small amount of movement of the arms into full elevation (Fig. 6.37 A).

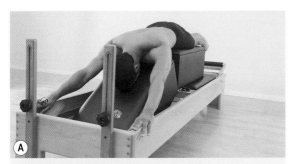

Figure 6.37 A
Prone arm lift on incline: start position

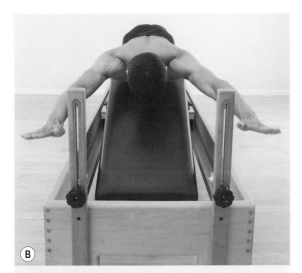

Figure 6.37 B
Lifting arms

Cue the client to lift the arms a small amount, almost unweighting the arms off the box. Notice the difference between the right and left sides and if and when a shift occurs in the thorax (Fig. 6.37 B).

Visualizing the ribs as concentric rings, the rings turn (rotate) and side bend. Observing the arms lifting, see where the rings are moving in order to achieve a lift of the arms. Then place the hands at that ring segment (let's say at the fifth rib), with one hand on the right side and the other on the left (under the armpit). Gently draw the rib ring in toward the spine, creating a feeling of stability.

Hold the ring and cue the client to breathe in and then exhale slowly to lift the arms again. Follow the breath with a light compression of the rib ring. The pulling in of the rib rings activates the local muscles to stabilize the thorax so the arms elevate without extra thoracic movement.

Repeat the movement three times with the hands-on. Practice the movement without the hands-on 2–3 times.

One arm movement and rib translation

Adding resistance from below and elevating the arm creates a lateral translation of the upper thoracic spine away from the lifting arm. The upper spine, the vertebromanubrial region (T1–T2 and manubrium) and the upper part of the vertebrosternal region, will produce a concavity on the same side of the elevated arm. The lower thoracic spine will translate in the opposite direction, with a convexity toward the elevated arm, creating a balance for supporting the weight. This also recruits the local stabilizers to support the thorax while elevating the arm. If there is a restriction or weakness in the area, the hands-on cueing will facilitate a change.

Load the push-through bar of the Cadillac from the bottom with a long yellow spring.

- The client sits sideways on the table with the arm to be elevated toward the push-through bar end.

- The client bends the working arm at the elbow, close to the ribs, with the palm up.

- The practitioner lifts the bar up for the client to hold (avoiding the client bending laterally and making too great an effort in a poor position to begin the movement).

- On the inhale, the client elevates the arm, extending the arm (Fig. 6.38).

- Slowly lower the bar, bending the elbow down close to the ribs a small amount.

- Repeat, lift the bar.

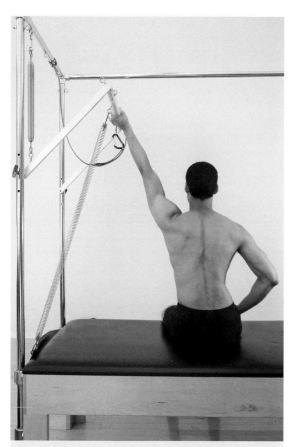

Figure 6.38
One arm lift with rib translation: arm extended

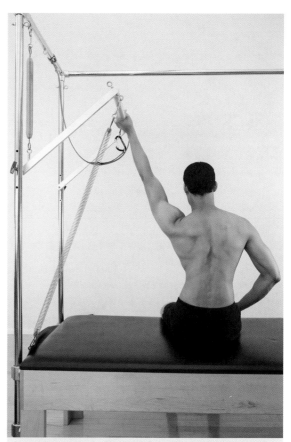

Figure 6.39
Dysfunctional movement of ribs

Practitioner note

Monitor the stability of the body from the pelvis throughout the thorax. Observe the scapulohumeral mechanics, cueing for any mis-movements.

Practitioner note
Hands-on

Observe the movement of the client to determine where your hands-on would best intervene with a dysfunctional movement and assist the client to feel the healthier movement choice. If elevating the left arm, the scapula will be fully upwardly rotated. If there is a trunk weakness, the lower thoracic spine may trans-

late away from the arm, causing a compression of the left side ribs (Fig. 6.39). A useful cue would be to place the left hand at the rib being translated away and the other hand at the attachment at the spine and verbally cue to "breathe into the my hand, translate the rib into my hand," using the right hand to encourage the right translation (Fig. 6.40).

One arm work on Reformer

The Pilates repertory has many arm movements involving the straps with whole body movement. To challenge the shoulder girdle, working with one arm variations requires the lateral and oblique connections to stabilize the motion of one arm.

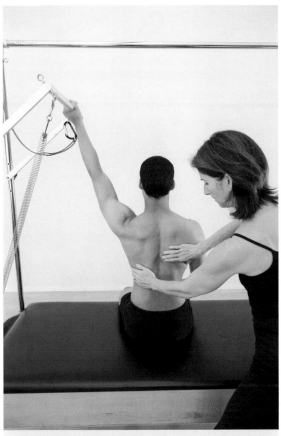

Figure 6.40
Hands-on guiding translation

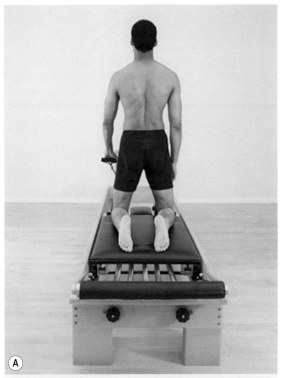

Ⓐ

Figure 6.41 A
One arm chest expansion: start position

One arm chest expansion

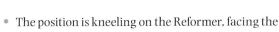

- The position is kneeling on the Reformer, facing the ropes; use one light spring.
- Hold on to one strap; the arm begins at about 20–25° toward flexion. Adjust the rope so it has a little tension to prevent it from having slack but not sufficient to pull the body forward (Fig. 6.41 A).
- Inhale in good kneeling alignment (side plumb line).
- Exhale and pull the rope to 5–10° shoulder extension (Fig. 6.41 B).
- Control the movement back to the beginning position.

- Observe for spinal instability (Fig. 6.41 C).

Serratus Arms

- The client starts seated on the Reformer, facing the foot bar, either on the carriage cross-legged if the knees are at the level of the hips or (better) on a box in the short position on the Reformer.
- One light or one medium spring is used; hold the handles with the palm down and the ropes coming underneath the arms, not on top of the forearm.
- Pull the ropes taut with the arms straight at 90° shoulder flexion; check the alignment of the position of the shoulder girdle and arms (Fig. 6.42 A).
- Cue the client to maintain the width of their back, stabilizing the scapula while moving the humerus into abduction with elbows bent; the hands are in

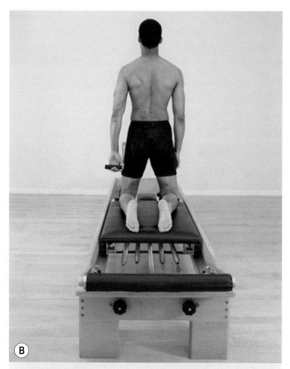

Figure 6.41 B
Movement action

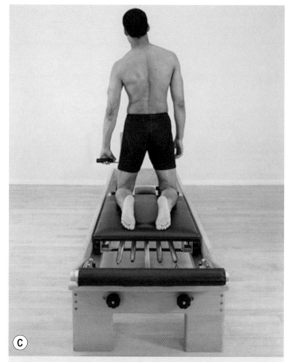

Figure 6.41 C
Instability of the spine during movement

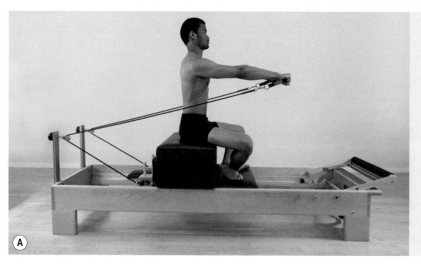

Figure 6.42 A
Serratus Arms: start position

alignment with the elbows so that the arms create a squared U shape (Fig. 6.42 B).

• Begin returning the arms to the starting position, initiating the movement from the lower edge of the scapula ("Scapula Reaches" exercise above),

activating the serratus anterior/oblique connection and feeling the length of the arm through the pinky side of the arm.

• Repeat the movement with awareness of the notes below.

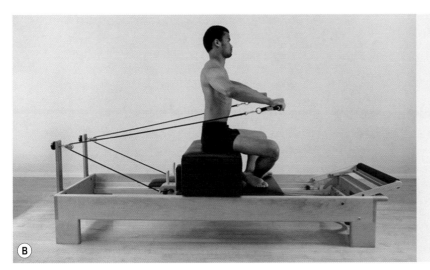

Figure 6.42 B
Movement action

B

Tip

The movement is active throughout the straightening and bending of the arms. The action of pulling the ropes is coming from a spiral going from the inferior edge of the scapula around to the inner upper arm, over to the outer lower arm and to the little finger. The bending is resisting the pulling of the Reformer by the outward action of the elbows creating the width of the back and creating space in the shoulder joint ("Coronal Arm Circles" feel). The wrists maintain their alignment with the radius and ulna; there is no deviation throughout the movement.

Practitioner note
Hands-on

Practice the arm movement without the straps prior to adding the ropes. With the arms straight, lightly place the palms of your hands at the client's lower arm, near the wrist and at the elbow (Fig. 6.43). Cue the client to press your hands away equally, maintaining pressure onto both hands. At the bent arm position (the squared off U), lightly touch the elbow and cue to reach outward, pressing the hands away, and feel how that creates width in the front and back of the shoulder. Instead of using straps another possibility is to add a pole through the loops to create a stable and single surface to press away. This is useful if one arm is stiffer or weaker. It assists in helping to coordinate both arms but more importantly, in recruiting the trunk in a balanced way.

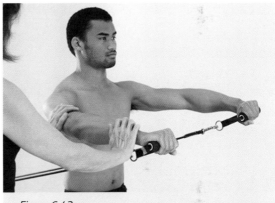

Figure 6.43
Hands-on Serratus Arms

Bridging to Chapter 7

Continuing to move and strengthen healthy movements of the upper spine and arms requires a variety of challenges, including weight bearing on the arms. Moving the arms freely with resistance, as when using the Pilates straps or free weights, is a specific training targeting the arms on a stable trunk. Weight bearing on the arms, either using a static position, as in a plank, or supporting the body with the arms moving the trunk on a piece of apparatus is challenging the stability of the arms on the trunk. In Chapter 7, the focus is the linkage from the hand to the trunk and the power the wrist contributes to movement of arm to trunk.

Weight bearing on the hands

"To touch the coarse skin of a tree is thus, at the same time, to experience one's own tactility, to feel oneself touched by the tree. And to see the world is also, at the same time, to experience oneself seen."

David Abram, *The Spell of the Sensuous*

Contemplative awareness: receptivity

Many cultures use the hand as a symbol, whether of the hand of God or as a sign of power, and for communication through a silent but expressive visual language. It is through the hands that we carry out the necessary actions for activities of daily living. The dexterity of our hands comes from the fine motor skills available to them, defining their difference from other joints in the body. The refined movements of the many small structures of the hand and wrist produce acts of expression as well as responses. When the hand is injured, ordinary tasks become extremely difficult and we may need someone else to help us. The hands manipulate objects and help us to navigate our path through the world using our sensations and complex mechanics.

Touch

Touching another person powerfully shifts the person. A warm embrace relaxes the receiver with a felt sense of peace and happiness. A soft stroke helps transfer kindness and love. Both giving and receiving positive feelings affect the brain's pleasure neurotransmitters for both the giver and receiver. The movement practitioner uses touch to effect change in the body through its structures and the nervous system. As described previously (Ch. 6, "Function and Form"), the hands contain many sensory neural receptors (Chaitow et al., 2012) and reside in a significant motor/sensory area of the body map in the brain. The brain–hand relationship is important not only for sensation but also for how the environment is interpreted. The interaction between the brain and hand enables us to know what is being felt by using our previous knowledge of whatever is being touched. To effectively touch, the more knowledge about the body and its anatomy we have, the more can be felt.

> **Practitioner note**
>
> A movement practitioner's touch objectives are:
>
> - tactile cueing
> - enhancing movement
> - adding resistance
> - sensing tissue tension
> - feeling release of tension in the tissue
> - evaluating symmetry in the positions of the body
> - evaluating range of motion and quality of the range of motion
> - sensing the space between client and practitioner.

Working with touch is similar to being in a meditative state, focusing in the moment and being aware of sensations without reaction. The practitioner's awareness of "noise" in the mind or physical tensions in the body is vital to filtering the information received by the hands. When the use of touch is unconscious, it disrupts the line of communication between client and practitioner. One's thoughts and feelings become disconnected from the purpose of the hands, palpating for information. The communication then becomes about the practitioner having distracted thoughts rather than the client, and it becomes difficult to clearly sense movement in the body. As a practitioner, working on one's own body and mind improves the quietude of one's own system. A distracted mind impedes perception and affects not only how the practitioner interprets the intention of the touch but also, more importantly, how the client interprets it. While the practitioner may be touching the client, however, it is also true that the client is touching the practitioner. Boundaries and grounding for the practitioner are important to the healthy and professional relationship between practitioner and client.

Listening with the hands

Having presence, a centered and grounded spirit, provides the opportunity of "listening" to the body. As defined by Frank Lowen (2011), "listening in the hands, the objective recognition of multiple sensations, the sorting out of what these sensations are and their categorization" may be diminished by empathy without boundaries. For a practitioner, a healthy, grounded presence is one where self-referencing is practiced and where one is comfortable in one's own body. Occupying one's space completely and being neutral during an interaction with the client helps with the ability to listen to the body's tissues. Lack of presence is a loss of the ability to perceive. The practitioner who is humble and maintaining the center will have the capacity to recognize the sensation of tissue changes.

Try it!

You will need a partner to work with.

- Stand behind the partner, who is seated.
- Place the hands so they are resting gently on top of the partner's shoulders.
- Think the following thoughts, one at a time, and ask for feedback from the partner of how it feels to them; the partner is to sense if it feels good, pleasurable, relaxing, if there is no sensation, if it is uncomfortable, or describe any other sensation experienced:
  - Have thoughts of anger; think of an event or person that causes you to feel anger.
  - Have thoughts of fear; think of something that is fearful.
  - Have thoughts of happiness; visualize a moment or person that brings forward the emotion of happiness.
  - Have thoughts of true love, not a sexual love but a loving, warm, heartfelt experience,
  - Have sexual thoughts.
  - Ground, self-reference (try saying your name inaudibly) and listen with the hands.

Each emotion will affect the partner's nervous system response in some way. Experience how the intention and emotion the practitioner feels is transmitted to the receiver and the receiver's perception. As a hands-on practitioner, be aware how the state of mind and emotions of the practitioner generate an impact on the receiver. Notice that no information from the partner's body was felt through the hands. Hopefully, at the last step, a sensation from the partner's body was apparent in the hands.

Practitioner note

"No one argues with the wine taster who, by using his palette, can tell us the characteristics of a wine – its region, its vineyard, or even its vintage. The education of touch can go at least as far" (Barral, 2007).

Useful listening techniques are the palpation tools developed by Jean Pierre Barral, D.O. The concept of listening is the sensing of global and local tensions by means of a sensitive hand. This enables the practitioner to perceive the condition of the body or of particular organs or vice versa. Listening touch inhibits the body's adaptation that allows the practitioner to feel where the primary source of dysfunction is centered in the body. This will be the area unable to compensate readily against gravity.

For the movement practitioner, the consciousness of touch is a powerful tool in guiding and enhancing a shift in movement patterning. Beyond the tactile cueing of direction changes of the body or tapping an area for more awareness, the conscious touch and clarity of the intention create a response in the client's tissue. The response may be better fascial gliding, a realignment of tissue, or a release allowing for more fluid movement. Or simply, the movement of a bone may be improved or structures brought into a more congruent relationship, such as the scapula, humeral head, and clavicle. The intention and clarity of where the hand is placed, of the landmarks, plus knowing the structure to be touched (the anatomy), is the basis for good manual skills. Differentiating structures takes practice and confirmation from another skilled practitioner.

Try it!

- Rest one hand on top of the opposite forearm.

- The palmar side of the hand is in contact with the skin.

- Relax the hand completely so that you can listen with it.

- Imagine viewing a movie screen.

- On the screen, place the structure to be palpated.

- First see the skin on the screen and sense the palm of the hand on the skin. Saying the name of the structure inaudibly helps bring the structure into the hands.

- Without changing any tension in the hand, see muscle on the screen; say "muscle" and listen with the hand for muscle contact.

- Notice a different quality or feeling of the hand. Did it change? Was the feeling one of a depth change as if an invisible elevator dropped into a lower floor?

- Next see the bone (ulna) and sense it with the hand.

- Maintain the visual and thought about bone.

- Did it feel as if the level underneath your hand dropped, as an elevator drops to a lower floor? Or did the bone move into the hand?

- Now visualize fascia; the depth changes again, this time up from the bone to the fascia.

- Play with different layers of the body and practice feeling the depth and quality changes of the hand without adding any tension or movement. Skin–fascia–muscle–bone.

Hand to shoulder interconnection

The neuromuscular connections from the hand to the trunk give the arms multiple qualities of movement. The limbs move freely, animating gesture from their root, the trunk. Limb movement potential relies on the support of the trunk to give the arms their freedom of movement.

The arms move either freely in space or in arm-supported movements in which stability and mobility are enhanced by intricate movements of the wrist to the shoulder. In both actions (one called open chain, the other closed chain), the interconnection of the arm through the shoulder into the trunk relates back to the center of gravity in the pelvis. Movement can occur as a whip, starting at the feet, travelling up the spine and rippling through the arm to a gesturing hand (imagine a baseball pitcher). And the body can move from the hand, traveling through the spine to the other hand (imagine Michael Jackson's dance moves). The possibilities are enormous. As in a wave motion, one end has to move to create the movement at the other end. The hand, to shoulder, into trunk connection has an interconnection of movement at all times. A movement restriction in any one of the joints will compromise the movement capacity of the others. The shoulder, as the dynamic base of support for the hand, links to the elbow, which enables the hand to move up close to and far away from the body, and the forearm, which adjusts the positioning of the hand.

Shoulder link

The vulnerable nature of the shoulder girdle, with its only bony attachment to the skeleton at the sterno-clavicular joints and its suspension by the myofascial network, provides a wide range of motion available to the hand (see Fig. 6.7). Movement becomes challenging when there is a need for a stable base to move from or against large resistances. The shoulder complex function necessitates a balance of both mobility and stability called a dynamic stability. The movement direction, anchor points, and contrasting poles of movement all interplay to create the dynamic stability. (Review Ch. 6, "Shoulder and Arm Continuations," making the connections of the dynamic stability of the shoulder girdle and trunk.)

Elbow link

The elbow complex serves the hand and provides mobility to the hand in space. There are two types of mobility required for moving the hand in space. One is shortening and lengthening of the arm, the flexion and extension of the elbow; the secondary motion to maneuver the hand is the rotation, pronation, and supination of the forearm. This ability to move in the two motions, the hinge and axial rotation, allows for manipulation of objects and bringing the hands toward the face. A restriction in the hinge joint affects daily living activities such as eating. Without rotation of the forearm bones (the radius and ulna), tasks such as typing, using tools, or cleaning oneself are compromised. If the elbow complex is compromised, then movement of the shoulder girdle is impacted and loses its movement rhythm (as described in Ch. 6). The shoulder complex would then accommodate the restriction of elevating the hand by moving the shoulder girdle as one unit. The loss of healthy shoulder girdle movement also diminishes the arm connection into the trunk. When training the upper body, always take into consideration the shoulder girdle, elbow, wrist, and hand mobility balance and the dynamic stability of the trunk.

Wrist link

The primary actions of the hand and wrist come from muscles that cross the elbow and provide stability and function to the wrist and hand. The stability and range of motion at the shoulder and elbow are important to the performance of the wrist and hand. The wrist is a complex of smaller bones (carpal bones) articulating at the radiocarpal joint, where the forearm (radius and ulna) joins the wrist. The carpal bones are in two arched rows, with four bones in each row (Fig. 7.1). The carpal bones act as an anchor to control the length tension of the intrinsic muscles of the hand and make fine adjustments of the hand such as gripping.

The movements of the wrist are:

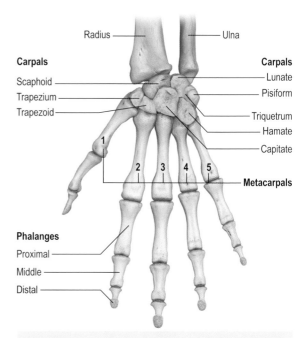

Figure 7.1
Bones of the wrist and hands

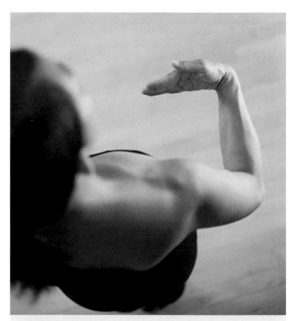

Figure 7.2
Wrist flexion

• flexion, which is when the fingers point toward the inner forearm (Fig. 7.2)

- extension, when the fingers point to the back of the forearm, as if holding a tray (Fig. 7.3)

- wrist deviation toward the thumb side (radial deviation or abduction) (Fig. 7.4) and toward the little finger side (ulnar deviation or adduction) (Fig. 7.5)

- the combination of all the motions, circumduction of the wrist, which is not a regular cone shape movement owing to the differences in the range of motion in each direction

- less range of motion in the wrist in pronation than in supination.

Most everyday activities involve placing the wrist in a mild extension (think of common motions performed every day and notice the wrist position). Over time, the wrist may become stiff, with limited movement. The inability to grip the hand or move the fingers cannot be made up for by using the elbow or shoulder joints (Norkin and Levangie, 2011). The lost of normal function of the wrist has little impact on the elbow or shoulder complex until the hand needs

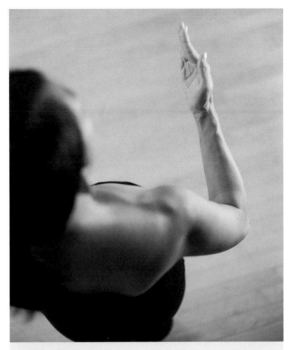

Figure 7.4
Radial deviation

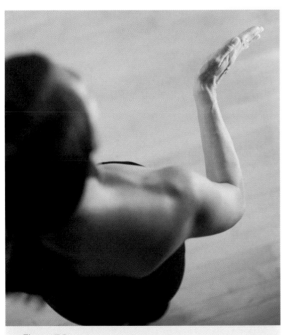

Figure 7.3
Wrist extension

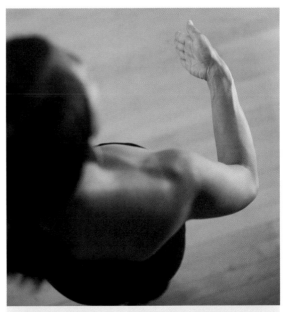

Figure 7.5
Ulnar deviation

to be in action. However, if using positions such as plank ("Front Support" in Pilates), wrist inflexibility and lack of carpal and radial bone movements will impede the execution of the position. Weight bearing on the arms is a whole dynamic of the body. To eliminate wrist discomfort and develop strength in the arm, the understanding and felt sense of how the arm links move in relationship to one another is the key to better wrists.

Bone shapes and movement of the lower arm

Hinge joint movement

To visualize movement of the arm, it is necessary to understand the bone shapes and structures in motion. The elbow joint is a side by side positioning of the humerus, ulna, and radius articulations with its ligaments and muscular attachments (Fig. 7.6). The apposition is necessary for congruency for the hinge joint motion. The moving joints of the lower arm are the humeroulnar and humeroradial joints, and the superior/inferior radioulnar joints. At the elbow, the lower end of the humerus has two articulating surfaces, the trochlea and the capitulum. The trochlea resembles a spool with a central groove and the capitulum, both a rounded shape and a hemisphere. The top of the ulna, the trochlear notch, articulates with the trochlea (the bottom of the humerus) and has a corresponding shape, a longitudinal ridge appearing similar to a sheet of corrugated steel. The posterior side of the trochlear notch is the olecranon, commonly called the elbow. The radial head's shape bears a resemblance to a wheel with a cupped surface, a concavity to meet the convexity of the capitulum (Kapandji, 1999). Two indentations are present just above the trochlea on the humerus, called the coronoid fossa and the radial fossa above the capitulum. During elbow flexion there is a sliding motion of the ulna around the trochlea into the coronoid fossa, and the radial head slides over the capitulum, entering the radial fossa. On the posterior side, the olecranon fossa receives the olecranon of the ulna with elbow extension. There is no contact between the articulating surfaces of the concave radial head and convex capitulum during elbow extension (see Fig. 7.6).

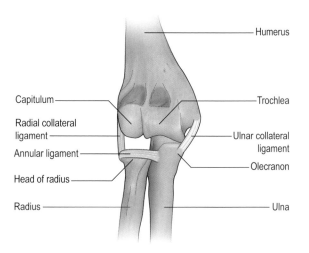

Figure 7.6
Bones and ligaments of the elbow

Radial rotation

The shape of the radius as described by Kapandji (1999) can be seen as a crank. The top has a bend, called the supinator bend, with the radial tuberosity medial to the bone. The radius bows outward creating another bend, called the pronator bend; pronator teres inserts at this level (Fig. 7.7 A). The bone bows medially to meet the distal ulna at the inferior radioulnar joint. The curved shape of the radius makes it possible for the bone to cross over the ulna during pronation (Fig. 7.7 B).

Rotation (supination and pronation) occurs at the superior and inferior radioulnar joints. These joints are mechanically linked, and therefore movement of one joint will produce motion in the joint at the other end. In supination, the ulna and radius lie parallel to one another. The radius crosses over the ulna with little to no movement of the ulna in pronation (see Fig. 7.7 B). When the radius moves relative to the ulna, it traces half of a cone shape with the top apex at the elbow and wide base at the wrist. The radial head, which is shaped like a wheel, moves about its axis within a ring formed by the annular ligament making a cuff around the wheel (see Fig. 7.7 B). The ligament holds the head in place and allows for some stretching during pronation. The head of the radius displaces

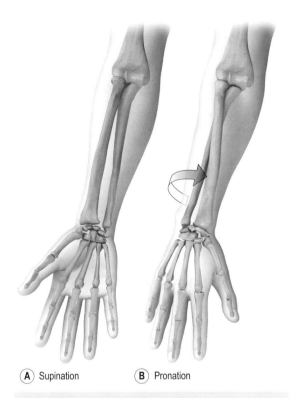

(A) Supination   (B) Pronation

Figure 7.7
A Supination of forearm: uncrossed radius and ulna
B Pronation of forearm: crossed radius and ulna

laterally to lie transversely, moving the medial tuberosity of the radius between the radius and ulna. The main movement is the rotational displacement of the lower end of the radius around the ulna.

Pronation and supination are easily distinguished from shoulder movement with the elbow in 90° flexion. The elbow position stabilizes motion of the humerus and disassociates the rotation of the radioulnar joint from the shoulder. In elbow extension, the active pronation and supination occurs with some rotation at the shoulder joint.

Try it!

Bend the elbow by the waist at 90°. Start with the thumb facing up (Fig. 7.8). Slowly rotate the hand into pronation, palm down (Fig. 7.9). Observe the

thumb of the hand. What is the angle of the hand? Horizontal to the floor is 90° range of motion. Without any shoulder motion, normal pronation range is 85°. Try with the arm extended. Extend the arm out in front with the palm up and elbow straight (Fig. 7.10 A). Hold the humerus above the elbow joint to stabilize it and slowly pronate the forearm. Feel for bone movement when the radius stops moving, or, feeling the first movement of the humerus, freeze the forearm in space (Fig. 7.10 B). The bones of the forearm stop moving, and the tissues will glide to force a horizontal position of the hand. Notice the difference between bone movement and the tissue gliding.

If the pronation range is less than 85°, the arm chain of movement will be altered from the thorax to the hand. Commonly, the shoulder takes up the motion. Investigating available motion of the upper spine, shoulder through wrist, is necessary to free up the restriction of the forearm.

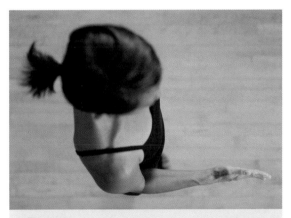

Figure 7.8
Try it! Elbow bent, thumbs up

When weight bearing or holding a handle or dumbbell, whether the palm position is facing down or up, there are changes in the related movements between the shoulder and the hand. In the supinated position, with the elbow flexed, palm up, the hand becomes horizontal to the floor with a range of motion 90°. The hand is flat. The palm will not become horizontal to the floor during pronation due to the range of motion being 85°. In order to meet the floor or a surface, the

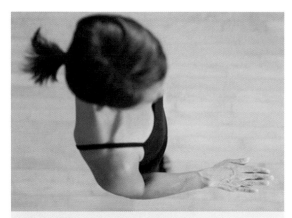

Figure 7.9
Try it! Elbow bent with pronation

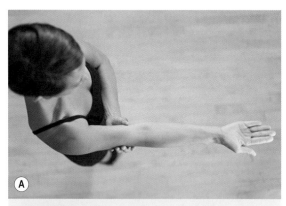

Figure 7.10 A
Try it! Elbow straight

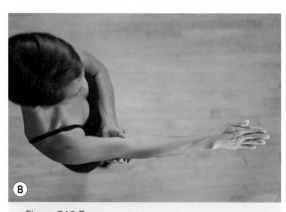

Figure 7.10 B
Elbow straight with pronation

humerus will rotate slightly with the pronation. If the range is less than 85°, then the restriction in pronation causes the shoulder to internally rotate excessively. Over time, the shoulder joint becomes tight in an internally rotated position, disrupting its functional movement range. When weight bearing on the arms, the placement of the hand and wrist in relation to the shoulder affects the movement at the elbow and pressure on the wrist.

Movement of the radiocarpal joint and the carpal bones

There are two joints, the radiocarpal joint (wrist joint) and the mid-carpal joint. The radiocarpal joint is between the radial head with its disk and the proximal row of carpal bones. The mid-carpal joint is between the two rows of the carpal bones (see Fig. 7.1).

Carpal bones (in order from the thumb)

(see Fig. 7.1)

Proximal row (articulates with the radial head):

- scaphoid
- lunate
- triquetrum
- pisiform.

Distal row (the mid-carpal articulates with the proximal row):

- trapezium
- trapezoid
- capitate
- hamate.

The bones of the proximal row form an arch, with the convex side articulating with the radius and articular disk. The concavity side forms a recess into which the distal row fits, particularly the projecting parts of the capitate and hamate. The shape of the hand has a gentle convex curve on the back of the hand and the palm side of the hand has a deep concavity. When the hand is pressed into the floor, it spreads out, making contact with the base of the thumb (thenar eminence) along the lower palm of the hand to the base of the little finger side (hypothenar eminence), along with all of the metacarpals and the pads of each finger. The space from the inner thumb to below the base of the second and third metacarpals does not make contact with the surface. The base of the fingers and the proximal phalanges make contact. This will be important to visualize when placing the weight on the hands.

Passive forces and gliding

Ligaments of the wrist provide support for the radioulnar and mid-carpal joints and contribute to motion by complex passive forces. Intercarpal ligaments prevent a separation or collapse of the arch of the hand. The primary function of the ligaments is to stabilize the carpal bones in their movements, which are supported and moved by the tension or relaxation of specific sets of ligaments. Passively, the carpal bones have micromovements in between each bone. The small articulations allow for the gliding of the two rows of carpal bones at the mid-carpal joint, to move into wrist extension.

Movement of the wrist joint (radioulnar joint) is a gliding of the proximal row of the carpus on the radius and radioulnar disk. The proximal row moves in opposition to the movement of the hand. During wrist flexion, the carpals slide back (dorsally) on the radius and disk (Fig. 7.11 A). In wrist extension, the mid-carpal bones move on a relatively fixed proximal row in the same direction as the hand motion (Fig. 7.11 B). When the wrist, the superior and inferior radioulnar joints are aligned where the inferior radius and ulna line up horizontally, and the wrist is at full extension, the ligaments pull the carpal bones together into a closed pack position, uniting all the carpal bones. The whole unit moves on the radius and radioulnar disk, reaching full extension. The sequence of wrist extension and flexion varies according to the individual's ligamentous qualities (loose or tight) and the locking of the intercarpal surfaces. Studies on wrist kinematics have drawn different opinions on the degrees of movement.

Synergistic action of wrist and hand

> **Try it!**
>
> Make a soft fist of the hand and flex the wrist by bringing the fist toward the inner forearm (Fig. 7.12 A). Relax the fist and straighten the fingers, then repeat the flexion of the wrist (Fig. 7.12 B). Notice the range of motion and the strength differences in the wrist movement. Try a soft fist and extended fingers moving into extension of the wrist.

The flexor muscles of the wrist work synergistically with the extensor muscles of the fingers so that when

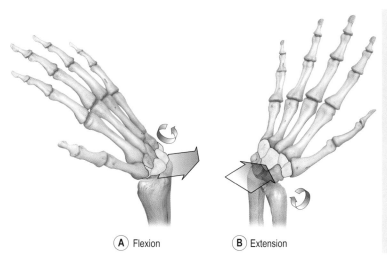

Figure 7.11
A Wrist flexion
B Wrist extension

(**A**) Flexion   (**B**) Extension

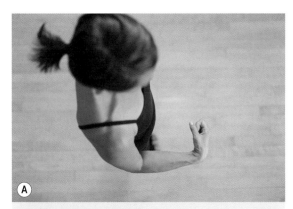

Figure 7.12 A
Try it! Soft fist wrist movement

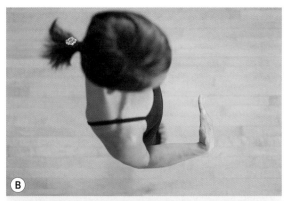

Figure 7.12 B
Hand extended wrist movement

the wrist is flexed there is an automatic response of the phalanx (finger) extensors. During wrist extension, the fingers automatically flex. The wrist extension places the finger flexor tendons at an advantage, being in a shorter position than when the wrist is in neutral or flexion. Using the action of the fingers can facilitate better wrist motion, especially when weight bearing on the hands.

Cueing to engage the finger flexors while weight bearing on the hands works to improve the support of the wrist and an optimal wrist position feeds into the chain of arm activity into the trunk. This helps to engage the hand to core connection and assists in relieving any unnecessary joint stress in an exercise or pose. For the movement practitioner, knowing how the bones move and the synergistic coordination of myofascia from the beginning to the end is relevant to guiding strong movement.

Fascia and muscle linking

In designing movement, one may begin to link the trunk through the hand (proximal to distal) or work distally (the hand) toward the trunk. In either direction, the connections determine how the arm musculature activates. Whether using resistance open chain actions such as arm work on the Reformer, reaching the arms in Virabhadrasana, or pulling a Theraband, the positioning of the whole chain, from the fingers to the trunk, activates the arm in a particular way. It is the continuity of the

myofascial expansions with the musculature that contracts simultaneously along its path of connection (review "Shoulder and Arm Continuation" in Ch. 6). And the path of connection as seen in embryology development, from the limbs buds to fully formed arms, divides the musculature into front and back divisions.

Flexor division of the arm to the hand

Connections are as follows (see Fig. 6.3 A):

- brachial fascia, continuous from above with the pectoral fascia; biceps brachii

- medial and lateral intermuscular septum from deep brachial fascia divides the arm into anterior and posterior compartments

- antebrachial fascia, continuous from brachial fascia, surrounds the forearm and thickens to form the palmar aponeurosis

- palmaris longus muscle connects into flexor retinaculum, the flexor carpi radialis, and thumb side of the palm (thenar eminence)

- muscular fibers of flexor pollicis longus directly insert to the palmar retinaculum (Stecco and Stecco, 2012).

Extensor division of the arm

Connections are as follows (see Fig. 6.3 B):

- expansions of the latissimus dorsi muscle and posterior deltoid merge into the brachial fascia

- triceps, medial head specifically continuous with the posterior portion of the antebrachial fascia

- posterior forearm, the extensor carpi ulnaris and abductor digiti minimi to the dorsal fascia of the hand (Stecco and Stecco, 2012).

To stimulate a flexor response in the arm, attention can be placed on the thumb side of the arm connection to the shoulder. For the extensor engagement, focusing on the little finger side of the arm connects the posterior side of the arm into the trunk.

> **Practitioner note**
> **Verbal cue**
>
> Cue for directing the energy of the arm from the trunk through the side of the arm with the intention of engagement. Example: as the client is pulling the arms forward from bent arms to straight ("Row Front 1" or "Serratus Arms on the Reformer"), cue "Reach through the little finger side of the hand," lining up the third finger in the center of the hand to place the wrist bones in a strong position for stability.

Interosseous membrane

The interosseous membrane of the forearm is an extension of the antebrachial fascia (Agur and Dalley, 2013) that lies between the radius and the ulna. The interosseous membrane and an oblique cord knit the ulna and radius together and divide the forearm into anterior and posterior compartments. The membrane is a broad thin sheet with oblique fibers oriented downward from the radius to the ulna. It extends a surface for attachment of the deep forearm muscles (Fig. 7.13). Circulatory vessels (the interosseous arteries) and deep nerves are woven onto and through the membrane and attaching muscles.

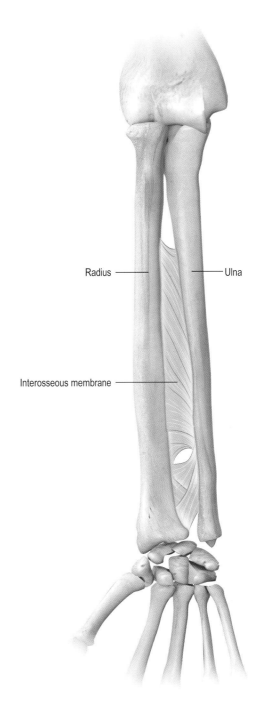

Radius — Ulna

Interosseous membrane —

Figure 7.13
Interosseous membrane

The interosseous membrane is part of the fascial matrix of the body and therefore has the same capacity as all fascia for resilience in movements of compressing and stretching. When the forearm is midway between pronation and supination, the membrane is taut. At full pronation and supination the membrane is slackened. The quality of the tissue is important, allowing for the radius to cross and uncross. The pronator and supinator muscles' normal length and ability to function depend on the quality of the membrane's tension. Bodyworkers, computer workers, factory line workers, carpenters, and any hand-orientated workers tend to have tight and immobile fascia of the arms. This can inhibit pronation and supination motion, affecting the whole arm. If the forearm is restricted, then the movement of the shoulder will be compromised and the hand will not be able to meet the floor. Releasing the interosseous membrane is one element in improving the whole arm movement sequencing.

Interosseous membrane release

- The practitioner sits next to the client and the arm to be worked.
- The client places the arm in 90° elbow flexion, with the upper arm next to the trunk, as relaxed as possible and with the thumb facing up.
- The practitioner holds the radius at the elbow and at the wrist (Fig. 7.14 A).
- Slightly supinate the forearm (approximately 5–10°) to slacken the membrane.
- Wait for 1–3 minutes, allowing gravity to separate the bones and creating a lengthening between the bones.
- Slightly pronate the forearm (approximately 5–10°) to slacken the membrane (Fig. 7.14 B).

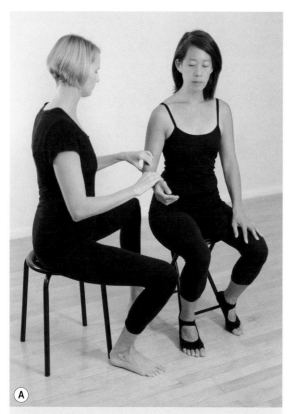

(A)

Figure 7.14 A
Interosseous membrane release: supination

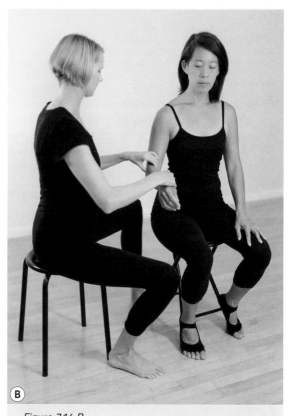

(B)

Figure 7.14 B
In pronation

- Wait for 1–3 minutes, allowing gravity to separate the bones and creating a lengthening between the bones.

Weight bearing on the hands

Synthesizing all the above information, the positioning of the pelvis–spine–shoulder girdle–humerus–forearm–wrist and fingers will maximize the ability to bear weight on the arms without increasing stress to the joints. The key is to see the individual's bone alignment and movement capability, and line up the anatomical landmarks for this particular individual. This is fine-tuning of the individual's form with awareness.

Aligning for weight bearing

Wrist alignment using the wall
VIDEO LINK V 7.1

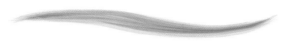

- The starting position is standing facing a wall.

- Stand in a whole body good form and place the hands flat on the wall's surface between 75° and 90° shoulder flexion with the elbows straight (Fig. 7.15).

- Look at the wrist joint and see a crease that runs along the wrist from thumb to little finger (Fig. 7.16).

- Notice if a prominent bone is appearing at the base of the little finger (styloid process and inferior surface of the ulna head).

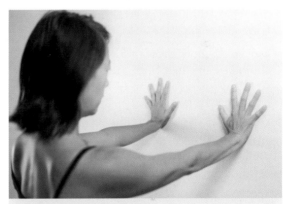

Figure 7.15
Wrist alignment for weight bearing on arms using wall

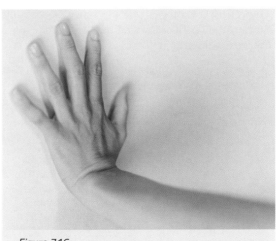

Figure 7.16
Close-up of wrist alignment

- Shift the hand so that the crease at the wrist is horizontal to the floor.

- Notice where the fingers are pointing; either the second finger or the third finger will be pointing vertically; the hand may seem slightly turned out.

- Maintaining the arms straight, slowly rotate the elbows in and out while watching the prominent ulna head bone.

- When the bone slips into place and virtually disappears, stop the rotation.

- Now the wrist crease is horizontal and the head of the ulna is in place.

- Notice that the superior end of the radius longitudinal axis is running more vertical; the superior end is over the center of the inferior end.

- Look at the inner elbow crease (eyes of the elbow) and notice the angle. Are the "eyes" cross-eyed? Are they looking at the wall? In most people, the elbow crease is cross-eyed.

- Maintaining the horizontal wrist crease and elbow crease angle, place more weight at the base of the thumb and second finger and on all the finger pads.

- Flex the finger pads slightly to engage the finger flexor muscles that synergistically work with wrist extension; keep the base of the fingers in contact with the surface.

- Be aware of the thorax spine and move the sternum away from the floor to bring the thorax in contact with the scapula.

- Observe for the congruency of the head of the humerus and posteriorly with the scapula.

Practitioner note

The crossing of the radius is important for aligning the radius from the elbow to the wrist to transfer the weight through the bones. The weight transfer stimulates a synergistic activity of the upper arms: the biceps and triceps; the pectoralis and latissimus; rhomboid–serratus anterior–external obliques (see Figs 6.3 A & B). Start at the wall with the bone alignment and whole arm engagement (see "Finding the Dynamic Engagement" below). Hold the position for a duration that challenges the muscle connections. Transfer to the quadruped position before plank. Try using finger flexion on the mat or wall for those who have difficulties in wrist extension.

Conflicting cueing exists in many movement classes around the wrist to spine relationship. A common cue for scapula stability is to overemphasize pulling the latissimus dorsi tight, followed by an external rotation of the humeral head. To believe scapula stability is achieved by using the latissimus dorsi and "opening" the front of the shoulder through external rotation of the humerus is to misunderstand the dynamic stability concept of the shoulder complex. The scapula is a part of the shoulder girdle and the latissimus acts primarily on the humerus as a depressor and internal rotator. By cueing the latissimus as a shoulder girdle stabilizer, a downward compression of the humeral head with internal rotation is created, thereby decreasing the thoracic outlet space. In addition, the client is then asked to externally rotate the humeral head and since this is opposing the direction of the latissimus, the person will compensate in the spine or movement of the scapula. The shoulder becomes vulnerable to stress. Starting with the alignment of the wrist to the elbow and shoulder joint will provide the support for the synergistic engagement of the arm and trunk. Cueing to isolate muscles without the understanding of whole body movement and relationship of the bones to one another limits the training effect for functional movement. A dynamic stability and engagement of the arm needs to be felt to imprint the position and movement in the body. Teach the client the smaller adjustments from the wrist into the trunk in order to feel the synergistic connections.

Finding the dynamic engagement of the arm in weight bearing

Teaching a felt sense of how to engage the body in a pose prior to moving in and out of the pose is a valuable tool. When people feel the body, it imprints into the brain and the muscle memory, rather than cueing a muscle or two. This felt sense exercise is performed with a partner first, then solo on the wall, followed by quadruped, then in the plank.

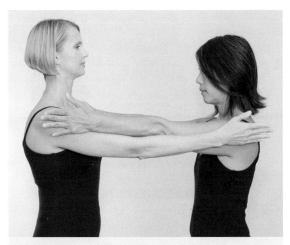

Figure 7.17
Partner work for feeling arm engagement

- Stand facing a partner (Fig. 7.17).

- With the arms straight, place the little finger side of the hand (hypothenar eminence) against the side of the humeral head.

- One person's arms are on top, the other from underneath.

- First press the hands into each other's shoulders.

- Feel how the forearm moves in toward the midline.

- Next, press the side of the shoulders into the partner's hand.

- Feel how the upper arm moves outward and the chest lengthens sideways.

- Now, with a balance of how hard to press, do both at the same time.

- The lower arm moves inward as the upper arm moves outward.

- Feel the pressure of the shoulder into the partner's hands as the lower arm is moving inward.

- Hold the engagement to feel the whole arm and trunk participation.

- Practice the plank or quadruped position with the arms engaged in this feeling.

Exercises

Arm supports and planks

In Pilates mat work, weight bearing of the arms occurs by supporting the body to the front, back, and side, similar to a variety of yoga poses. In each direction, awareness of how the hand is placed in relation to the radius and ulna lines and finger engagement will set up the ability to hold the pose with strength.

"Front Support" in Pilates mat exercises is a plank (Fig. 7.18). First practice the placement of the hands and the wrist to shoulder alignment in a kneeling position. Then move into the plank, maintaining the arm stacking, with the lower arm moving inward as the upper arm moves outward, and the widening of the collarbones. Hold the position as one leg lifts up without disturbing the plank position, moving from an extended hip motion.

"Back Support" is a reverse plank similar to Purvottanasana in yoga except for the head placement. In Pilates, the focus is forward and in the yoga pose the focus is back (Fig. 7.19). The wrists in this pose

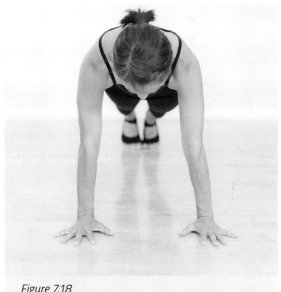

Figure 7.18
Front Support

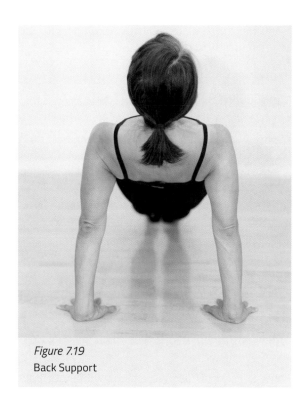

Figure 7.19
Back Support

remain similar to the front placement. The fingertips are facing the feet, placing the shoulders in a more internal direction than would be the case with fingers facing to the side or the back. The humerus is best supported when its position is as if the arm were hanging by the side of the body with the thumbs forward – a neutral placement. The pronation of the forearm is the movement that achieves a healthy shoulder position when the fingers point toward the feet. When the fingers are facing to the side, it places the humeral head in a more externally rotated position. It may be easier to place the weight on the first and second bases of the fingers; however, when moving into the extended body pose, the shortening of the latissimus dorsi and pectoralis major fascial connections pulls the humeral head downward, inhibiting the necessary work of the shoulder girdle myofascia network (i.e. rhomboid–serratus anterior–obliques). The restriction does not allow for the upper thorax to move with the roll of the clavicles upward as the trunk lifts. A disconnect of the arms in this way lessens the core support and lightness of the lifted trunk. Creating the lightness will decompress the body weight into the wrists.

In one arm supports, as in the "Mermaid" or "Twist" in Pilates, the fingers are pointed away from the body. Prior to moving into the straight arm side plank, set the arm bones with the wrist crease in a straight line and the diagonal line of the radius. The motion of the ribcage is what moves the body up and over the wrist. Inhale into the side of the ribcage, moving in the direction of the ceiling, and move the ribcage up into the side plank position. This action is very different from pressing the hand into the floor to lift. The energy of the trunk moving on the arm signals the trunk musculature to produce the movement while engaging the support of the whole arm.

> **Try it!**
>
> Practice moving the ribcage over the arm by placing the forearm on the floor, and perform a side plank (Fig. 7.20).

Bend to straight

Weight bearing through alignment of the hands and wrist, along with the contrast of inward spiral of the lower arm and outward widening of the upper arm, provides great support and continuation of the trunk core work. Once a bending of the elbows occurs to

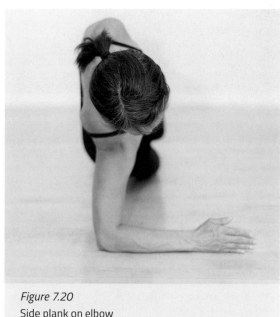

Figure 7.20
Side plank on elbow

lower the trunk toward the floor, the weight on the hand and action of the arms changes.

As in the knee bend to squat or plié, the initial action is to unlock the intermediary joint, the knee, or in this case, the elbow, creating the unscrewing action of the rotation of the arm. The weight shifts to the little finger side of the hand as the radius and ulna change position at the elbow. When the arms are straight, the radius is crossed over the ulna – the pronation position. To bend and lower the body, the radius at the elbow moves back toward the supinated relationship. Due to the wrist being fixed, the shift off the radius and ulna is felt at the little finger side of the palm of the hand (hypothenar eminence). To straighten the arms, the weight is transferred toward the base of the first and second fingers (Figs 7.21 A & B).

Try it!

Place yourself in a quadruped or plank position and practice, with straight arms, the alignment and engagement principle described. Slowly bend the elbow without changing the body in space (meaning no lowering of the trunk). It is a small movement, giving the feeling of stabilizing the body in space and then of the weight transfer to the little finger side of the hand. Lengthen the arms by moving from the outer edge of the hand to the base of the thumb and second finger. Practice the small bend of the elbow joint without trunk movement. Then fully lower the body to the floor but only to the place where scapula stability is on the edge of being lost. Consciously begin a shift of weight in the hand toward the base of the thumb and second finger and cross the radius and fully straighten the arms. Notice how the change of weight in the hands helps in the strength of the push up.

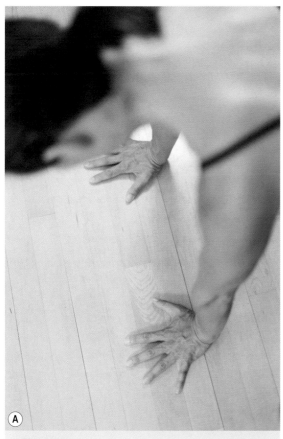

(A)

Figure 7.21 A
Push-up

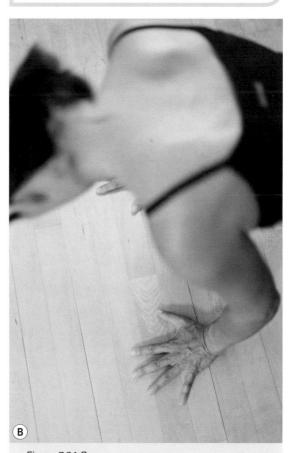

(B)

Figure 7.21 B
Close-up of weight transference at the wrist during elbow flexion

CLIENT STORY

Personal story

Typical of most professional dancers, during my dance career in the 1980s I survived many foot, spinal, and shoulder injuries. In modern dance, it was the artistic expression of the times for women to be able to move like male dancers and perform tasks that typically a male dancer is expected to perform, such as lifting a partner. The 1980s was a decade when societal molds and expectations were being challenged. I was the tallest woman in the company, and the choreography inevitably had me catching men, lifting other women, and supporting the weight of men. The day after a major performance before an audience of 3000, I woke up unable to move my right arm without pain. Luckily, the performances were over and I had a period of rest to heal. Even after healing, that shoulder was tight and a bit dysfunctional but it did not immediately cause me problems. Fast forward 30 plus years, and the same shoulder resurfaced as an issue for me. I am a hands-on practitioner and overuse can become a problem. There was no single incident that caused the problem to arise again. I believe that the body can hold it together for a long time until, one day, it shifts and can no longer maintain the compensation. My body time was now spent focusing on moving in ways that would ease up the shoulder and re-educate the trunk to shoulder patterns. I went from not being able to reach behind my back at waist level to reaching up to almost bra height. I noticed I was still more restricted than before. I was 85% better but I wanted that missing 15% back so I could continue progressing my physical practice. I turned my attention to my wrist. I noticed that my right ulna was very prominent (more than I remembered as my normal). The alignment of my radius and ulna was off and they were not moving well, sliding over one another. I had no pain but weight bearing on my hands was uncomfortable and I felt I could not sustain a balance. I sought out a colleague who knew the osseous release technique and did hands-on movement of the wrist bones, since it is impossible to do this to oneself. I added neural stretches and release as well, performed on my own. After that I began moving my wrist more with the hand fixed and placed on a wall, observing when the ulna dropped into place. From this place, I introduced more of my body weight onto the arms through the quadruped position, then plank. I used the Reformer, with arm-supported work on the foot bar and with the shoulder rests always monitoring the wrist alignment. Eventually, I added handstands against the wall to challenge the range and the load to the wrist. I eventually recovered fully, with 100% return of function of my whole arm to trunk. I feel my new shoulder will never revisit that 1980s shoulder tear.

Movement releases for the nerve lines

Radial nerve line

- Begin by standing with the straight arm hanging down, palm facing outward, and fingers elongated and open (Fig. 7.22 A).

- Fold the thumb in toward the palm of the hand then curl the other fingers over the thumb to make a fist.

- Turn the whole arm inward, into internal rotation, and flex the wrist (knuckles toward the inner arm) (Fig. 7.22 B).

- Notice if tension is felt in the arm and if so, reverse the motion of the flexed wrist.

- Repeat several times until no tension is felt.

- If no tension is felt, then assume the position and abduct the arm, moving it away from the body.

- Maintain the internal rotation of the arm and flexion of the wrist; check the wrist (it is easy to be unconscious of the wrist position).

- Hold the position and side bend the head toward the arm and elevate the humeral head toward the head (Fig. 7.22 C).

- Move the head and shoulder away from each other (Fig. 7.22 D).

- Repeat, tilting toward the elevated shoulder and away from the lowering shoulder.

- The motion is easy, as if flossing the nerve in between the neck and arm.

- Repeat the flossing motion 3–5 times.

- Center the head and release the position.

> **Tip**
>
> Play with the position of the arm to find the line of tension. The arm may need to be slightly extended and abducted. The arm may not be too high. Move slowly into the arm position, feeling for the "sweet spot" of the line. Floss the sweet spot for best results.

Ulnar nerve line

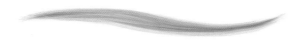

- Stand with both arms hanging down by the body.

- Turn the arm to be worked outward, bend the elbow, lifting the hand as if you are a waiter (wrist is extended, palm up, and fingertips away from the shoulder) (Fig. 7.23 A).

- Pronate the forearm so that the fingertips are now touching or pointing toward the shoulder (Fig. 7.23 B).

- Place the other hand on top of the hand being worked and press the palm to increase the wrist extension (Fig. 7.23 C).

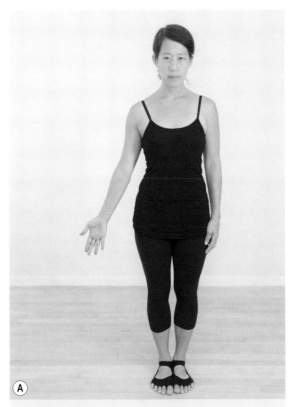

(A)

Figure 7.22 A
Radial Nerve Stretch: start position

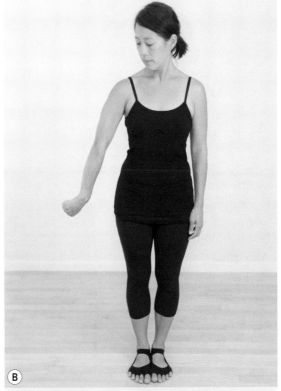

(B)

Figure 7.22 B
Internal rotation of arm and flex wrist with hand in fist

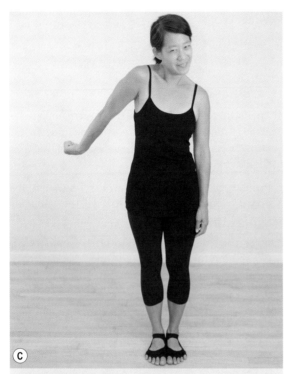

(C)

Figure 7.22 C
Flossing the Nerve: moving head toward the shoulder

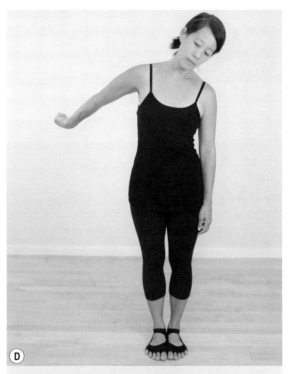

(D)

Figure 7.22 D
Flossing the Nerve: moving head away

- If tension is felt here, hold it for three breaths and release; repeat that 3–5 times.
- Or continue the movement by lifting the elbow up as high as possible without overpressure on the shoulder.
- Be aware of any tension or pain; if the line is tense or if pain or nervy sensations are present, stop, rest and repeat 3 times.
- To continue further, place the palm of the hand over the ear (Fig. 7.24).
- The final pose is to make a mask with both arms, demonstrating a fully elongated ulnar nerve (Fig. 7.25).

Coracobrachialis and median line

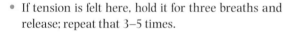

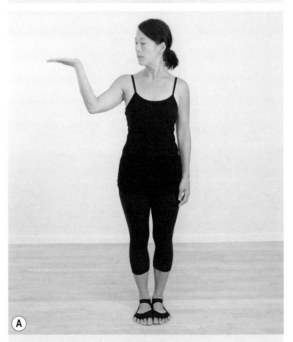

(A)

Figure 7.23 A
Ulnar Nerve Stretch: start position

- Stand with both arms hanging by the body.
- Turn the arm to be work outward.

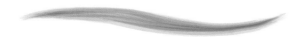

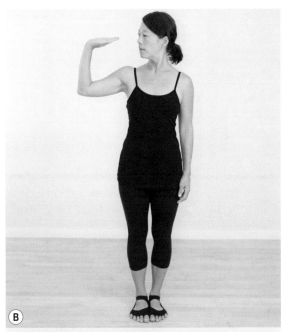

Figure 7.23 B
Turning fingers inward

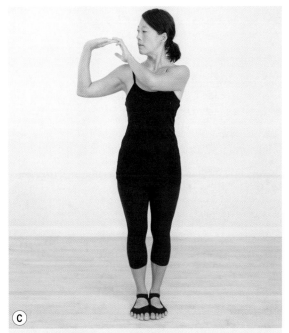

Figure 7.23 C
Adding stretch

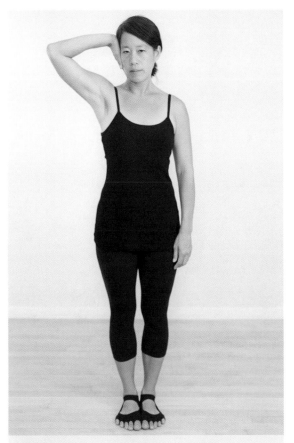

Figure 7.24
Increasing the stretch of the ulnar nerve

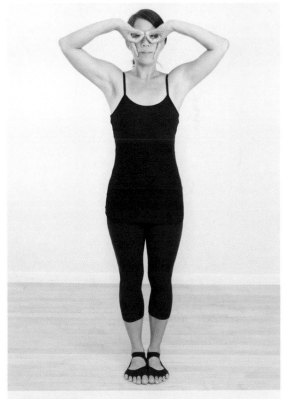

Figure 7.25
Full ulnar nerve length position

- Reach the arm up into a back diagonal (abducted and extended approximately 90–105°) with the wrist extended (Fig. 7.26).

- Make a small circle of the shoulder to find the placement of the scapula and the "sweet spot."

- Side bend the head toward the shoulder to release the tension at the thoracic outlet.

- Move the head away.

- Hold and breathe for 5–20 seconds.

Clasped Hands: moving in and out

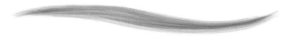

- Stand and clasp the hands in front and relax the arms.

- With soft elbows, gently reach the clasped hands toward the floor with the elbow creases (inner elbow) facing each other (Fig. 7.27 A).

- Turn over the palms by turning the thumbs in toward the body and down to the floor, spread the palms and spiral the arms inward (Fig. 7.27 B).

- Inhaling, reach the hands forward, maintaining the inner elbows facing inward and palms spreading.

- Reach higher (as long as there is no shortening of the clavicle line across the chest).

- Exhale and lower; this is called the "In" movement of the clasped hands.

- The "Out" movement reverses this by turning the palms out, with externally rotated arms and soft elbows (Fig. 7.27 C).

- Release the thumb grasp, spreading the thumbs wide, and spread the palms, reaching for the floor.

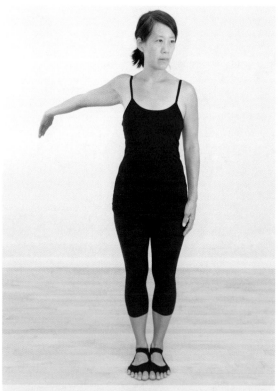

Figure 7.26
Corobrachialis and median line lengthening

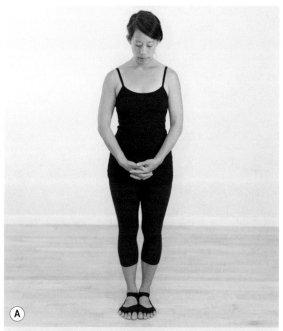

(A)

Figure 7.27 A
Clasped Hands mobility: start position

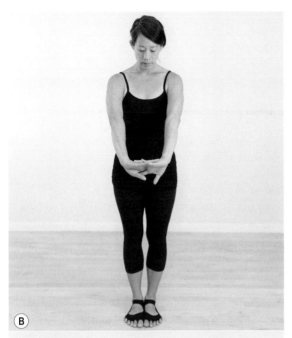

B

Figure 7.27 B
Turning thumbs over

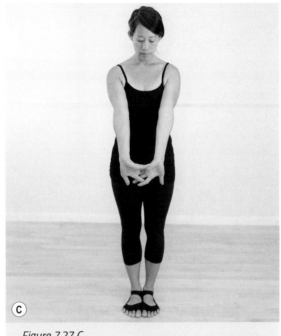

C

Figure 7.27 C
Moving outward

- On an in breath, move the "out" position upward (as long as there is no shortening of the clavicle line across the chest).

- Exhale and lower.

- Repeat the movement with the breath and easy feel in all of the joints from the shoulder girdle, elbows, and wrists.

- The feeling is one of sliding and gliding of the tissues and joints, with no locking out in any of the links along the arm.

The nerves of the arms are continuous from the cervical plexus. Addressing the neck is vital for any issue of the arm. Chapter 8 covers the neck with the continuation of the tissues from the head to wrist, adding "Supple Neck" movements to a practice that is focused on fine-tuning the upper limbs and trunk.

Upper Arms on the Cadillac

This movement is a staple for the elongation of the trunk into the arms, followed by a bridging to

lengthen the other end of the trunk. It is placed in this chapter because of its movement from the hands, through the arms, into the trunk.

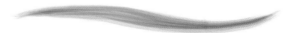

- Lie underneath the top loaded push-through bar so that the arms holding the bar are at 90° flexion (Fig.7.28 A).

- Legs are bent and prepared for bridging action.

- On an inhale, draw the bar downward as the arms widen across the clavicle line, elbows to the side, armpits opening (slight internal spiral motion) (Fig. 7.28 B).

- Exhale and externally rotate the arms as the bar moves overhead until the arms are straight (outward spiral of the shoulder moving toward anatomical neutral) (Fig. 7.28 C).

- Inhale and reverse the path of the arms, returning the bar to the beginning position.

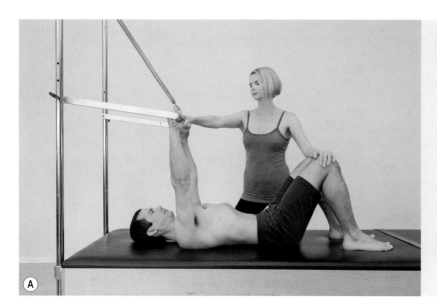

Figure 7.28 A
Upper Arms Cadillac: start position

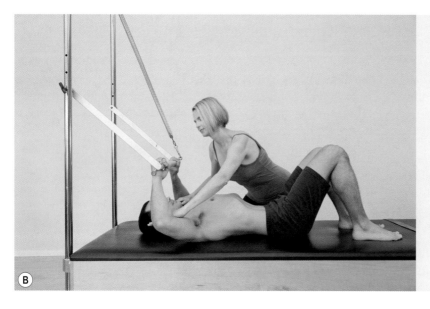

Figure 7.28 B
Pulling bar down

- The arm path is one of external rotation and widening of the chest followed by a internal rotation to extend the arms to the starting position.

- The top loaded bar will pull the arms beyond the scapulohumeral congruency; control the bar by activity of the scapula stabilizers.

- On an inhale, perform a bridge (Fig. 7.28 D).

- Exhale and return the bridge to the starting position.

- Repeating this portion is useful for the purpose of the upper arms and trunk movement patterning.

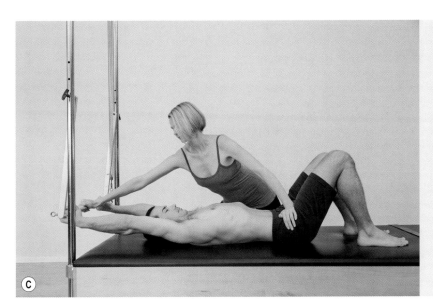

Figure 7.28 C
Bar overhead

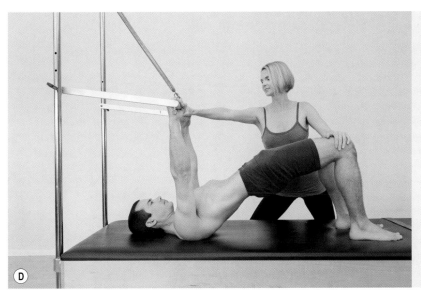

Figure 7.28 D
Bridge

Practitioner note

The full "Upper Arms" includes following the bridge with a torso lift, pressing the bar upward. The torso lift may be extension by lifting from the sternum and extending through the spine to sitting up, or rolling from the top of the head, moving from flexion into a neutral seated position with the arms fully flexed overhead. It can be mirrored as a mini "Teaser" position.

Practitioner note
Hands-on

- Stand next to the table, near the client.
- As the client pulls the bar down, use both hands to assist the elbow bend wide, intentioning the pectoralis and clavicular line width (see Fig. 7.29 B).
- Change the hands to the upper arm and enhance the external rotation motion of the humerus as the bar transitions from the downward direction to overhead.

- Cue that the elbows do not drop or lift; the elbows maintain a space hold as the rotation occurs.

- Stand in a lunge position with the front of the thighs pressing into the table and move the hands, one to the bar and the other to the right hip, where the thigh meets the pelvis.

- Feel the grounded lunge position; inhale as the space between the hands lengthens by pressing the bar away and the top of the femur at the pelvis in the opposite direction (see Fig. 7.28 C).

- Feel the lengthening of your own body between the arms, along the pectorals and clavicle lines, and listen to the client's body for the gliding of the tissues, specifically the thoracolumbar fascia into the pelvic fascia.

- On the reverse movement of the arms, repeat the widening of the elbows as the transition occurs from the bar overhead to the upward position of the bar.

- Place the forearm across the femurs just above the knees to facilitate a lengthening of the femurs in the direction of the feet.

- Prior to the lowering of the bridge, place the hands on the pelvis at the upper rim to enhance a lengthening of the pelvis away from the ribs as the pelvis is lowering.

- Repeat the hands-on 2–3 times.

Arm Press on Cadillac bottom loaded push-through bar

The purpose is to train the shoulder in a functional internal rotation and pronation of the forearm to facilitate strengthening the connection of shoulder girdle to arm movements. The action of straightening and bending works the triceps and biceps synergistically.

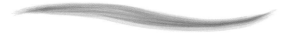

- Set up the push-through bar with the safety strap and one bottom loaded red spring, or one red and blue for more resistance.

- Lie underneath the bar where the arms are able to be at 90° shoulder flexion when the elbows are extended.

- Place the hands on the bar with the fingertips toward one another and full contact of the palms of the hand; the shoulders are internally rotated, the elbows bent wide to the side (Fig. 7.29 A).

- Press the bar up, extending the arms (Fig. 7.29 B).

- Repeat 8–10 times.

Practitioner note

The purpose of the internal rotation of the arms is to work with the scapula on the ribcage positioning, maintaining the position, to activate the shoulder girdle muscles as the stabilizers with the armpits open, and to strengthen the triceps/biceps action of straightening and bending the elbow. It is crucial that the bones are in congruency with their relationship to one another as described in Chapter 6, "Shoulder and Arm Continuations."

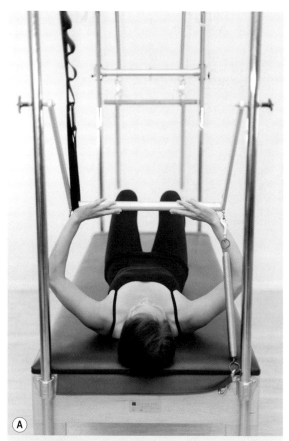

Ⓐ

Figure 7.29 A
Arm Press on Cadillac: start position

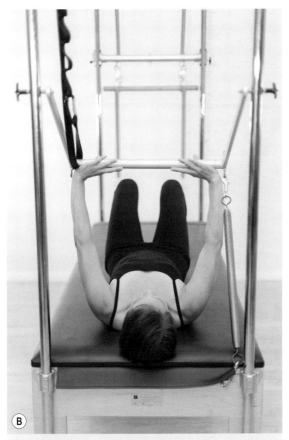

B

Figure 7.29 B
Pressing up

Arm supports on the Reformer

Performing the movements of the shoulder girdle prior to adding arm supports is helpful to activate the musculature patterning and mobility for placement of the scapula on the ribcage. Prior to arm weighted "Down Stretch," 5–8 repetitions of the "Forearm Supported Knee Stretch" in Chapter 6 is a good sequencing.

Down Stretch

"Down Stretch" is a very different exercise. Once the client has the ability to find a lifted ribcage with good scapula motion, this exercise challenges the motion of the shoulders in extension and flexion while maintaining an extended and lifted trunk. The breathing pattern is the same as that used in "Knee Stretches," which makes the sequence lovely to connect.

The proper position requires a balanced synergistic recruitment of rhomboids to serratus anterior through obliques and the back and hip extensors to achieve the placement of the ribcage with the scapulae. This is difficult to achieve if there is restriction in motion of the upper thorax, sternum, and scapulohumeral rhythm. The arms need to be able to extend without scapula motion. As the movement progresses, the scapulae will upwardly rotate to match the degree of flexion of the arms. On the return of the carriage, the scapulae move back but do not pass the placement of neutral. This maintains the training effect of the balanced synergy. This is an advanced position to be able to move into.

- Start by kneeling on the carriage, as in "Knee Stretches."

- From the quadruped position, lift the spine up and extend the hips so that the body makes a shape like the figurehead of a boat (Fig. 7.30).

- There should be a good side plumb line from the ear through the shoulder, the mid ribs, above the greater trochanter to the knee; the chest is open, clavicles wide.

- The scapulae are in a neutral position (not in adduction).

- Inhale and press out to about 60–90° of humeral flexion.

- Exhale and pull in by lifting the torso up.

> **Practitioner note**
>
> "Down Stretch" is sometimes part of the "Knee Stretch" series (p. 237) and is placed at the end of "Knee Stretch 2" to create a continuous loop of movement from "Knee Stretch 1" (neutral spine) to "Knee Stretch 2" (flexed or rounded spine) to "Down Stretch." Try repeating one movement 10 times, flowing into the second movement, repeating it 10 times, followed by "Down Stretch," 10 repetitions.

Control Front

This full body plank position is an advanced movement. Once a plank has been mastered, one challenge is the

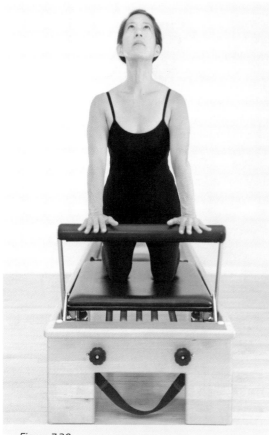

Figure 7.30
Down Stretch

- Carefully stand to the side of the Reformer and place the hands on top of the shoulder rests.

- Place one foot at a time on top of the low bar or on top of the wooden frame.

- Move into a plank position with straight arms (Fig. 7.31).

following, which adds flexion and extension motions of the arm while maintaining the plank. The hand position is different than that used for weight bearing on a flat surface. The hands are on top of the shoulder rests, with the fingers flexed. Use the action of the finger flexors to ease the wrist extension. The alignment of the wrist to shoulder is the same arrangement being practiced here. It is important to maintain the contact between the thorax and scapulae. The scapulae will glide along the ribcage as the arms flex and extend.

Set the bar up or down, depending on the level of challenge desired. The bar up position requires the feet to be perched on the metatarsals, adding a level of instability from the feet and thus requiring more trunk stability. The feet may be placed on the wood frame for more support from the feet.

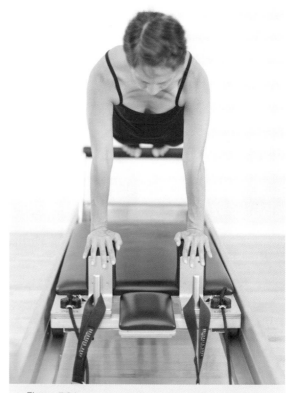

Figure 7.31
Control Front

- Align and activate the arms; be fully engaged in the body prior to moving the carriage.

- On an inhalation, press the carriage away without moving the trunk.

- On the exhalation, return the carriage to the home position.

- Repeat 5–8 times.

- Variation: standing on one leg, as in "Front Support" (p. 259) on the mat.

Side arm kneeling plank

Once the position of a side plank on the mat is established, challenge the movement by transferring it on to the Reformer. Set the Reformer with a low bar and one medium spring. Spring resistance may vary, as described above.

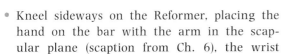

- Kneel sideways on the Reformer, placing the hand on the bar with the arm in the scapular plane (scaption from Ch. 6), the wrist aligned and the hand wrapped around the bar (Fig. 7.32).

- Lean the trunk at an angle that ensures the weight falls primarily on the knee next to the bar (if holding with the right arm then it is the right knee); the other knee is slightly lifted off the bed of the Reformer, allowing the pelvis to be level.

- Inhale and feel the side elongation.

- Exhale and press the carriage away.

- Repeat the movement 8–10 times on each side.

"Side Arm Kneeling" is a preparatory exercise for the advanced "Star" movement, which is a side arm support on one leg. Practice a side plank balancing on one leg, with the opposite leg next to the standing foot but not in contact with the mat, or with the leg lifted as in yoga pose "Vasisthasana." "Star" incorporates the pose in motion. Once in the pose of "Star," the body presses the carriage out and in. It is a moving "Vasisthasana."

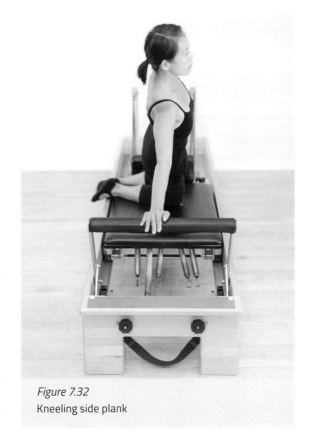

Figure 7.32
Kneeling side plank

One arm push-up on Wunda Chair

The classic one arm push-up on the Wunda Chair is performed in a plank position. The following version is done in kneeling to focus on the stability of the shoulder girdle as the arm is working. Arrange mats on the floor in front of the chair so that when the client kneels in the quadruped position the shoulders with straight arms and the pelvis are level.

> **Practitioner note**
>
> As above, the spring set-up will vary to match the client. If the bar is too heavy then it will be difficult to move with scapula and spine stability. It needs to feel just right for the client to control the bar up and down.

- Place a mat on the floor next to the bar end of the chair.

- Kneel in a quadruped position with one arm on the bar so that the arm is at 90° flexion; the arm is aligned as practiced, with fingers facing forward (Fig. 7.33 A).

- Press the bar down to start (Fig. 7.33 B).
- Check for alignment of the spine and the scapula position on the ribs.
- Allow the bar to come up, bending the elbow without changing the position of the trunk and scapula on the ribs.
- Press the bar down without a change in the trunk.
- The spine is maintaining elongation throughout the movement.

Practitioner note

Focus on the balance of work between the rhomboids and serratus anterior oblique connections.

Rotating Swan

The "Swan" is another classic Pilates extension exercise. Adding thoracic rotation using the push/pull action of the Wunda Chair serves the synergistic work of the whole spiral of the thoracic area (as described in the weave of trunk rotation in Ch. 4, "Superficial and Deep"). In addition, training the arm connection into

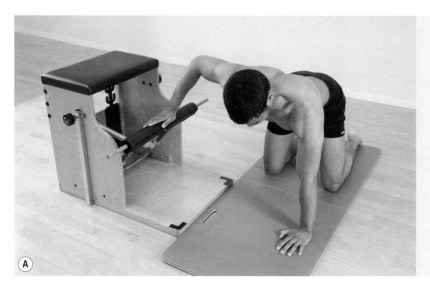

Figure 7.33 A
Wunda Chair one arm push-up: start position

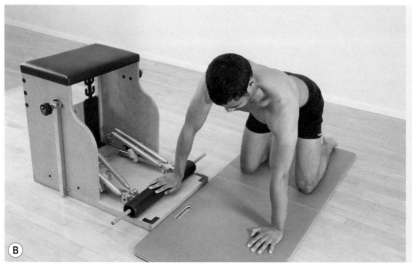

Figure 7.33 B
Pressing bar down

the spine with the scapula stability/mobility concepts blends all of the movement into an integrated whole.

- Wunda Chair set-up: the bar is weighted with one spring on each side in a middle place; the resistance should be the same and just sufficient to facilitate the rotational movement; too much resistance will not allow the client to work correctly.

- Lie prone, placing the pelvis on top of the chair with the navel at the edge; the hands are on the bar; the spine is long and neutral; the bar is not touching the bottom. To assist in stability of the legs, place the chair against the Cadillac so the client can lie on the table, or near a wall, to place the feet.

- The practitioner stands to the side of the client (or at certain times at the head).

- First perform three Swans with no rotation to warm up the extensors.

- Inhale and feel elongation and proper form.

- Exhale to lower the bar as the spine moves into flexion.

- Inhale and lift the spine into extension as the bar moves up.

- Repeat 3 times.

- To add rotation, pull the dowel out to split the bar; on an inhale, press the right arm down and elevate the left slightly as the spine rotates to the left; the arms remain straight throughout the movement (Fig. 7.34).

- Exhale and return the spine to neutral.

- Repeat on other side.

Practitioner note

The arms are actively pressing one bar down, and at the same time resisting the bar pressing up into the body. It is a push and resist feel. The rotation is occurring in thorax and not transferring into the lower spine and pelvis. The pelvis remains in firm contact with the chair.

Practitioner note
Hands-on

- Stand at the head of the client.

- Cue a small rib ring translation in the opposite direction of the rotation, i.e. translate left to rotate right.

- Hold the sides of the ribcage at about T6 to guide the translation and rotation (Fig. 7.35).

- Observe for the length at the sides of the body.

- If one side shortens into side bending, the translation is lacking. Encourage the side to lengthen by an elongating cue, with the hands providing a light traction.

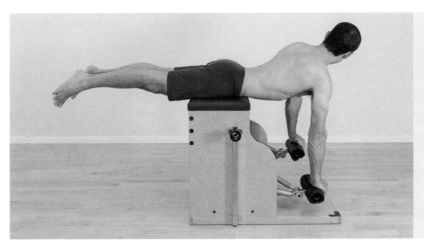

Figure 7.34
Swan on Wunda Chair in rotation

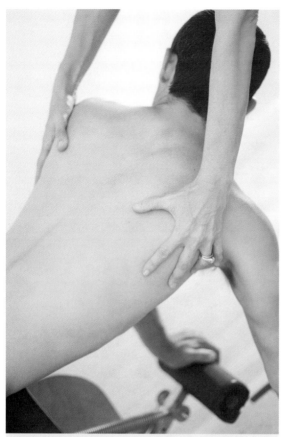

Figure 7.35
Hands-on Swan on Wunda Chair

Swan movement in all planes

- Move the spine in a circular way from a rotation left, pressing down into spinal flexion (bar handles are now level at the bottom) with the thorax in flexion.

- Press the left arm down as the right elevates, rotating the spine to the right; lift the spine into extension as the bar levels out in the up position.

- Repeat 2–3 times then change direction.

Bridging to Chapter 8

The thoracolumbar fascia, connecting from the back around the trunk and arms, along with the pectoralis fascia continuum with the abdominal and brachial fascia, is the root system for movements of the upper trunk, arms, and head. Developing strong pathways from the center of the trunk into the arms and head provides freedom of movement with strength. The expressive upper part of the body connects with the world by communicating, giving, and receiving. The neck moves the head so we can perceive the environment around us, respond to the senses, and nourish the body.

Movement of the head and neck

> *"Our heads are round so that our thinking can change directions."*
>
> Francis Picabia (1879–1953), in *I Am a Beautiful Monster: Poetry Prose, and Provocation*

Contemplative awareness: communication without words

The neck moves the head, tilting it softly when leaning in to listen or aggressively moving the face forward to "be in someone's face." Humans express themselves through communication, touch, and body movement. The expression is interpreted by seeing, feeling and sensing, and the movement and positioning of the head are instrumental in signaling a variety of messages to others. How we move and hold ourselves, both consciously and unconsciously, is communication without words. Both verbal and nonverbal messages are expressed through the face, head, and neck.

Most of our primary sense organs are located in the head. Responses to stimuli from the eyes, ears, mouth, and nose drive the movements of the head and neck, stimulating motion throughout the body. The neck synergistically works with the eyes to maximize our field of vision, increase spatial awareness, and present the face for expression. Neck muscles play a role in our facial expression through movement of the head and connections to the jaw. The neck and muscles of the face contribute to the functions of our senses and jaw tension, speech, and breathing. It is hardly surprising that neck muscles are constantly at work. In dysfunction, tension or stiffness in the neck causes pain and discomfort for many and affects the ability to live with a sense of vitality.

Gravity and the head

Gravity plays a significant role in the stabilization and balancing of the head. As a counterbalance to the forces of gravity, the neck muscles are in tension most of the time. Gravity will pull the head forward and increase cervical lordosis (Mayoux-Benhamou et al., 1992). The center of gravity for the head is situated near the sella turcica, a saddle-shaped depression in the skull that houses the pituitary gland, and the fulcrum of the head is just in front of the occipital condyles (Fig. 8.1). The posterior neck muscles

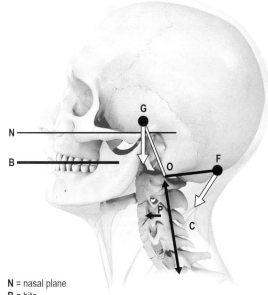

N = nasal plane
B = bite
O = fulcrum of occipital condyles
G = weight of head through center of gravity
F = force produced by posterior neck muscles
C = concave cervical column
P = perpendicular midpoint

Figure 8.1
Balancing of the head on cervical column

produce the force to counterbalance the head. The anterior and posterior neck muscles act synergistically with one another, depending on the neck–head position, to produce an anterior–posterior stabilization. There are different patterns of neck muscle activities due to the bone and ligamentous motion available, postural alignment of the head, spine, and neural control. For example, when the head moves backwards, the posterior cervical muscles become less active whereas the anterior cervical muscles are maintaining the head position. As the head moves forward, it elongates and engages (eccentrically) the posterior cervical muscles, especially the upper trapezius, and prevents the head from falling. At the same time, the anterior cervical muscles (especially the longus colli) are acting to maintain the cervical curve. The cervical spine and its joints, ligaments, and myofascia all contribute to head and neck movement.

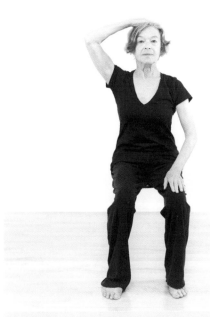

Figure 8.2
Elongation of spine

Try it!

Sit in an elongated spine position; place one hand on the crown of the head and simply press the crown up into the hand (Fig. 8.2). Practicing "Elongation: Narrowing of the Body" from Chapter 4 along with this upward movement of the crown places the head in a better place. Feel the neck muscles change tension:

- Interlace the fingers and place the hands behind the head at the occiput.

- Move the head behind the vertical axis, looking up with a minimal O/A extension (chin dropped with the top of the head back) (Fig. 8.3).

- Hold the position for three slow breaths, relax the upper shoulders, and rest the head in the hands.

- Return to the upright position; repeat 3–4 times.

- Notice what you feel (possibly less tension in the upper trapezius or tone change in the front of the neck).

Practitioner note

Practicing the "Head Float" exercise from Chapter 4 activates the deep anterior cervical muscles prior to curling the head off the mat.

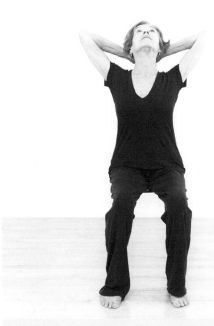

Figure 8.3
Head behind vertical axis

Characteristics and movements of the cervical spine

The cervical spine has two regions that are anatomically and functionally varied. The upper part, the suboccipital segment, is made up of the articulation of the occiput on the first cervical spine, the atlas (C1) and the axis (C2). The inferior segment is the remainder of the cervical spine, C3 to the top surface of T1. The vertebrae overlie one another in an oblique way, downwards and backwards, supported by the body of the vertebra. The planes of the facet joint angles change slightly, C2–C3 having 40–45° compared to C7–T1 with 10° (Kapandji, 1974), following the normal lordotic curve (Fig. 8.4). The cervical spine has no neutral position due to its lordotoc curve.

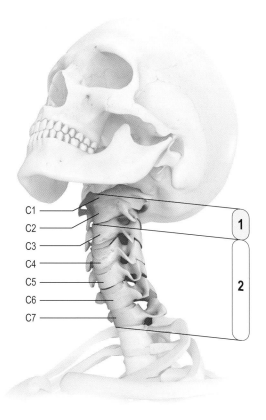

Figure 8.4
Bones of the head and neck

C1
C2
C3
C4
C5
C6
C7

1

2

Practitioner note

The articular facets (also known as the zygapophysial joints) are synovial joints that lie between the superior articular process of one vertebra and the inferior articular process of the vertebra above it. The articular facets are flat and oval shaped. The superior facets face backward, upward, and slightly medial. The inferior ones face forward, downward, and slightly lateral.

An upper vertebra can only move relative to the lower one. The movement passes from the lower to the upper cervical in a cumulative way. Imagine links of a chain where one link, when moved, will translate the motion through the following links. The structure of the cervical vertebra and the ligament system limits pure rotation and lateral flexion but produces combined movements of rotation and lateral flexion with an element of extension.

The two regions of the cervical spine are functionally complementary and rely on the compensatory movements. When looking sideways and up, the motion moves up from the base of the column. In the lower column, the side bending is a combination of lateral flexion and rotation. As it moves up the vertebrae chain to the suboccipital segment, the motion changes into nearly pure lateral flexion. The dance between the segments is a compensation of the suboccipital segment for the combined movements of the lower column. The mechanism of the suboccipital segment eliminates unwanted movements, maintaining the vertebral centers of movement stacked so that the eyes remain horizontal for balance and better vision. Starting at the base of the column, these centers of movement move upwards and forwards, following the contour of the normal cervical lordosis (see Fig. 8.4).

Architecture and movements of the suboccipital region

The suboccipital segment is a complex of three axes and three degrees of freedom. The unique shape of the occiput, C1, and C2 allows for almost pure rotation or lateral flexion. The occiput glides on the rocker-shaped facets of C1. Imagine a sphere gliding on the articular surfaces of the atlas (C1). The shape of the surface is oblique and lower at the back. The axis (C2) has a bony protuberance or peg (the odontoid process or dens) that rises perpendicularly from the upper rim of the bone. The odontoid joint (dens) articulates with the atlas and acts as a pivot for the atlantoaxial joint that holds the head. There are three mechanical links of the atlas and axis, the atlanto-odontoid joint and two lateral joints, the atlantoaxial joints. The combined motions of all three act like a swivel joint (Fig. 8.5).

Flexion and extension of suboccipital segment

Flexion or nodding of the head occurs as both sides of the occiput move together, sliding posteriorly and opening the space between the posterior occiput–atlas and then atlas–axis (Fig. 8.6 A). Flexion is limited by the articular capsule of the facet of the atlas, and the tension created by stretching the posterior ligaments, the posterior atlanto-occipital membrane, and nuchal ligament. In extension, the ring of the atlas becomes closer to the occiput as the occiput slides anteriorly and approximates the spinous processes of atlas and axis. The impact of the three bones limits the movement of extension (Fig. 8.6 B).

Rotation and lateral flexion of the suboccipital segment

In rotation, one side glides forward as the other side glides back. Due to the shape of the facet, the forward movement will rise up and the backward one sink down, creating a tilt in the vertebrae. The rotation is not in a pure transverse plane. It is as if it were moving on a slant. When the occiput rotates to the left, the left side moves back and sinks down as the right side moves forward and uphill. And the lateral atlanto-occipital ligament will cause the occiput to slide and left translate, causing a small right rotation (DiGiovanna et al., 2005). Rotating and side bending at the O/A joint occurs in the opposite direction to the other segments of the cervical spine. This slight displacement of the occiput is maintaining the foramen magnum over the center of the vertebral canal. Any rotation at the occiput is secondary to the rotation occurring at the axis (C2), with the center of the rotation at the dens (see Fig. 8.5). The atlantoaxial joint (C1 and C2) is the "real" axis for nearly pure rotation.

The alar ligaments, two bands from each side of the tip of the dens to the inner sides of the occiput,

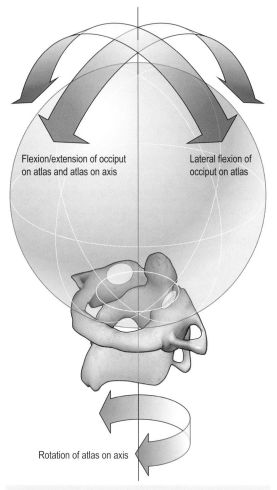

Flexion/extension of occiput on atlas and atlas on axis

Lateral flexion of occiput on atlas

Rotation of atlas on axis

Figure 8.5
Occiput C1 and C2; swivel joint of O/A, C1 and C2

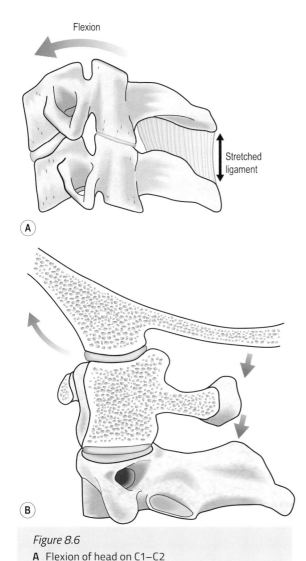

Flexion

Stretched
ligament

A

B

Figure 8.6
A Flexion of head on C1–C2
B Extension

the left transverse process will rise. The atlas has considerable motion, and it is possible for the atlas to be stuck or locked in a rotation. A rotated atlas will position the head in a slight side bend, which can be seen by comparing the levels of the zygomatic arches (cheekbones).

The combined motion of the suboccipital segment is a helical or spiral motion and functions as a swivel joint. Moving the suboccipital segment in the combined movement of a horizontal figure eight helps ease the holding of the head in a tilt.

This suboccipital articulation is a place where the body adjusts and compensates for dysfunctions occurring below. The reason is the righting reflex of the head, to maintain the eyes level for better vision. Some somatic practices consider this articulation as the key to unlocking dysfunctional issues throughout the rest of the body. Freeing up the movement in this area certainly helps to achieve change in tissue tension as far away as the sacrum.

> **Try it!**
>
> - Find the atlantoaxial joint by palpating the occiput where it meets the spine.
>
> - Feel the condyles of the occiput, behind the ears, and follow the lowest part of the occiput to the center.
>
> - Then palpate the center of the occiput and begin to slide the fingers down along the center of the cervical spine.
>
> - Almost immediately, feel the first prominent bone, the spinous process of C2.
>
> - Move above the spinous process into the space just below the occiput.
>
> - Follow the bones laterally to the side of the neck before the sternocleidomastoid (SCM) attachment at the occipital condyle.
>
> - Visualize (use the movie image for clear palpation in Ch. 7) the fingers over the transverse processes (though feeling them is considered very difficult).

restrain lateral flexion of the axis (C2). This causes the axis (C2) to rotate toward the side of lateral flexion. The four facets that articulate at the atlas and axis (the superior facets of the axis and the inferior facets of the atlas) are convex, producing a wobbling motion. During rotation of the axis on the atlas a swing is created of the atlas to the opposite side of the rotation. It can be felt with the hands at the transverse processes of C1 as a rise up of the axis on the opposite side of the rotation. If rotating to the right,

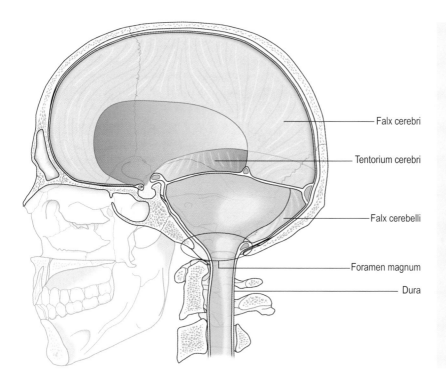

Figure 8.7
Dura mater

Falx cerebri

Tentorium cerebri

Falx cerebelli

Foramen magnum

Dura

- Hold the fingers in this position and with the hands move the bones in a rotation.

- Move the bones in a horizontal figure eight.

- The motion is only at the suboccipital level.

- The helical micromovement allows for freeing up unconscious holding of this area.

Combined movements

(Kapandji, 1974)

- Flexion of the head and neck involves:

  - full flexion of atlanto-occipital joint (sphere rolling back on atlas)

Practitioner note

There is a connective tissue bridge between the dorsal spinal dura at the occiput and C1 with the rectus capitis posterior minor, a suboccipital muscle (Zumpano et al., 2006). The dura mater is a thick inelastic fibrous membrane surrounding the brain and spinal cord, keeping in the cerebrospinal fluid; it adheres to the periosteum of the inner cranial bone (Gray, 2012). It has an internal architecture consisting of three folds of the dura mater, one running from back to front (falx

cerebri) that resembles a sickle and one on each side of the falx (tentorium cerebelli), also running from back to front parallel to the floor (if the head is upright standing straight). The dura attaches to the foramen magnum and upper cervical vertebrae. It surrounds the spinal cord and descends to attach to the sacrum at the second sacral segment (Fig. 8.7). The release of the upper cervical segment and suboccipital movement helps release tension and restores flow throughout the spine from the head to sacrum.

- flexion of the atlas on the dens
- full flexion of all the lower cervical vertebrae.
- Extension of the head and neck involves:
  - extension of the atlanto-occipital joint (sphere rolling forward)
  - extension of the atlas on the axis
  - extension of all the lower cervical vertebrae.
- Rotation of the head and neck involves:
  - rotation of the atlanto-occipital joint to the same side
  - side bending of the atlanto-occipital joint to the opposite side
  - rotation of the axis on the atlas to the same side
  - all lower vertebrae in rotation, side bending (lateral flexion) to the same side and extension.
- Side bending involves:
  - lateral flexion of atlanto-occipital joint
  - rotation of the atlantoaxial joint to the opposite side
  - both rotation and lateral flexion, slight flexion at the atlanto-occipital joint to compensate for the extension in the lower cervical column.

Architecture and movement of the lower cervical spine

This segment of the cervical spine adapts to the mobility and stability required for the great range of motion of the neck. In a normal cervical lordosis, the facet joints of C3–C7 face midway between the horizontal (rotation) and frontal (lateral rotation) planes. In the neck, rotation is always coupled with lateral flexion with a small amount of extension (Kapandji, 1974). When the head is tilted back, the facets are more orientated in the frontal plane, so therefore side bending is the primary movement. Forward bending of the head brings the facets into the horizontal plane allowing for rotation as the major motion.

> **Try it!**
>
> Sit upright with an elongated spine and the head on top. Bring the head behind the central axis, then look up at the ceiling, bringing the cervical spine into extension. Try to rotate the neck, followed by side bending of the neck. Notice which direction has more ease. Nod the chin and roll the head forward, in front of the central axis; try both movements again.

Flexion and extension of the lower cervical column

The head moving forward (to look down) is cervical flexion and backward (to look up) is cervical extension. However, the motion at the level of the vertebrae is not simply flexion and extension. Due to the complexity of the architecture of the cervical spine and its combined movements, a single vertebra may move in a greater range in one direction while the whole column exhibits movement in another direction.

During movements of both flexion and extension, the overlying vertebral body tilts and slides, compressing the intervertebral disc. In extension, the tilt and slide occurs posteriorly with the facets gliding inferior, widening the interspace between the bodies anteriorly. The superior articular facet closes by sliding inferiorly and posteriorly. The intervertebral space is compressed posteriorly, driving the nucleus pulposus slightly anterior and stretching the anterior fibers of the annulus. The facet joints are approximating and this congruency makes for a very stable position (see Fig. 8.6). The extension movement of the bone is limited by the tension in the anterior longitudinal ligament being stretched, and the impact of the posterior bony surfaces moving together.

During flexion, the reverse happens; here the tilt and slide is anterior and the interspace between the articular facets opens posteriorly. The facets glide superiorly and the ligaments of the joint capsule become taut, making the joint less stable. The top vertebra's lower plateau slides past the superior plateau of the lower vertebra due to the plateau's shape. The nucleus of the disc is driven posteriorly, stretching the posterior fibers of the annulus. Flexion is not limited by bony impact but the tension in the posterior longitudinal ligament, the capsular ligaments, ligamenta flava, interspinous septa, ligamentum nuchae, and posterior cervical ligament (see Fig. 8.6). In full flexion the neck is less stable and requires muscle action for support of the structure.

Practitioner note

It has been found that during whiplash, in the the timing of compressive forces, the movement begins at the hips and trunk as the body moves forward in an upward thrust, compressing the spine. Thus the thrust extends the head back, creating a buckling effect. After extension, there is compensatory flexion, hence whiplash. An abnormal extension occurs in the individual vertebrae, causing compression of the posterior components, especially at the facets. Fractures here have been noticed in cadavers as well as in living patients after motor vehicle accidents.

Uncovertebral Joints

Two small additional joints, the uncovertebral joints (also known as joints of von Luschka), located at the lateral edge of vertebral bodies C3–C7, are synovial joints continuous with the intervertebral disc. During flexion and extension, the uncovertebral joints guide the movement of one vertebral body relative to the other in the anterior and posterior directions. These specialized joints primarily prevent a sideways slipping of the vertebral body in rotation and lateral flexion (DiGiovanna et al., 2005). During side bending and rotation of one vertebra on another, there is a lateral translatory motion away from the direction of side bending. When the spine rotates and side bends to the right there will be a left lateral translatory motion (Fig. 8.8). Without the uncoverterbal joints, the vertebral body would slip laterally (a subluxation of the joint). These additional joints help maintain the balance of stability with mobility needed for the complex movements of the neck.

Better alignment, movement adaptability, and proper muscle activations of the cervical spine are necessary for long-term health of the neck. Lack of integrity and healthy support may cause instability of the cervical spine. Along with instability, other conditions, such

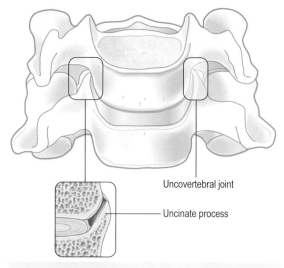

Uncovertebral joint

Uncinate process

Figure 8.8
Uncovertebral joints

as bone loss, disc degeneration, osteoarthritis, and other spinal issues, cause osteophytes or bone spurs to develop. The body is constantly naturally fortifying the spine by laying down more bone. In the cervical spine, bone spurs tend to develop at the uncovertebral joints. The channels where the nerve roots exit (foramina) are located at the uncovertebral joints. When a bone spur grows in the confined space near a foramen, it causes a compression of the nerves, or possibly the spinal cord. Foraminal stenosis is a condition characterized by narrowing of the foramina caused by bone spurs at the uncovertebral joints (and there are other causes for this condition). Head and neck positioning, stability, and mobility balance are important throughout life to ensure healthy necks.

When the cervical spine is positioned well, with its slight lordosis and balanced head, there is a good passive stability from the facet joints and supporting ligaments. The passive stability is able to bear approximately one third of compressive forces of the spine. If the cervical lordosis is excessive or the cervical curve is reversed, the passive stability is lost. The segmental muscles of the cervical spine go into constant contraction to stabilize the spine and the compressive forces are now borne by the discs, causing flattening and excessive pressure in addition to the potential of osteophytes developing.

Lateral flexion and rotation of the lower column

As stated above, the structure of the cervical spine innately produces the coupled movement of lateral flexion–rotation–extension. The orientation of the facets changes the angles from more horizontal 10° at C7–T1 to 45° at C3. The more horizontal facets at C7–T1 allow for nearly pure rotation. Higher up the chain, the 45° angle produces almost equal amounts of lateral flexion and rotation. The coupled movements are more significant as the motion passes from the lower vertebrae to the next.

The lower column is harnessed with a myofascial network to support the composite movement. The network weave of connective tissues runs an oblique course posteriorly, laterally, and inferiorly. The suboccipital segment is controlled by smaller fine-tuning muscles and the facial network. The fine-tuning ability is made possible by the synergistic–antagonist action that eliminates unwanted movements of the head deriving from the lower column.

Myofascial network for movement and support

The neck fascia has its layers and continuum with the fascia of the rest of the body. In Chapter 4, the section "Superficial and Deep" describes the whole body connection of the myofascial system with movement directions. Refer to that section to link the cervical muscles with the layers of the neck and its connections to the layers of the trunk.

Layers of cervical fascia and muscles

Fascial divisions of the neck (Fig. 8.9):

- superficial: fascia colli superficialis
- middle: fascia colli media
- deep: fascia colli profunda.

Superficial

The superficial fascia runs around the neck 360° and is situated below the skin. It runs from the mandible to the sternal notch and manubrium sterni where it is now called the pectoral fascia. Its wide spread covers the clavicles and extends to the shoulder (acromioclavicular or AC joint) and down the arm. It lies under the cover of the platysma and encloses the SCM, which glides freely in its covering. During respiration, the rise and fall of the sternum alters the fascia length as it moves with the breath. Follow the fascia at the AC joint over the posterior cervical triangle and upwards, continuing to the upper trapezius muscle as it wraps around and up to the mastoid process. It reaches as high as the superior nuchal line.

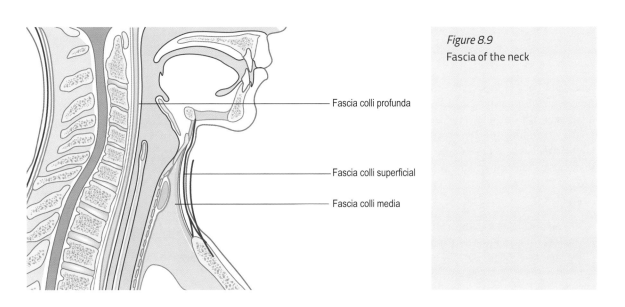

Figure 8.9
Fascia of the neck

Fascia colli profunda

Fascia colli superficial

Fascia colli media

Practitioner note

The platysma is a superficial muscle lying close to the skin. It extends from the lower neck and upper chest to the lower border of the jaw, lower face and mouth. It depresses and wrinkles the skin in an oblique direction of the lower face and mouth. An expression of melancholy or grimacing contracts the platysma.

Middle

The middle layer of cervical fascia envelops the "strap" muscles, which are the muscles attached to the hyoid bone (sternohyoid, sternothyroid, omohyoid) (Fig. 8.10). It is only found anteriorly and laterally on the neck. It starts at below the hyoid at the infrahyoid muscles and inserts into the posterior edge of the clavicle, scalene tubercle, and posterior sternum. It ties into the subclavius fascia, continues with the clavipectoral fascia, and on into the axillary fascia down the arm (refer to Ch. 6, "Shoulder and Arm Continuations"). This layer forms the carotid sheath, surrounds the large veins of the neck, and gives traction to the jugular vein, keeping it open. The mobility of this layer is important to venous drainage of the neck.

Practitioner note

Use the exercises in Chapter 6 for the shoulder area, specifically the "Pectoralis Fascial Stretch" and "Side Lying Ribcage Arms" followed up with a home program using the self-release "MET in Doorway" to improve the hydration and gliding of the cervical fascial layers.

Hyoid bone

The hyoid bone is suspended in the middle layer of the fascia, with its muscle attachments from above. Superiorly, the muscles run from the floor of the mouth, including the tongue. Another suspension point is an anchoring from ligaments from the styloid processes of the temporal bones.

Try it!

Find the hyoid bone. It is in front of C3 and above the larynx. Make a U shape with the thumb and index finger of the same hand. Gently place the fingers over the hyoid bone. Place the other hand on the back of the cervical spine. Swallow and feel for the movement of the bone. Wiggle the bone in a small side to side range to feel the sides of the bone. Notice if one side feels more prominent than the other. It may indicate the suspended bone is rotated. Since it is suspended, there are many possibilities for what has caused the rotation. Now try moving the hyoid bone forward and down, then back and up on an oblique angle toward the ears. Feel for the movement and position of the head and neck in both directions. Try rotating the neck, thinking of turning your head. Next focus on the hyoid and turn the neck from the hyoid. The motion changes in the cervical spine. Feel the difference in the quality of movement. There is more freedom to move the neck when the intention is placed on moving from the hyoid bone.

Hyoid movement for neck and head alignment

Hyoid bone for head balancing
VIDEO LINK V 8.1

A head forward mouth breather exhibits a forward and down position of the hyoid bone (Fig. 8.11 A). Moving the hyoid bone posteriorly and superiorly balances the head on top (Fig. 8.11 B). First practice by manually moving it, then use it as movement imagery; focus on the hyoid movement to elongate and balance the head on the neck. Practicing this motion, followed by holding the placement, gives a felt sense of where the head and neck balance in relation to gravity. It releases the unwanted tension of the neck muscles and allows for easier breathing. Clients with chronic neck tension find relief in this movement.

Tip

Cue a curl-up from the supine position beginning with the hyoid bone:

- "On an inhale, elongate the spine through the crown of the head" and

- "Think of unweighting the head" (Ch. 4, "Head Float").

- "Exhale and imagine the hyoid bone sliding back on a diagonal up toward the ears."

- "Sink the base of the neck into the floor as the head floats off the floor as the sternum softens."

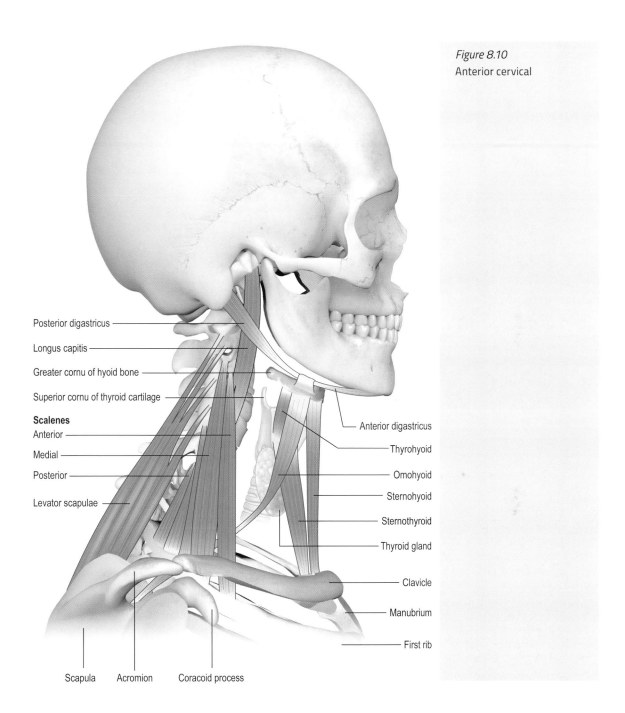

Figure 8.10
Anterior cervical

Posterior digastricus

Longus capitis

Greater cornu of hyoid bone

Superior cornu of thyroid cartilage

Scalenes
Anterior

Medial

Posterior

Levator scapulae

Scapula   Acromion   Coracoid process

Anterior digastricus

Thyrohyoid

Omohyoid

Sternohyoid

Sternothyroid

Thyroid gland

Clavicle

Manubrium

First rib

Deep or prevertebral fascia

The deep fascia is a continuation of the endothoracic fascia, transversalis, and pelvic fascia (Ch. 5, "Fascial Continuum" and "Three Diaphragms"). It is fixed to the base of the skull, the anterior ligament of the cervical spine, with a strong attachment to the scalene tubercle. The deep fascia surrounds the vertebrae, the deep anterior and lateral cervical muscles, and the brachial plexus. It ties into the endothoracic fascia and contributes to the attachment of the pleural domes of the lungs (Breul, 2012) (see Fig. 5.2).

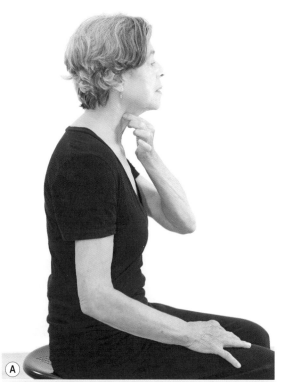

Figure 8.11 A
Head position with hyoid forward

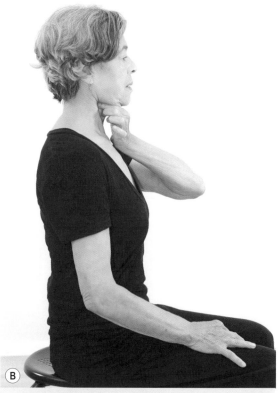

Figure 8.11 B
Hyoid in place

Practitioner note

The pleural dome is suspended by the costo-pleuro-vertebral ligament, which is attached to the first rib and to the transverse processes of C6 and C7. Another suspensory ligament of the lung connects the apex of the dome to the middle scalene muscle (Barral and Mercier, 2007). The heart in its fascial covering (the pericardial sac) is suspended within the thorax by the ligaments attaching C7–T4 and underneath the sternum. Stiffness or pain in the low cervical or mid thorax may be produced by strain in this deep fascial area (Barral and Mercier, 2007).

The light side of these attachments is cueing movement through the organs:

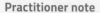

- For flexion:

- "Soften your heart"
- "Let your heart drop back as the head curls up"
- "Exhale and feel the lungs folding in toward the heart as the clavicles stay wide".

● For extension:

- "Lift the heart up and forward"
- "Feel the lungs unfolding away from the heart"
- " Inhale and fill the domes of the lungs as you look up".

● For side bending (from the lungs and heart, one can also cue all the abdominal area organs as well):

- "Bending to the right, inhale into the left lung"
- "Side bend around the heart".

● For twisting:

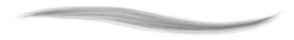

- Rotate to the right: "breathe into the left lung as the torso turns to the right"

- "Rotate around the heart".

- Play with initiating movement from all the organs. It places the intention to the deeper structures of the body and has a quality change to the body's ability to move without locking down.

Patterns and synergistic–antagonistic muscle relationships

There are more muscles in the back of the neck than in the front. Acting synergistically, the posterior muscles hold up the head and the anterior muscles support the curve. The lateral muscles maintain the head in the center. Imagine a telephone pole as a neck and the guy wires are the lateral muscles. The connections of the muscles of the middle cervical fascia inhibit not only shoulder girdle muscles but also the deep neck flexors of the deep fascial layer. A typical pattern of head forward posture (especially today, with so much time spent looking down at mobile devices) is overworking the posterior neck muscles and inhibiting the anterior neck muscles.

The following are the posterior neck muscles that extend the cervical spine and head, divided into three groups:

1. Arising from the thorax, running obliquely to the transverse processes (Fig. 8.12 A):
   a. splenius cervicis
   b. semispinalis cervicis
   c. longissimus cervicis
   d. iliocostalis cervicis
   e. levator scapulae.

2. Fibers running obliquely inferiorly and anteriorly (Fig. 8.12 B):
   a. on lower cervical column: transversospinalis (rotatores and multifidus)
   b. occiput to lower cervical: longissimus capitis, splenius capitis, semispinalis capitis.

3. All the muscles that bridge the cervical column connecting the occiput to the scapula (Fig. 8.12 C):
   a. trapezius
   b. sternocleidomastoid.

Unique synergy

Two common muscles that are in constant tension, sometimes causing discomfort and compression in the neck, are the upper trapezius and the SCM

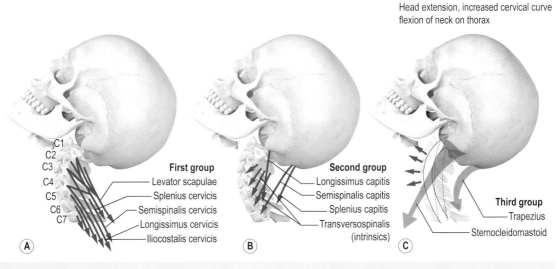

Head extension, increased cervical curve flexion of neck on thorax

First group
— Levator scapulae
— Splenius cervicis
— Semispinalis cervicis
— Longissimus cervicis
— Iliocostalis cervicis

Second group
— Longissimus capitis
— Semispinalis capitis
— Splenius capitis
— Transversospinalis (intrinsics)

Third group
— Trapezius
— Sternocleidomastoid

C1
C2
C3
C4
C5
C6
C7

(A) (B) (C)

Figure 8.12
A Three groups of neck extensors: group 1
B Group 2
C Group 3

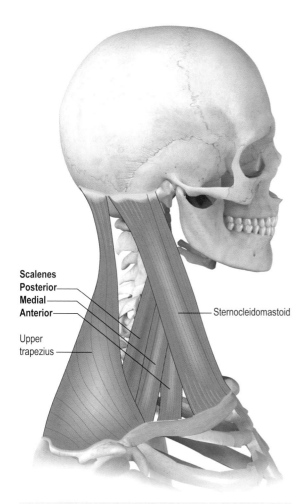

Scalenes
Posterior
Medial
Anterior

Sternocleidomastoid

Upper
trapezius

Figure 8.13
Synergy of SCM and upper trapezius

The SCM shortens with increased activity that compresses the cervical spine. This occurs frequently when performing a curl-up on the mat (flexion of the spine starting with the head lifting). The sequential movement from the top of the head through the cervical spine prevents the shortening of the SCM. If the movement of the head lifting off the floor is performed without the sequential movement of the atlanto-occiput flexion (the nod), flexion of the lower column, and combined with the cumulative movement of the cervical and sternal motion, then the increased tension of the SCM and upper trapezius causes stress in the neck. The increased tension then inhibits the support of the front of the neck via the engagement of the anterior cervical muscles. Head movement and positioning are important to facilitate proper muscle patterning for strength of the neck into the core. This habitual pattern of lifting the head off the floor creates restrictions of the SCM and prolonged shortening of the muscle. Releasing the SCM, strengthening the anterior cervical muscles, and practicing the movement pattern of cervical motion sequencing prior to holding the head up for longer periods of time is a healthy approach to re-patterning the neck. (See below for re-patterning movements.)

The SCM within the superficial fascia is a continuation of the pectoral fascia into the abdominal fascia.

(sternocleidomastoid) (Fig. 8.13). These muscles work synergistically along with the rectus capitis lateralis, superior, oblique and the splenius capitis in side bending of the head. (In Ch. 3, "Lateral Bending of the Trunk" describes the whole body network for side bending.) If the head is balanced over its center of gravity, these muscles have a normal resting length of support. When the head is forward of the axial center, then the upper trapezius is elongated while contracting and the SCM is shortening, pulling the mastoid (back of the ear), its attachment, toward the sternum. The SCM extends the head on the occiput, flexes the cervical column on the thorax, and extends the cervical column on itself, heightening the cervical lordosis.

In addition to learning how to move the head and neck, the release of the fascial areas related to the neck, the pectoral and clavipectoral fascia, will further assist the head to find its balance. Chapter 4's "Release Techniques for the Trunk" gives ways to restore the glide to the fascia of the trunk.

Self fascial movement for SCM

- Start by sitting in an elongated position looking forward.
- If this is the first time, looking in a mirror will help see the SCM.
- Feel for the "meat" of the SCM by placing the pad of the thumb on the back edge of the SCM, half way down, where the muscle is thick, and the inner edge of a flexed index finger on the front side of the muscle (a pincer grasp) (Fig. 8.14 A).

- Gently squeeze the muscle and follow it through its entire length.
- Start at the top of the left side muscle near the ear and hold it firmly (do not squeeze but hold firmly).
- Slowly turn the head on easy exhale to the right as the index finger is moving the muscle away from the direction of the turning (Fig. 8.14 B).
- Repeat this for the entire length of the muscle.
- The muscle may flip out of the hold if the grasp is too tight, or the hold is only on the top of the muscle, or if the fascia is stuck to the other layer.
- Move in a range feeling the muscle gliding away (it may be small at first).
- Repeat on the other side.

Deep cervical muscles

The prevertebral level of the neck is the deepest and most profound area. The anterior and lateral muscles, when active, support the neck and decrease the

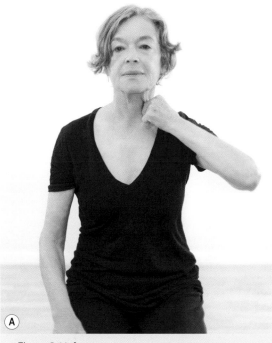

(A)

Figure 8.14 A
Self-release of SCM: start position

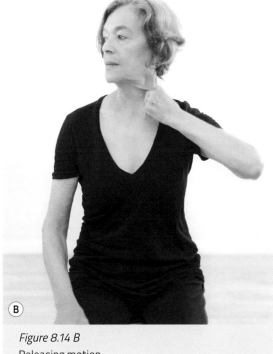

(B)

Figure 8.14 B
Releasing motion

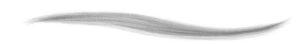

fatigue of the posterior muscles. The anterior cervical muscles are active when we reach the crown of the head up (elongation), roll the head prior to curling the head (supine flexion of head), or move the head behind the center of gravity (extension).

The following are the anterior cervical muscles for support of the neck (Fig. 8.15):

- longus capitis
- longus colli (primary)
- rectus capitis anterior.

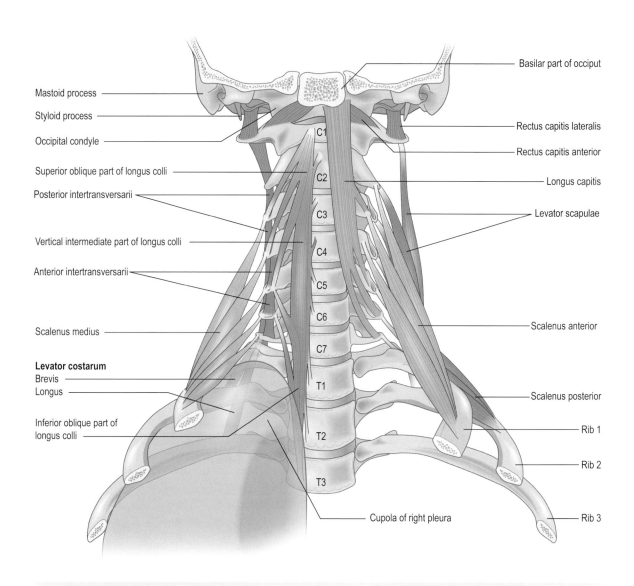

Figure 8.15
Deep cervical muscles

Muscles for flexion of the head on the cervical column and the neck on the thoracic column are:

* rectus capitis anterior for atlanto-occiput flexion

* longus colli and rectus capitis anterior at lower vertebral column

* suprahyoid muscles (mylohyoid, anterior digastric)

* infrahyoid muscles (see Fig. 8.10)

* hence the effectiveness of the hyoid bone cueing for neck flexion.

Scalene muscles (anterior, middle, and posterior scalenes) may be seen as the cranial continuation of the intercostal muscles with attachment at the first and second ribs and the cervical column (see Fig. 8.13). In breathing, the scalenes assist the intercostal muscles in the pump handle motion of the first two ribs. They lift the first and second rib upward in the front. In movement, a unilateral contraction creates a lateral bending of the cervical column to one side. The brachial plexus passes between the anterior and middle scalenes under the clavicle, pectoralis minor, and into the arm. Sustained tension or alignment dysfunction of the lateral neck causes an impingement of the plexus along with the circulatory and lymphatic vessels. It is a critical area to maintain ease and movement of the arm and cervical spine.

Fine-tuning muscles of the nape of the neck

The suboccipital muscles deep to the upper trapezius at the base of the head are considered the fine-tuning muscles vital for head positioning. These muscles are also responsible for righting the head, adapting for the three planar motions of the lower cervical column and working with the fast phasic head movements such as orienting to gaze shifts (Fig. 8.16). They are:

* rectus capitis posterior major

* rectus capitis posterior minor

* obliquus capitis posterior

* obliquus capitis superior.

> **Practitioner note**
>
> The superficial neck muscles have fast twitch muscle fibers (fast glycolytic), which are good for speed but fatigue easily. The deeper muscles have the fast oxidative glycolytic and slow oxidative fibers. The slow twitch fibers are the postural muscles with great resistance to fatigue. If a client is using more of the superficial neck muscles, such as the upper trapezius and SCM, these muscles fatigue easily, causing tension and pain. Teaching clients to move from the deeper muscles to support the spine and control fine movements in a balance with the superficial muscles is a recipe for happy necks.

Other short muscles of back of the neck

Primarily these muscles act as the postural muscles of the neck. They participate in the motion of the column. The multifidus and interspinales produce extension, whereas the multifidus along with the intertransversarii move in lateral flexion. When the multifidus partners with the rotatores, rotation occurs (see Fig. 8.16).

Activating the postural muscles in movement improves the whole movement pattern of the body (see "Common Patterns" below). Whether working with an issue or preparing for moving with greater range and resistance, waking up the postural muscles allows the body to tune as a whole organism.

Preferential movement through the movement of the eyes

An interaction of eye–head–trunk motion is linked to controlling gaze. The suboccipital muscles are the righting mechanism of the head, to keep the focus of the eyes on a point. The brain translates visual cues into movement and orienting the body in space. This is done through the vestibular system. If someone is running for the bus, the head is bouncing around while the focus is on the bus. The vestibular system sends the message to the brain on the speed and direction of the body to adjust the position of the eyeballs and the head placement. The gaze direction is achieved through the equilibrium of the focal point, which is the bus.

The link goes deeper into the back of the eyes to a structure called the superior colliculus. The superior colliculus is thought to play a role in integrating sensory

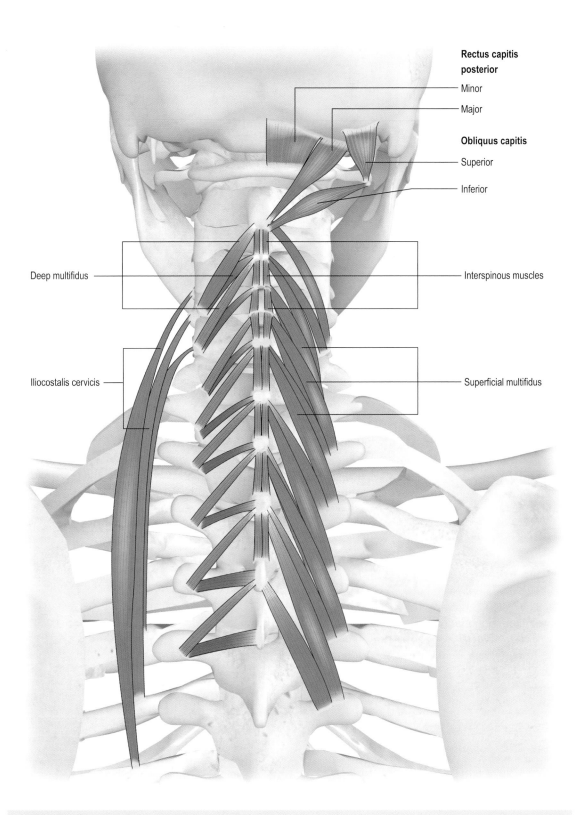

Rectus capitis posterior
Minor
Major

Obliquus capitis
Superior
Inferior

Deep multifidus

Interspinous muscles

Iliocostalis cervicis

Superficial multifidus

Figure 8.16
Suboccipital muscles and deep posterior cervical muscles

information into motor signals that help orient the head toward the stimulus. A pathway of responses from the eyes to the muscles of the neck turns the head toward the target. A continuous map is created by the active neurons crossing both sides of the superior colliculus corresponding to an equilibrium state to determine gaze direction (Goffart et al., 2012).

> **Try it!**
>
> Lightly place the pads of the fingers at the base of the neck over the suboccipital muscles. Move the eyes to the right and left. Feel how the six small muscles contract and release with the side to side movement of the eyes.

As a movement practitioner, cueing the gaze to follow or to begin the direction of movement establishes an internal motor control optimizing the training of the mind–body connection and improves range of motion.

Eye movements and the neck muscles

Sit in an upright position and place one hand on top of the head for a feeling of elongation. The other hand covers the front and sides of the neck. Use the hands for listening to the activity of the neck muscles. Close the eyes. Move the eyes inside the eye sockets, as follows:

- Float the eyes up and down.
- Move the eyes forward, as if looking out, and backward, deep into the back of the sockets.
- Roll the eyes in toward the nose (cross-eyed) and then roll them apart.

- Look on the diagonals: upper right corner to left lower corner; upper left corner to right lower corner.

Sensing the neck muscle activity while performing a variety of eye movements provides valuable awareness of the connection between the two; additionally, the exercise helps release held tension. Cueing to soften one's gaze allows for a balance of the sympathetic (fight-or-flight mode) and parasympathetic (at rest, nonreactive mode) nervous systems.

Neck rotation range and peripheral vision

The range of motion for cervical rotation is relative to the range of peripheral vision. If the peripheral vision is limited on one side, then the motion of the neck is increased since the neck will turn further to accommodate a restriction of vision. Cueing the eyes with the movement direction of the head and scanning the horizon improves the range of rotational motion of the neck. Look to the right with the eyes first, then follow the movement of the head, neck and trunk.

> **Try it!**
>
> Stand facing a partner. The partner walks to one side, as the eyes follow without moving the head. Signal the partner to stop at the point where they almost step out of view. Repeat it on the other side. Observe the difference in the range of peripheral vision from side to side. Now test the range of motion of the cervical spine. Compare how your neck rotation range of motion relates to the peripheral vision. The eyes tend to compensate for the lack of range of motion of the neck. Close the eyes and scan the horizon from one side to the other in the direction where the neck was restricted in rotation. Repeat for 30 seconds, open the eyes and test the rotation.

CLIENT STORY

Neck movement often becomes limited in elderly people as the cervical spine stiffens with age unless you work on keeping a healthy and mobile spine. A 70-year-old female client, who is active and practices Pilates twice a week, was noticeably losing rotation range in her neck. Driving the car was becoming difficult when she needed to look over her left shoulder as she turned left. Our sessions became focused on more mobility in the thorax with special attention paid to how to rotate the whole spine to look over the shoulder. What made an immediate and powerful change was the work with her eyes. Closing the eyes and scanning the horizon repeatedly to the left improved her range. The peripheral vision work restored her rotation to a range in the neck where she was able to see when looking to turn left. The combination of whole-spine movement, improved cervical rotation, and the consciousness of moving the eyeballs to the left then moving the whole spine improved the rotational pattern to the left.

Restoring ease of motion to a stiff neck

Specific directed movements to the segments of the head and neck that are restricted, done gently, ease neck tension, increase flow, and shift the nervous system to a calmer level.

Cervical release with towel

A thick bath towel is rolled up and draped around the neck with both ends crossed in front of the chest (Fig. 8.17 A). The client holds the crossed ends and pulls the towel taut. The towel fills the space between the top of the shoulders and the base of the head. Using gravity and the weight of the head, the client simply rolls the base of their skull around the towel in a slow manner, maintaining contact with the towel (Fig. 8.17 B). At points along the way the neck may feel tension. Pause at this point, breathe and allow the head to be weighted. Continue the circle of the head.

Elbow walking of the head

In a seated position, clasp the hands behind the head on the lowest area of the occiput and support the head (Fig. 8.18 A). Walk the right elbow up and back as the left elbow moves forward (Fig. 8.18 B). Reverse the direction, so the left elbow moves up and back as the right elbow moves forward. Feel the base of the hand on the occiput moving the head in rotation. The arm

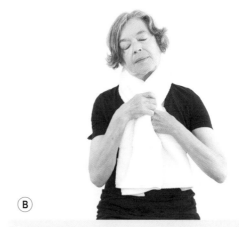

B

Figure 8.17 B
Movement in circle

movement is generating the movement of the head. There is minimal effort and specific motion at the sub-occipital segment.

Stabilizing chin and head movements

In a seated position, hold the chin with both hands to stabilize the mandible (Fig. 8.19 A). Nod the head up and down on the jaw, focusing on moving the skull away from the mandible (Fig. 8.19 B). It is a strange feeling to open the mouth this way rather than the mandible moving down and up as in talking. Focus on the motion at the O/A joint rather than the chin.

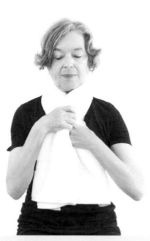

A

Figure 8.17 A
Cervical release with towel: start position

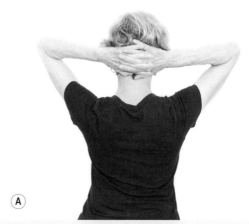

A

Figure 8.18 A
Elbow walking of the head: start position

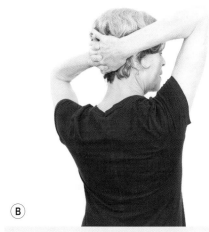

B

Figure 8.18 B
Moving elbows and head

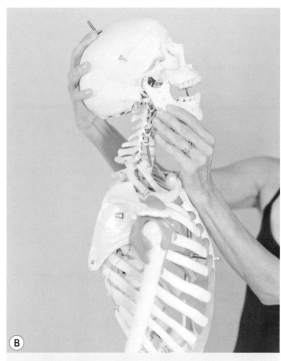

B

Figure 8.19 B
Moving head

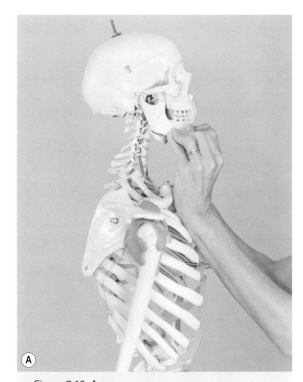

A

Figure 8.19 A
Stabilizing chin to move the head on C1 and
mandible: start position

Adding lip and tongue movements with a stabilized
mandible shows how often the temporomandibular
joint (TMJ) is moving with the lips and tongue motions.
Isolating the muscles of the face lets the TMJ joint take
a break from its normal work of moving all day. Hold
the chin to stabilize it in space (a space hold) and try
to move the lips on diagonals. Try it with the teeth
together and slightly apart. With the teeth apart, move
the tongue on diagonals without the TMJ moving.

Stimulating the head and face

Using a light touch and with a small circular motion,
gently massage:

- the back of the neck, over the head to the bridge of
  the nose
- the eyebrows at the top, starting from the center
  and moving across to the ears

- under the zygoma (cheekbone) near the nose, across to the ears

- underneath the jaw line at the center of the chin, along the mandible to the inner ears

- around a relaxed open mouth, expanding the cavernous mouth

- with closed eyes, around the orbits, with a sense of expanding

- with the fingertips placed around the ears, on the temporal bone, intentioning an anterior (forward) rotation of the fingers and ears

- with eyes closed, around the eyes, stroking gently from the center outward.

Relationship between shoulder girdle and head–neck tension

Expanding out from the specific segments of the head and neck, the spine and shoulders affect the alignment of the head. Working on the spinal movements, especially on the upper thoracic and shoulder strength, alleviates the effort of balancing the head on the spine. A connected core and good breathing skills support the head and neck. Restoring the thorax by improving the natural kyphosis through movement and breath is important to a whole-body approach when addressing neck issues.

Eve Gentry's neck and shoulder releases

Eve Gentry was a dedicated student and teacher with Joseph Pilates from 1942 to 1968. She moved to Santa Fe, remaining there until her death in 1994. She taught her students how to move, understanding the concepts and principles rather just learning exercises. Eve enriched the Pilates Method with her wisdom and healing gifts.

Nose Circles

Lie supine with the head supported by a small folded towel. Imagine a paintbrush on the tip of the nose and paint small circles on the ceiling. Imagine a small halo in front of the nose and trace the circle with the nose. This is a simple and effective release of the suboccipital segment. Add this movement when feeling neck tension (it can be used even when seated).

Practitioner note

If teaching group classes, especially on the mat where the head is held up, causing tension, use the nose circles or small figure eights to quickly release the tension. Teach clients this micromovement as a home program for relief.

Alternating shoulder blade glides

- Sit in an elongated spine.

- Inhale and shrug both shoulders toward the ears (Fig. 8.20 A).

- Exhale and drop the shoulders.

- Repeat 2–3 times.

- Add rotation of the shoulders; inhale, shrug and turn both shoulders to the left; the left shoulder moves back as the right shoulder moves forward (Fig. 8.20 B).

- The eyes remain focused forward.

- Exhale, bringing the shoulders to the center.

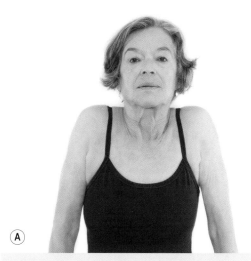

(A)

Figure 8.20 A
Alternating shoulder blade glides: shoulders up

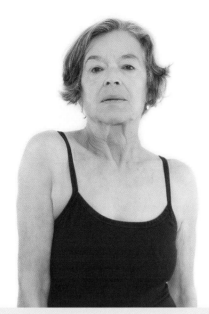

- Feel this shoulder girdle as a whole unit moving on the ribcage.

Elbow Circles

- Sit with the elbows lifted in the scapular plane (scaption) and with fingertips resting on top of the shoulders (Fig. 8.21 A).

- Circle the elbows forward and around (Figs 8.21 B & C).

B

Figure 8.20 B
Turning shoulders to left

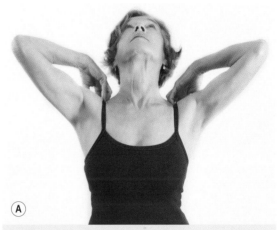

A

Figure 8.21 A
Elbow Circles: start position

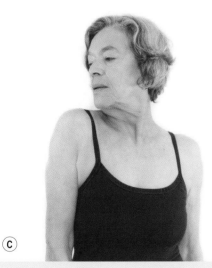

C

Figure 8.20 C
Adding head rotation

- Repeat in a circular way 3–4 times leading to the right, then change to leading to the left.

- Add a head rotation; turn the head, looking toward the shoulder that is up and forward (Fig. 8.20 C).

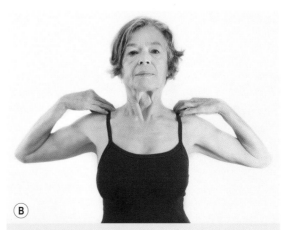

B

Figure 8.21 B
Moving shoulders in circle

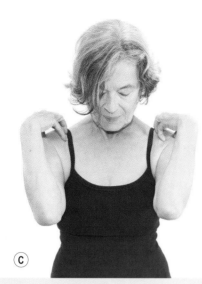

(c)

Figure 8.21 C
Circling motion

- Circle in reverse.
- Add head, neck, and upper back flexion on the forward direction of the circle.
- Look upwards with a smooth movement and extend the upper spine as the elbows circle back.
- Inhale on the upward motion.
- Exhale on the downward motion.

Common patterns

Patterns of movements can be described as a preferred way of moving and a non-preferred way. The neuromuscular system automatically selects the most efficient movement patterns for the given conditions (for example the person's health, physical conditioning, or movement organization skills). In order to excel in a particular sport, a preferred movement pathway is developed and practiced. Since culture and emotions also influence human movement patterns, however, they are highly variable from person to person. A particular pattern may work for one person but would not be efficient for another. Sometimes a preferred movement pattern may become dysfunctional and therefore develop into a non-efficient pattern. In centering the body for balanced movement

potential, becoming aware of a person's preferred and non-preferred way of moving is valuable information for planning a session.

> **Practitioner note**
>
> When assessing a client, observe simple movements such as how the head and neck rotate from side to side. This provides information on the balance between the preferred side and the non-preferred side. Every person has a way they prefer to move. However, if the non-preferred side is unable to perform a range of movement, then movement in one direction (preferred) is greater than the opposite direction (non-preferred), creating an imbalance. For example, if the neck is able to rotate well to the right, the neck will prefer to rotate to the right. In this case, the non-preferred side is the left side. Work to improve the left rotation will balance the tissue pulls on the spine, alleviating potential stress in the area.

Head forward

The most common neck and head pattern is holding the head slightly in front of the midline. The constant use of cell phones and work on computers in our culture means interacting with a device is more common than interacting with the outside world. Thus the head and neck forward pattern has become more exaggerated than ever. The posterior neck muscles are lengthening and working, eccentrically contracting, developing strong, sore, and bigger muscles. The skeletal muscles fatigue when required to work in a sustained way. This may be felt as achiness, pain, or soreness of the neck. Simultaneously, the muscles in the front of the neck are shortening since gravity assists the head tilting down position. This pattern contributes to the elongated and overactive muscles of the posterior neck and weak anterior cervical muscles.

Changing the pattern movements

- Practice moving the head backwards in space and then pressing the top of the head upward (the "getting tall" feeling of axial elongation, Ch. 4).

- Practice the "Head Float" in Chapter 4.

- Balance the posterior neck muscles with support from the anterior neck muscles.

- Perform the extension exercises in Chapters 4 and 5.

- Practice activating the anterior cervical myofascia on the roller (below) and strengthen.

Activating the anterior cervical myofascia using a roller

Cervical rotation using the roller
VIDEO LINK V 8.2

Lie prone on an elevated surface such as large yoga bolsters or the Pilates arc plus bolster. Place a roller crosswise to the bolsters and rest the forehead on the roller. The spine and pelvis position is neutral, with hips released over the bolster.

- First, feel the atlanto-occipital (O/A) joint motion of nodding by rolling the roller away and toward the body (Fig. 8.22 A).

- Repeat the O/A motion, coaching the person to find a natural cervical lordosis.

- Maintaining the position, slowly lift the whole head off the roller without changing the position of the cervical curve (Fig. 8.22 B).

- Hold for 2–3 breaths and lower down to rest the forehead on the roller.

- Repeat 5–8 times.

Practitioner note

Notice how the person lifts the head off the roller. Many times, the upper back extensors will concentrically contract and dominate by extending the spine to lever the head up. The thorax remains stable, allowing for the work of the stabilizers of the thorax and the synergistic contractions of the anterior and posterior neck muscles.

If lying prone is not possible, then another option is to stand in front of a wall. Take a 5–6 inch (13–15 cm) ball and place it on the wall at the level of the forehead. Place the forehead on the ball and roll it up and down the wall (Figs 8.23 A & B). Be careful to stand with the diaphragms stacked and put enough pressure on the ball that it does not fall, but not so much as to cause over-effort of the neck.

Head Float with a pole

- Lie supine with the knees bent.

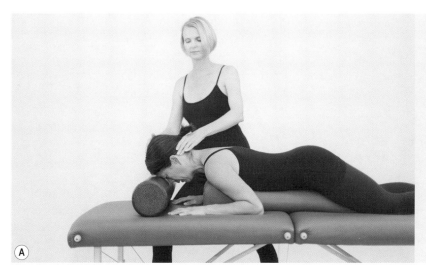

Figure 8.22 A
Activating anterior circles with roller: start position

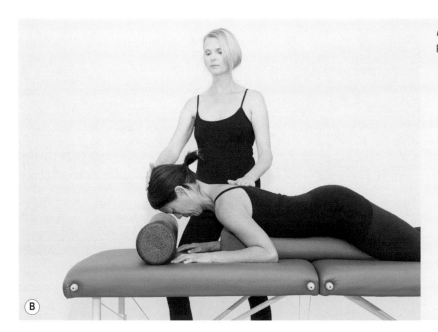

Figure 8.22 B
Floating head off roller

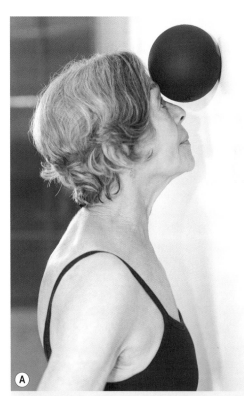

Figure 8.23 A
Standing cervical motion using a ball: start position

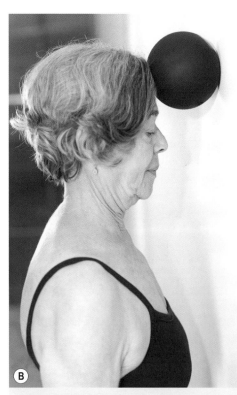

Figure 8.23 B
Rolling ball to move neck

- Hold a pole so that the occiput rests on the pole (Fig. 8.24 A).

- Maintain a chin to sternum alignment – no nodding in either direction.

- Float the head up, resting the head on the pole (Fig. 8.24 B).

- Hold the position for three continuous breaths.

- Lower the head down and rest.

- Add rotation; after the "Head Float" up, hold the "Head Float" and press gently into the pole as the head rotates from side to side.

Looking cute

When being photographed many people pose by tilting the head to one side. For some people, the head is in a side bend much of the time. Remember, with the side bending there is the coupled rotation. In the side bending presentation, one side of the neck is shortened and the opposite side is elongated. This pattern develops overactive muscles on the long side of the neck. One also sees that some people present one side of their face more to the front than the other (a rotation presentation). This pattern contributes to shortened and overactive diagonal muscles (SCM and upper trapezius).

Changing the pattern movements

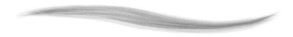

- Practice elongating the shortened side of the neck:

  - bring the ear upward and away from the shoulder (Fig. 8.25)

  - then cue "Listen to the ceiling with your ear".

- Practice tilting the entire upper body toward the long, more active side of the neck:

  - hold the tilt of the body

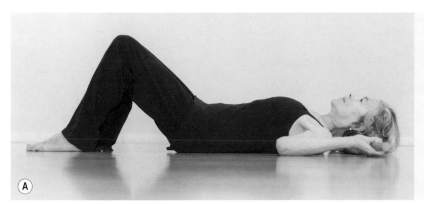

Figure 8.24 A
Head Float using a pole: start position

(A)

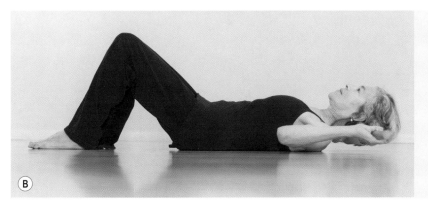

Figure 8.24 B
Floating

(B)

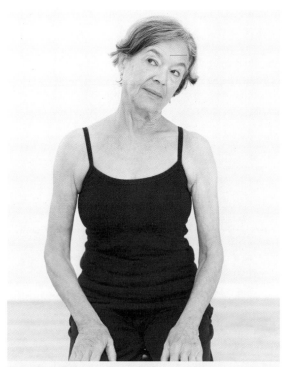

Figure 8.25
Listening toward the ceiling to elongate shortened side

- slowly lower the head toward the ground on the long side (Fig. 8.26 A)

- then raise the head back up (Fig. 8.26 B)

- and repeat several times to elongate and activate the muscles on the opposite short side against the pull of gravity.

- Practice rotating the head to the non-preferred side against resistance of the hand:

  - if facing to the right and presenting the left side of the face forward

  - place a hand on the left side of the face (Fig. 8.27)

  - then resist with the hand as the head rotates to the left

  - and repeat 10 times on the one side.

- Work with the peripheral vision (above).

- Practice "Cervical Rotation on the Roller" (below).

Cervical rotation on the roller

 Cervical rotation using the roller
VIDEO LINK V 8.2

- Lie prone on the elevated props as above, so that the head and neck are aligned in an optimal way for the client (the head may begin slightly forward).

- Place the roller vertical relative to the head.

- Place the most medial part of the cheekbone (zygoma) on the roller, very close to the nose (Fig. 8.28 A).

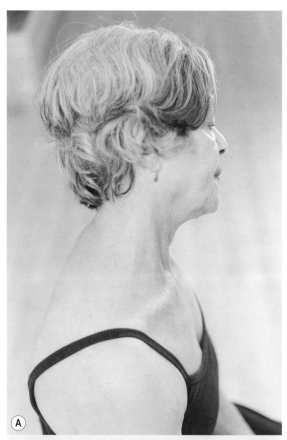

(A)

Figure 8.26 A
Using gravity, side tilt body: tilting body

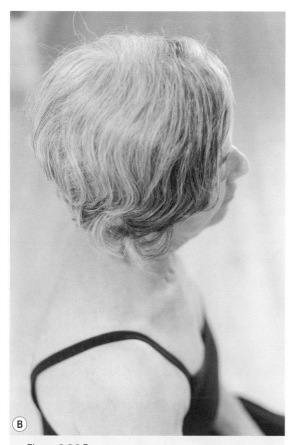

Figure 8.26 B
Moving head against gravity

- Be mindful that the head is in alignment with the spine.

- Rest the head on the roller.

- Gently press the roller along the zygoma, rolling the roller toward the ear (Fig. 8.28 B).

- Slowly roll the along the zygoma back toward the nose.

- Repeat 3 times and change to the other side.

Resistance for strengthening and balancing the neck muscles

Resistance for strengthening and balancing the neck muscles
VIDEO LINK V 8.3

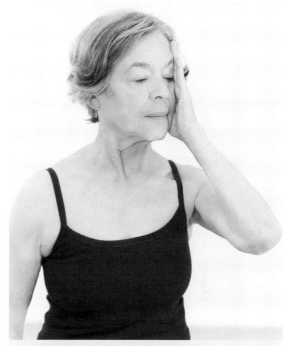

Figure 8.27
Self-resistance for rotation of neck

Release of posterior neck and activation of anterior neck

- Find the vertical axis in a seated position.

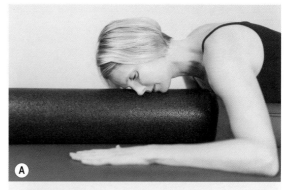

Figure 8.28 A
Cervical rotation on roller: start position

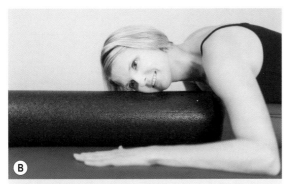

Figure 8.28 B
Rotating head and neck

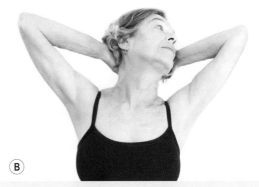

Figure 8.29 B
Adding rotation

- Clasp the hands behind the head, with elbows forward so the arms are in scaption.

- Arch the head behind the vertical axis (Fig. 8.29 A).

- Press the head against the resistance of the hands.

- Allow the upper spine to arch as the head presses back so that the muscles engage in the back of the neck.

- Rotate the head from side to side, resisting, always pressing backward (Fig. 8.29 B).

- Bring the head to the center.

- Take the weight of the head off the hands.

- Feel the anterior neck muscles engage.

- Repeat 3–5 times.

Arching with resistance: anterior cervical spine

- Place the palms of the hands on the forehead.

- Press the forehead into the palms (Fig. 8.30 A).

- Maintain the resistance and arch the upper spine back, allowing gravity and the forehead-to-palm pressure to create resistance of the anterior neck muscles (Fig. 8.30 B):

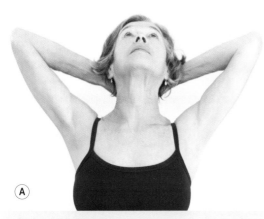

Figure 8.29 A
Release of the posterior neck muscles: start position

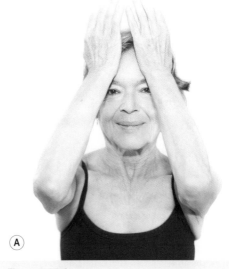

Figure 8.30 A
Activating anterior cervical muscles: start position

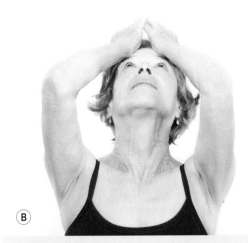

B

Figure 8.30 B
Resisting behind vertical axis

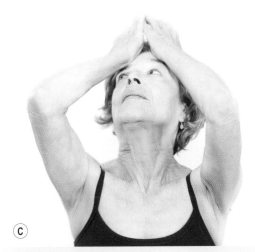

C

Figure 8.30 C
Adding rotation

- rotate side to side (Fig. 8.30 C)
- return to upright.

Lateral neck

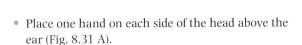

- Place one hand on each side of the head above the ear (Fig. 8.31 A).

- Move the head sideways and press with the hand above the ear of the same side, resisting the movement (Fig. 8.31 B).
- Stay on the same side and resist with the opposite hand (Fig. 8.31 C).
- Rotate the head to look down against the resistance of the hand, keeping the head tilted to the side (Fig. 8.32 A).
- Rotate the head keeping the head in the same side tilt, resisting with the other hand (Fig. 8.32 B).

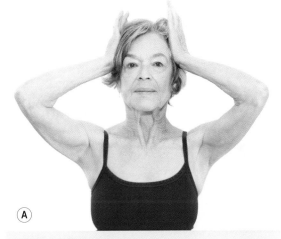

A

Figure 8.31 A
Lateral neck: start position

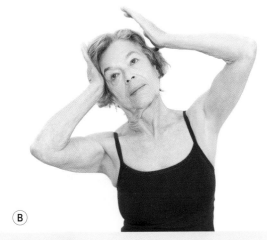

B

Figure 8.31 B
Side resistance

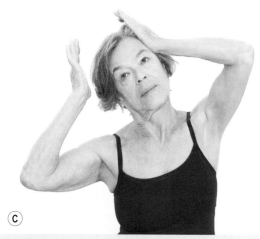

Figure 8.31 C
Opposite side resistance

- Bring the head to the center, take the weight of the head off your hands, and feel the top lateral muscles engage.
- Repeat 3 times.
- Change to the other side.

Diagonal sequences

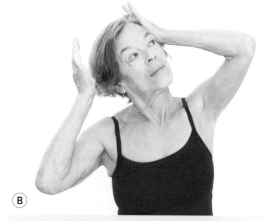

B

Figure 8.32 B
Same tilt resisting with other hand

- Look down under the right armpit and up over the left shoulder (Fig. 8.33 A).
- To add resistance, place the right hand on the right side of the forehead and the left hand at the back of the head on the left side.
- Repeat the movement, looking under the armpit and over the opposite shoulder. (Fig. 8.33 B)
- Add resistance in both directions.
- Alternate the sides, repeating 3–5 times.

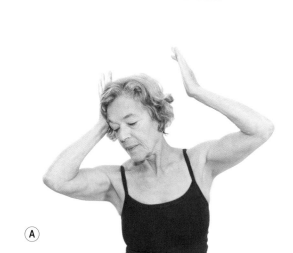

A

Figure 8.32 A
Lateral neck adding rotation: resisting into the rotation looking down

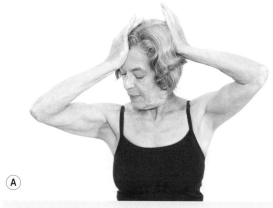

A

Figure 8.33 A
Diagonals: looking down

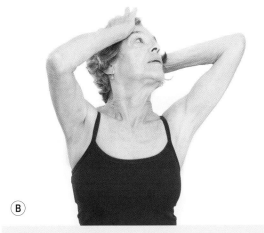

(B)

Figure 8.33 B
Looking up

Prone positions: mobility and strength of the neck

Chest Float

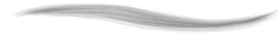

- Lie prone with the hands stacked on top of one another and the forehead resting on the hands.

- Neck movement 1. Float the forehead off the hands, unweighting the head but maintaining the axial elongation (Fig. 8.34 A); move the forehead to the side, as if the forehead is brushing along the hands (Fig. 8.34 B).

- Neck movement 2. Float the head up; look to the right with your eyes and rotate the head to look at the right elbow; do both sides (Fig. 8.35 A):

  - add an oppositional leg reach; if looking to the right, the left leg is in dorsiflexion and reach back; this can also be done against a wall, pressing the foot firmly into the wall (Fig. 8.35 B).

- Neck movement 3. Hands behind the head; float the upper body up off the mat, leading with the eyes, look to right upper diagonal and left diagonal (Fig. 8.36):

  - advanced movement with arms straight overhead.

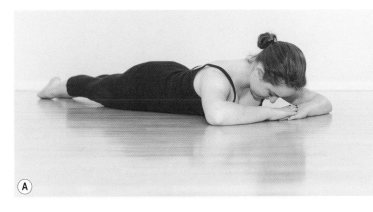

Figure 8.34 A
Prone Chest Float: start position with head floating

(A)

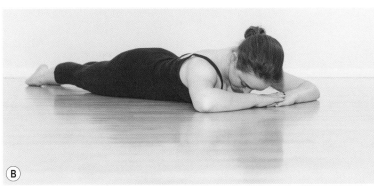

Figure 8.34 B
Side bending head on neck

(B)

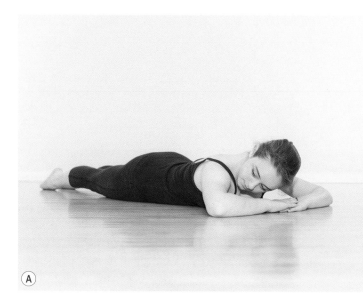

Figure 8.35 A
Prone Chest Float: head and neck rotation

(A)

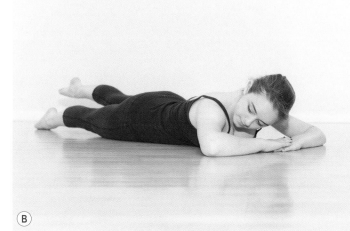

Figure 8.35 B
Adding oppositional leg lift

(B)

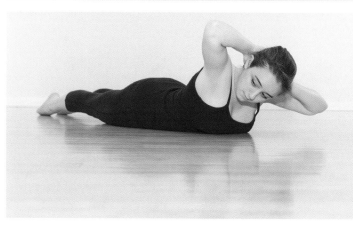

Figure 8.36
Advanced prone Chest Float

Enhance challenge of mat position by reducing kyphosis with equipment set-up

Double Leg Stretch on a long box

- Lie supine with approximately T6 at the edge of a Reformer box in the long position so that the head and upper trunk can extend over the edge (Fig. 8.37 A).

- Begin in "Double Leg Stretch" position:

  - supine with hips flexed and knees bent into toward the chest in slight abduction of the hips, heels together and close to the buttocks, sacrum anchored

  - upper spine in flexion, arms wrapped around the outer thighs in toward the shins to reach to the top of the ankles

  - press the inner edges of the feet together as if stuck there with a strip of Velcro

  - at the same time press the outer thighs into the wrapped arms.

- Inhale and exhale as the legs extend out, maintaining the contact of the spine with the box and the

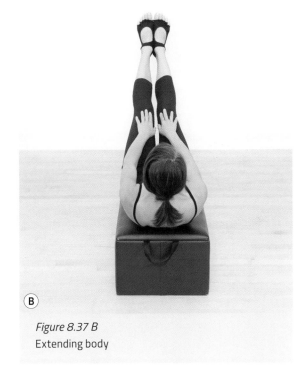

B

Figure 8.37 B
Extending body

sacrum anchored (Fig. 8.37 B).vvThe arms reach to touch the tops of the knees, legs straight.

- Inhale, and move the arms overhead.

- Extend the upper back over the box (Fig. 8.37 C).

- Exhale, circle the arms to the side, and curl the head up.

- Fold the legs in and hold the ankles in the starting position, then inhale.

- Repeat the sequence 5 times.

Long sit-up

The Cadillac table set-up is using the push-through bar in the bottom loaded position with a blue or red spring. Match the person's size, strength, and movement control in choosing the spring.

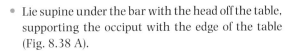

- Lie supine under the bar with the head off the table, supporting the occiput with the edge of the table (Fig. 8.38 A).

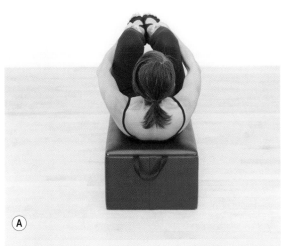

A

Figure 8.37 A
Double Leg Stretch on box: start position

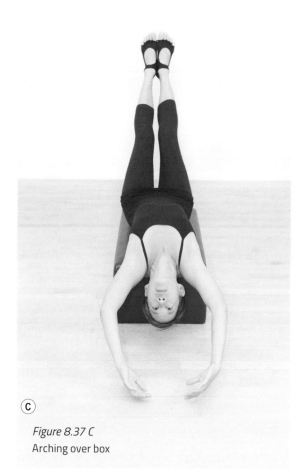

C

Figure 8.37 C
Arching over box

- Hold the ends of the bar.

- The legs are straight and together.

- Inhale in the starting position.

- Exhale, roll the chin toward the throat, and press the bar away, straightening the arms (Fig. 8.38 B).

- Roll up into a seated, upright position, with arms extended over the head (Fig. 8.38 C).

- Inhale in the extended position.

- Exhale as the elbows bend and bring the bar down and behind the head (Fig. 8.38 D).

- Inhale and press the bar overhead, fully extending the arms (see Fig. 8.37 C).

- Exhale and lift both legs up into a V; sit and lower legs (Fig. 8.38 E).

- Inhale, press the bar up, and begin to curl the coccyx.

- Exhale, continue curling down through the pelvis and spine (see Fig. 8.37 B).

- Inhale as the head extends over the table (see Fig. 8.37 A).

- Repeat 5 times.

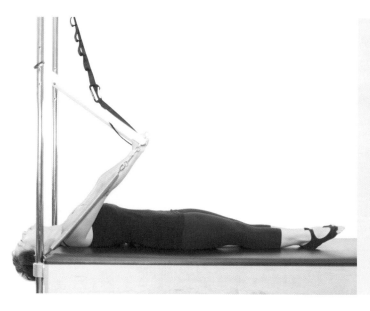

A

Figure 8.38 A
Long sit-up on Cadillac: start position

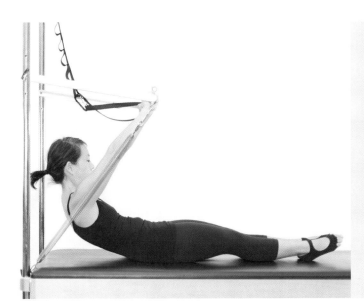

Figure 8.38 B
Rolling up

B

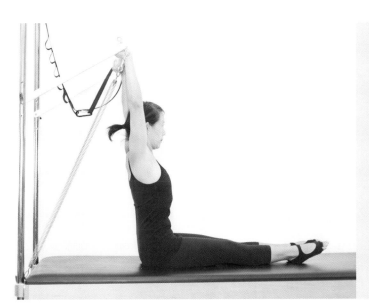

Figure 8.38 C
Upright against resistance
of bar

C

Practitioner note
Hands-on

Stand behind the head of the client. Place both index fingers under the occiput and guide the head in the rolling motion. Change the hands to the scapula and encourage the contact of the scapula on the ribcage. When the legs lift, the pelvis remains in its position; do not allow the pelvis to posteriorly rotate. Cue the client to continuously press the bar upward during the roll down phase. The cue is creating a contrast of movement of the upward motion of the bar with the flexion of the spine, creating a nice fascial glide and prohibiting a collapse of the spine, engaging the elongation feeling of the body.

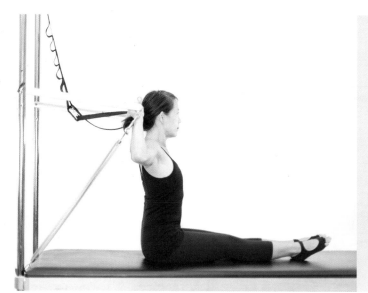

Figure 8.38 D
Arms behind head

D

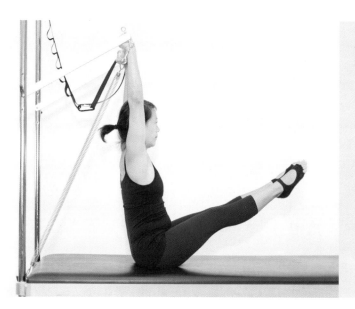

Figure 8.38 E
Teaser

E

Overhead reach on Small Barrel

Sit with the ischial tuberosities on the edge of the Small Barrel step (called the lip). The spine is in an elongated neutral, and the arms are reaching forward at 90° shoulder flexion, with the palms facing each other (Fig. 8.39 A).

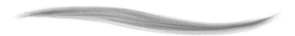

- Inhale and curl the coccyx as the arms continue to reach forward.

- Exhale to continue the flexion motion through the spine (Fig. 8.39 B).

- Inhale and extend over the barrel, with the head resting on a box at the end of the barrel or on the barrel itself (Fig. 8.39 C).

- Simultaneously, the arms move from the forward position to overhead.

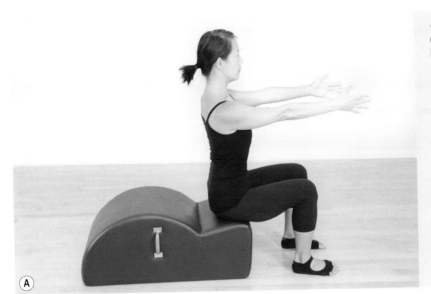

Figure 8.39 A
Overhead reach on Small Barrel: start position

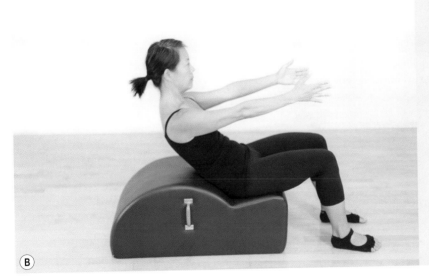

Figure 8.39 B
Rolling back

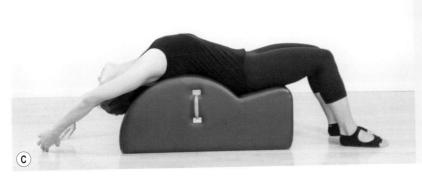

Figure 8.39 C
Arch over

- Using a long continuous exhale, the arms move from overhead to a T position with the palms up.

- At this point, the head rolls, chin toward the throat, and flexion continues through the spine with the xiphoid–pubic bone connection.

- Articulation is through the spine until the shoulders are over the pelvis in a bowed spine.

- From the crown of the head toward the ceiling (vertical axis), elongate the spine to the upright seated position.

- Repeat 3 times then reverse the path of the arms 3 times.

Variations at this point may match your client's ability:

- For a client who is having difficulty smoothly curling and keeping the feet grounded:

  - Allow the arms to move to the forward 90° flexed position as they are curling up off the arc of the barrel and hold their hands to provide a minimal assist.

  - Progress to the same arm position but not assisted.

  - A more advanced version is to curl up with the arms overhead throughout the spinal motion.

  - An option is to hold Magic Circle or a pole as the arms reach forward and up.

Pulling Straps with Rotation

This is a variation of the Pilates Reformer exercise "Pulling Straps," but adding the eye motion and upper spine rotation. The box is placed in the long position with one blue or red spring. Ropes are shortened to match the length of the client's arms. Have the client reach out toward the risers, and adjust the straps. If the straps are not adjustable, then simply pull up on the ropes so that the arms are straight and the ropes taut.

- Lie prone on the long box with head facing the risers.

- Begin looking down under the right armpit (Fig. 8.40 A).

- Inhale, and smoothly pull the straps, so the spine extends long (Fig. 8.40 B).

- The eyes scan the path from the floor up through the center and then look over the left shoulder.

- The arms are fully extended next to the trunk, the spine in extension with a left cervical rotation (Fig. 8.40 C).

- Exhale and reverse the path, scanning to the floor under the right armpit.

- Lower the body to the starting position.

- Repeat 3–5 times on one side then switch sides.

"Pulling Straps with Rotation" is a version of the "Tom Swan" adding more range from flexion into extension and resistance from the springs. Cue the scanning of the eyes throughout the movement.

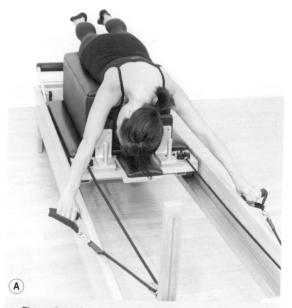

(A)

Figure 8.40 A
Pulling Straps with head and upper spine rotation: start position rotated to one side

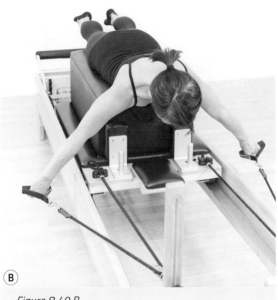

(B)

Figure 8.40 B
Moving through center

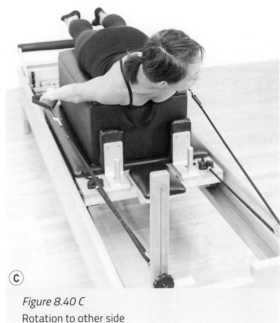

(C)

Figure 8.40 C
Rotation to other side

Bridge to Chapter 9

The journey we have taken through *Centered* has moved from the ground or "roots" of the body, through the center connections, and back to another "root," namely the crown of the head. The head represents the "crown," our place of knowing, communicating, sensing, and expressing. Movement gives the body and the self an avenue of energy to live the way we choose in this one body. Learning and embodying an awareness of how

uniquely – and not so uniquely – the body moves provides a way of being, to self-help the body to realign itself toward the center. From a center, life seems less muddled. There is space to breathe even among chaos, or during times of change and disruption. The body is adapting to the environment, and to physical and emotional health. When moving is fully integrated with integrity and respect for the body, with a mindful connection, it is a healing and rewarding practice.

Part 4

The whole body conclusion

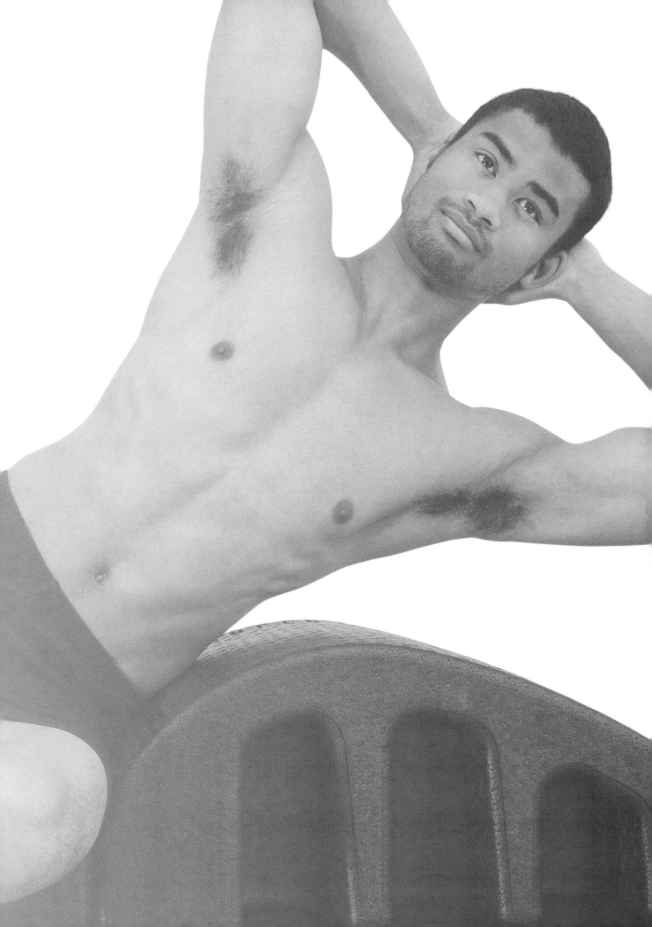

Perception and felt sense

"It's not that I don't get off center. I correct so fast that no one sees me."

Morihei Ueshiba, O Sensei

Contemplative awareness: equilibrium

To be alive and thriving is to be moving, breathing, and feeling. The living body is not static: it is in constant motion, for even when standing still, it is adjusting and righting itself to maintain a balance of all systems. These continual changes and adaptations add to the quality and type of movement patterns seen in the body's tissues. An important influence on the righting reflexes is the exposure to the environment, both externally and internally. Movement is altered when the body is out of balance: it has been found, for example, that inflammation of the intestines affects movement of the abdominal wall and its ability to contract efficiently (Beach, 2010). How the body is treated, the food that is eaten, or a lack of exercise, for example, impacts health and health affects movement.

The body, including the brain, is made up of an extensive network of systems that interact with one another to maintain a healthy equilibrium. A change in one system will generate a shift in the others. The body's natural healing capacity comes from its ability to restore equilibrium. Problems occur when the body's systems are disrupted as a result of stress, threat (fight or flight), pain, and/or distress. Each system has to balance the constant input from the environment in order to preserve a fundamental homeostasis that maintains or boosts one's state of health. Think of the story of "Goldilocks and the Three Bears" (Southey, 1837). The first bowl of porridge was too hot and the second too cold, but the third was "just right." The set point, that "just right" feeling, is based on an individual's body, an important point for balance.

Each body regulates the constant disturbances to its balance caused by the ever changing environment. The stronger and more balanced the body's physical conditioning is, the more capable it is of adapting, minimizing how far away it is from homeostasis.

Why is it important to move well?

In a healthy body, the capacity to adapt to life or to athletic challenges requires a process for normalization. When the body is stressed, whether by choice or not, a short amount of time to recuperate is a sign of good health. Each person has a different ability to adjust and acclimate to stress. For some people, no outside intervention is necessary and the body heals over time. If the adaptive capacity is exhausted, however, or balance is elusive, then introducing an appropriate external intervention can help the body return to its equilibrium. Many people find that help from a body-based practitioner can accelerate the body's ability to return to homeostasis.

Physically, the body's structure will appear altered from its relative normal movements when disequilibrium is present. The best way to see compensated movement is to observe someone walking. If a leg swings around to the side rather than moving efficiently through the hip as the leg leads with the knee orientated forward (normal hip flexion with knee bent and extending the lower leg forward), this reveals abnormal mechanics in the hip. In short, the hip is compromised. The gait pattern has veered away from normal movement, thereby disrupting the effort of walking and turning the pattern into a stressed one. The stressed effort affects not only the hip joint itself, but impacts all the structures, including the movements of the diaphragm, so breathing will be altered. If breathing is altered, then the process whereby all the systems adapt toward a multisystem equilibrium will change and have a negative impact on biomechanical factors and the body's biochemistry (Chaitow et al., 2014).

It is important to maintain good function and a healthy structure to minimize any unnecessary stress. Whether strolling down the street or exercising, the relationship between the movements performed and total health is an important connection to understand. Moving well increases the vitality of health.

Mind to move

Today's fitness world is beginning to incorporate complementary practices within the gym. It is now being recognized that an element of release work versus stretching and movement awareness should be included in the fitness model. A body that is only

stressing itself through the fast and hard practice typical in workouts is not sustainable over a lifetime. Many orthopedic injuries in people over the age of 45 are due to years of overuse and lack of functional healthy movement. Once upon a time, the disciplines of the gym and the dance studio were far apart from each other, and each was unaware of what the other had to offer. Today, however, the worlds of fitness, movement studies, and science are drawing closer.

Practice of the practice

The practice of an integrative movement practitioner is the ability to synthesize knowledge, embody it, and apply the senses of seeing, touch, and hearing while working with a client. This is the process work of the practitioner where one's presence and clarity are available for decisions that are made in the moment. Each practitioner has his or her own presence and individual way of perceiving and communicating. Developing the skill to see a client's movement patterning and structure takes education, experimentation, and

---

CLIENT STORY
Personal story

Discovering my dream to become a professional dancer started me on a difficult path toward making it a reality. The life of a professional dancer involves complex physical challenges, accepting criticism, being strong in who you are, and 90% practice. The commitment to improving my technical and performance skills opened the door to a variety of movement teachings such as Rolfing, somatic movement techniques, and the use of balls. In the late 1970s and early 1980s, the modern dance world integrated these alternative movement practices to increase proprioception, interoception, and kinesthetic awareness. By doing these complementary practices in addition to dance training, I learned to move efficiently for balancing the strict demands of classes in dance techniques. Becoming more aware of moving included not only the coordination of body parts but also a sense of body systems in movement, such as the organs,

fascia, and fluids (interoception). My responsiveness expanded to feel where unconscious tension was being held and was limiting my ability to fall to the floor, turn multiple times, or suspend a jump in the air. Learning the mechanics of movement, such as how the hip spins, I would visualize and feel for the bone movement to increase a leg extension or use the imagery of organs moving the pelvis. The more I understood the mechanics, the clearer my visualizations were, helping manifest movement qualities and skills in my dancing. With practice, the visualizations were no longer necessary because the movement became second nature, developing into an unconscious conscious awareness. This awareness is the mastery place for movement, where the body moves itself, without thoughts directing every moment. Practice had imprinted the new movements that allowed for my body to move differently.

guidance from a skilled teacher. As practitioners, we are creating the environment that can help someone shift less than desirable movement habits to achieve "normal" functioning and a strong body.

The practitioner's professional skills

In the body movement training profession, it is vital to teach people the importance of fine-tuning the body to meet the daily needs of movement for a lifetime and see how it enhances the athletic endeavors. This requires from the movement professional:

* the knowledge and physical experience of moving soundly

* the ability to communicate to the client the observations of the client's relative normal movement

* identifying non-efficient movement patterns

* teaching the skill of sensing one's state of being

* presenting sound movement skills to facilitate a felt sense for healthy movement

* using touch, breath, and movement to direct awareness

* hands-on guidance tools for redirecting the body toward balance

* educating the client for awareness of daily movement habits such as sitting to standing or walking

* challenging the client's physicality by meeting their edge, pushing it when ready, and varying the movement training plan

* balancing the somatic approach of awareness with physical training for developing balanced strength.

The process and technique

Communication, touch, and specific techniques in combination with the appropriate timing are elements of the training process involved in organizing the body prior to integration and strengthening. The starting point is to investigate the client's strategy for movement by observing it and identifying the pattern. Ask, is this strategy a helpful one for optimal movement or

is it potentially one that is (or will be) destructive? The mastery of this work is the ability to identify the strategy, then coach the person to move with function. It may require a hands-on guidance or adding an apparatus technique shown in *Centered* to reorganize the restricted movement into a healthy one.

Communication through words

Choosing words that will elicit the desired response in the body is important to the mental part of the training. Feeling, rather than seeing, words imprints the movement on the body map. Carefully chosen words give a person a sensation experience while moving. As an example, try using "soften" for bending the knee or "elongate and narrow" to extend the length of the body. Use action words that convey the quality of the movement, such as "float" rather than lift, "slide" in place of straighten, "sink" for dropping the shoulder or hip. There is an endless and creative pool of possible imagery for the body to feel and direct the sequencing of movement. Here are some examples:

* For lumbopelvic side bending movements, imagine the pelvis as a steering wheel and turning the wheel to the right and left.

* Imagine the foot as a tongue, and lick the floor as the foot lifts up.

* To give the sense of how to feel the shoulders and to inhibit holding shoulders up, imagine the shoulders are the mantelpiece resting on the fireplace.

* Place a heavy velvet cloak around the neck and let it hang off your shoulders down the back, to feel upright.

* There is a pile of sand on top of the pubic bone; slowly pour the sand into the navel then reverse the process, pouring the sand back onto the pubic bone in pelvic tilts.

* Shine a laser beam from the middle of the sternum to the right, in thorax rotation.

"Cueing" (see Ch. 4) uses the bone movement, wheels, loops, and other sentences for effective wording for movement directions. Throughout the exercise sections, there are other possible cueing series to improve the client's mental connection to feeling the movement sequences desired.

Touch and techniques

Word cueing is effective for guiding clients through smart movement sequences and allows for the practice to imprint into their consciousness. However, the body that has a strong holding pattern requires assistance through a manual cue (touch), or techniques such as the muscle energy techniques (MET) used in this book.

Observe, for instance, the steering wheel motion of the pelvis turning right (the right side of the circle moves down as the left side moves up). The unrestricted normal "right turn" action is when the right ilium drops downward (a "Hip Drop"), creating a left side bending of the lower spine and left hip abduction and right hip adduction. If there is a restriction, the right side of the pelvis will not move downward and the left side will not be able to move upward. The tissues and structures between the ilium and lower ribs on the right side are shortened and those on the left elongated. The hip joint is off its central position in the joint, sitting in a hip sway to the right. With this observation, then choose a movement sequencing and/or hands-on work to enhance the movement of the hip joint from side to side (the hip sway and medial spins are in Ch. 3). Additionally, the balanced side bending and twists and exercises for integration of lumbopelvic motion from Chapter 3, combined with the hip spins, will change the lack of right hip drop. In Chapter 4, the "Resetting the Trunk" exercises will re-establish and balance the spine in its side bending and rotation balance. This approach of sequencing movements for structural change with the techniques presented in *Centered* effectively teaches a client new movement skills and the feeling for optimal movement.

Proprioception and felt sense

When we start to learn a new movement, the body's sense and coordination are not fully organized. Individuals seeking to learn new movements are required to concentrate actively and go beyond their current ability. Improvements are accomplished by mental focus, allowing the brain and nervous system to adapt to these changes (Ericsson et al., 2006). The integrated movement practice cannot be performed mindlessly. Over time and repetition, the brain maps and imprints movement information, developing a strong sense of the movement pattern. The new pattern is formed and the movement becomes second nature. Elite movers such as professional dancers and athletes, who practice complex motor skills day in and day out, seeking perfection, develop superior proprioception skills interacting with all the senses.

Proprioception (from the Latin word *proprius*, meaning one's own or individual) is considered an addition to the primary senses. It is part of the somatosensory system, which is the system that detects touch, pressure, pain, temperature, joint and muscle positions. It is this sense that allows feeling the body's position, its orientation in space, and the movement of the body as a whole and of its parts. Current ideas concerning the role of fascia in proprioception suggest a conscious and subconscious sensing of limb position, measuring the stretch and tracking the rate of movement in each joint. When the fascial structure has a mechanical connection with the muscular or skeletal component, it is able to contribute to the mechanoreceptive stimulus necessary for proprioception (van der Wal, 2012).

Visualize picking up a small rock. The body determines the weight of the rock prior to actually lifting it and coordinates the proper muscle recruitment necessary to perform the action. The body judges the right amount of effort needed. Fine touch skills, such as typing or using fine tools, are examples of the position and location information relayed by the skin, fascia, joints, bones, and muscle receptors and brain maps.

Proprioception has an effect on equilibrium. Feeling the limb positions and the movement of the body is called a felt sense. The brain's representation of body parts gives the feeling of ownership of the body (Héroux et al., 2013). Closing the eyes and touching the index fingers together without looking, for example, demonstrates the proprioception sense and ownership of the fingers. This is possible because each body part is mapped in the brain (see Ch. 6, "Function and Form"). In addition to the body's anatomy, the surrounding environment is also mapped onto the brain tissue (Blakeslee and Blakeslee, 2007). The many maps in the brain interact with one another,

Practitioner note

Proprioception has two distinct pathways of neural connections: one is exteroception (the body relating to the outside world) and the other interoception (a sense of the physiological world, including sensations from viscera, muscular effort, tickling, and sensual touch). The two are processed at different locations in the brain, with interoception being processed in the insular cortex rather than in the somatosensory cortex (Schleip and Jaeger, 2012). It is always related to the homeostatic needs of the body. When working with the body, support interoceptive sensations by drawing attention to feeling the sensations while moving. In an inversion there is an opportunity to experience visceral movement or emphasize a warm sensation of blood flow, for example after using the Small Ball foot exercise of creating friction (Ch. 1)

making it possible to move about and interact with objects. These body and sensory maps are changed through practice.

Practice improves motor skills, which increase the activity of proprioception and the body maps on the brain. It has been found that the areas of the brain activated through practice have an increase in gray matter density even after short daily practice sessions (Duerden and Laverdure-Dupont, 2008). Changes correspond to the area of the brain specific to the movement practiced. Deliberate practice is necessary for effective training to stimulate this growth and bring about changes to the body map. Subsequent continued practice brings the changes into a new phase of long-term structural change: "The skill becomes better integrated into your maps' basic circuitry, and the whole process becomes more efficient and automatic" (Blakeslee and Blakeslee, 2007).

Embodying felt sense

First, the client needs to know where their body is when it is beginning this process of change. Is there awareness of the parts of the body that move reciprocally or in synchronization? Is there the ability to move the legs independent of the pelvis? Is there a sense of how it feels to be connected to the trunk through the center? If the client is unaware that when lying on the floor the right side of the pelvis is more weighted than

the left, there will be no reference point for directing the movement or assessing a change. Guiding a client through movement awareness techniques teaches where the body is in this moment, the felt sense of the body, and allows easier access to strength.

Self-assessment

Noticing the body in the moment provides both client and practitioner with information about how an individual's body is organizing itself. From this moment, a practitioner chooses the beginning point for starting the process of organizing the body, followed by strengthening it. To make an impact on the client's consciousness, the client needs to feel and recognize how their body is at this moment. Teaching the client to self-assess and feel the body will help progress the client more quickly. Choose to direct the self-assessment skill in standing, lying down, or seated. Ask questions as the client scans and feels for the answers. The self-assessment can be referenced during a session while executing a movement exercise.

Practitioner note

After working with the client, use the self-assessment, comparing the difference from the start of the session to the end and noting the changes. Verbalize to the client, e.g., how only one side of the back was in contact with the floor and now notice how it has changed since both sides of the back are in contact.

Standing scan

Ask the client to stand without giving any specific direction to alter the stance. Begin a series of questions bringing attention to the stance. Since the only physical contact point is the bottom of the feet, begin there. Remind the client to remember the answers to the questions for reference later. At the end of a session or movement class, return to this process for assessing how the body has shifted through the movement practice.

These are example questions as a suggestion (create observations relating to the class and your teaching environment):

* Sense the bottom of the feet with the floor:
  * Where is the weight placed primarily?

- o On the heels?

- o Where on the heels?

- o Is there weight on the toes?

- o Is one foot more weighted than the other?

- Is the floor cold?

- Scan to feel the whole leg:

  - Where is there more tension?

    - o In the front of the thigh?

    - o One hip more than the other?

  - Is one knee locked more than the other?

  - Do you feel standing on one leg more than the other?

- Pelvis and spine:

  - Can you sense which direction the pelvis is facing?

    - o Is it facing more right or left?

    - o Try to feel the pelvis's position.

  - Is there tension in the spine?

    - o What area do you feel more tension?

  - Do you feel movement in the trunk while being still?

    - o Is it the breath?

    - o Is it breakfast?

  - Shoulders and neck:

    - o Which side feels more at ease?

    - o Can you sense which direction your chest is facing?

    - o How are the arms hanging?

    - o What are you seeing with your eyes?

Lying scan

Simply lying on the floor can provide a sensory feedback for the body's position. Try lying on a soft foam roller for specific spine rotation awareness.

- Lie on the floor with the legs straight, arms to the side (approximately 60°) with the palms up (if on a roller, the knees are bent with feet on the floor, arms resting on the floor palms up).

- Notice the areas of the body that are in contact with the floor and feel weighted.

- Start at the feet and legs:

  - Where are the heels in contact? Outer edge or inner side?

  - Do you feel the contact of the back of the leg? What parts?

  - More on the right or left?

- Feel the back of the pelvis, the buttocks' contact with the floor:

  - Is one side more weighted than the other?

- Feel the back of the body on either side of the spine:

  - At the sacrum, is there more weight toward the tail or higher up?

  - From the sacrum upward, where is the next place to have contact?

- Feel the back of the shoulders for the contact points.

- Where on the back of the skull is it touching the floor?

Seated scan

Sit in a chair or on the floor. People are often asked to sit on the floor but this is a difficult position for most people to maintain while remaining comfortable and balanced. An exercise can include the awareness of the body in the uncomfortable seated position. Draw attention to the limitation of the breathing capacity while in this position. Suggest a change of position, such as sitting on top of a block or a folded blanket, and notice the change in breathing and comfort.

Listening to the body

Offering a way to experience how the body adapts to daily life and is reflected in its structure will be valuable for people to experience. People want to be fixed, to have a permanent change, and are always looking for the "one pill" quick recovery. Clients look to the outside, to the professional, or to the inner critic for feedback. Teaching a person to feel and self-assess turns the attention to listening to and feeling one's body. Listening to the body sends a different message to the brain, enhancing the potential change of the body maps.

After a session, a client may ask, "will the changes last?" My answer is another question, "What lasts in this world?" What is permanent? Maybe plastic is! The body is a living, biological being, and is changing all the time. Being present to one's needs today and choosing the training approach appropriately and the appropriate method of training will develop the body into a stronger and healthier one.

Summary

Continue to grow and learn as a practitioner. Being a teacher of movement is a nonlinear process. To evolve into a higher level of expertise is a life commitment of practice. Life is practice and practice is life. The learning process is an individual experience. Is it studying the science, experiencing the movements, the analytical process, or is it the ability to see and assess that inspires effective work? Trust that, as a practitioner, the teacher is within.

The essence of this work is deep in one's consciousness and connected to those teachers who came before. This life's work is built upon the gifts of these teachers who were 100% committed to studying, exploring, and discovering ways to improve the human body. We build upon their gifts. And today, a valuable resource is aligning oneself with like-minded practitioners and educators. Seek out those who inspire you.

Centered was a challenge to write, maintaining a multifocus approach, looking closely at both a specific area and the relationships with the three-dimensional, whole-body phenomenon. As a practitioner in this field, this is how I work, focusing in and expanding out. It is all about movement and the connection of movement to the self. The work is analogous to being a sleuth who investigates the moving body to discover the key to unlocking the mystery of the movement to help others move for a lifetime. Teaching movement and working hands-on with the body is an acquired skill, with heart. *Centered* is a source to be re-read and practiced, to become confident and to balance the intellectual mind with an intuitive sense of working with the body.

References

Introduction

Ridley C. (2006), *Stillness,* North Atlantic Books, Berkeley, CA, p. 190.

Chapter 1

Beach P. (2010), *Muscles and Meridians,* Elsevier, Edinburgh, p. 149.

Dowd I. (1995), *Taking Root to Fly,* Irene Dowd, p. 75.

Gorman D. (1981), *The Body Moveable,* vol. 3, Ampersand Press, Ontario, pp. 114–119, 148–149.

Kapandji I.A. (1987), *The Physiology of the Joints,* vol. 2, 5th edition, Churchill Livingstone, Edinburgh, pp. 174, 180, 208, 224.

Kessler R.M., Hertling D. (1983), *Management of Common Musculoskeletal Disorders,* Harper and Row, Philadelphia, pp. 468–469.

Myers T.W. (2009), *Anatomy Trains,* Elsevier Health Sciences, Edinburgh, pp. 154, 199.

Schoenwolf G., Bleyl S.B., Brauer P.R. et al. (2009), *Larsen's Human Embryology,* 4th edition, Churchill Livingstone, Edinburgh, p. 617.

Stecco C., Stecco A. (2012), "Deep fascia of the lower limbs", in R. Schleip, T.W. Findley, L. Chaitow et al., *Fascia: The Tensional Network of the Human Body,* Churchill Livingstone, Edinburgh, ch. 1.5 (pp. 31–36), p. 33.

Wearing S. 2012, "Anatomy of the plantar fascia", in R. Schleip, T.W. Findley, L. Chaitow et al., *Fascia: The Tensional Network of the Human Body,* Churchill Livingstone, Edinburgh, ch. 5.9 (pp. 253–262), pp. 253–254.

Chapter 2

Casasanto D., Dijkstra K. (2010), "Motor action and emotional memory", *Cognition* 115: 179–185.

Fairclough J., Hayashi K., Toumi H. et al. (2006), "The functional anatomy of the iliotibial band during flexion and extension of the knee: implications for understanding iliotibial band syndrome", *Journal of Anatomy* 208: 309–316.

Gracovetsky S., interviewed by A. Templier: inhttp://www.somatics.de/Gracovetsky_Interview.pdf (accessed April 14, 2015).

Hoppenfeld S. (1976), *Physical Examination of the Spine and Extremities,* Appleton-Century-Crofts, New York, pp. 187–188.

Kapandji I.A. (1987), *The Physiology of the Joints,* vol. 2, 5th edition, Churchill Livingstone, Edinburgh, pp. 84, 98, 114, 122, 164.

Myers T.W. 2001, *Anatomy Trains,* Elsevier Health Sciences, Edinburgh, p. 123.

Schoenwolf G., Bleyl S.B., Brauer P.R. et al. (2009), *Larsen's Human Embryology,* 4th edition, Churchill Livingstone, Edinburgh, pp. 626–628.

Stecco C., Stecco A. (2012), "Deep fascia of the lower limbs", in R. Schleip, T.W. Findley, L. Chaitow et al., *Fascia: The Tensional Network of the Human Body,* Churchill Livingstone, Edinburgh, ch. 1.5 (pp. 31–36), p. 32.

Chapter 3

Anderson L. (1990), "Walking and Falling", *Big Science* (album).

Feldenkrais M. (1944), *Judo,* Penguin, USA, p. 27.

Gibbons S.G.T. (2007), "Assessment and rehabilitation of the stability function of psoas major", *Manuelle Therapie* 11: 177–187.

Gracovetsky S.A. (1988), *The Spinal Engine,* 2nd edition, Springer-Verlag, New York/Vienna, pp. 244–246.

Hu H., Meijer O.G., van Dieën J.H. et al. (2011), "Is the psoas a hip flexor in the active straight leg raise?", *European Spine Journal* 20: 759–765.

Lee D. (2011), *The Pelvic Girdle,* 4th edition, Churchill Livingstone/Elsevier, Edinburgh, pp. 86–87.

McGill S.M., Patt N., Norman R.W. (1988), "Measurement of the trunk musculature of active males using CT scan radiography: implications for force and moment generating capacity about the L4/L5 joint", *Journal of Biomechechanics* 21(4): 329–341.

Mitchell F. (2001), *The Muscle Energy Manual,* vol. 3, MET Press, East Lansing, MI, pp. xxiv, 21–26.

Sahrmann S. (2002), *Diagnosis and Treatment of Movement Impairment Syndromes,* Mosby, St. Louis, pp. 134–135, 318.

Schultz L., Feitis R. (1996), *The Endless Web,* North Atlantic Books, Berkeley, CA, p. 38.

Snell R. (2012), *Clinical Anatomy,* 9th edition, Lippincott Williams and Wilkins, Baltimore, p. 254.

van Wingerden J.P., Vleeming A., Buyruk H.M. et al. (2004), "Stabilization of the sacroiliac joint in vivo: verification of muscular contribution to force closure of the pelvis", *European Spine Journal* 13(3): 199–205.

van der Wal J.C. (2012), "Proprioception", in R. Schleip, T.W. Findley, L. Chaitow et al., *Fascia: The Tensional Network of the Human Body,* Churchill Livingstone, Edinburgh, ch. 2.2 (pp. 81–89), p. 81.

Vleeming A. (2012), "The thoracolumbar fascia", in R. Schleip, T.W. Findley, L. Chaitow et al., *Fascia: The Tensional Network of the Human Body,* Churchill Livingstone, Edinburgh, ch. 1.6 (pp. 37–44), pp. 38, 40.

Yerys S., Makofsky H., Byrd C. et al. (2002), "Effect of mobilization of the anterior hip capsule on gluteus maximus strength", *Journal of Manual and Manipulative Therapy* 10(4): 218–224.

Chapter 4

Beach P. (2010), *Muscles and Meridians,* Elsevier, Edinburgh, p. 96.

Bogduk N. (2005), *Clinical Anatomy of the Lumbar Spine and Sacrum,* 4th edition, Churchill Livingstone/Elsevier Health Sciences, Edinburgh, p. 99.

Breul R. (2012), "The deeper fasciae of the neck and ventral torso", in R. Schleip, T.W. Findley, L. Chaitow et al., *Fascia: The Tensional Network of the Human Body,* Churchill Livingstone, Edinburgh, ch. 1.7 (pp. 45–52), pp. 50–52.

Gentry E. http://www.pilatesanytime.com/workshop-view/1129/video/Workshop-Breathing--Michele-Larsson (accessed April 14, 2015).

Grenier S., McGill S.M. (2007), "Quantification of lumbar stability by using 2 different abdominal activation strategies", *Archives of Physical Medicine and Rehabilitation* 88: 54–62.

Kapandji I.A. (1974), *The Physiology of the Joints,* vol. 3, *Trunk and Vertebral Column,* Churchill Livingstone, Edinburgh, p. 200.

Lee D. (2001), *The Thorax,* 2nd edition, Diane Lee Physiotherapist Corporation, South Surrey, British Columbia, pp. 27, 44–49.

Lee D. (2011), *The Pelvic Girdle,* 4th edition, Churchill Livingstone/Elsevier, Edinburgh, pp. 36–38, 78–82.

Lundon K., Bolton K. (2001), "Structure and function of the lumbar intervertebral disk in health, aging, and pathologic conditions", *Journal of Orthopaedic and Sports Physical Therapy* 31(6): 291–303; discussion 304–306.

Malouin F., Richards C.L., Jackson P.L. et al. (2003), "Brain activations during motor imagery of locomotor-related tasks: a PET study", *Human Brain Mapping* 19(1): 47–62.

Myers T.W. (2001), *Anatomy Trains,* Churchill Livingstone, Edinburgh, p. 78.

Richardson C., Hodges P., Hides J. (2004), *Therapeutic Exercise for Lumbopelvic Stabilization,* Churchill Livingstone, New York, pp. 31–57.

Stecco C. (2014), "Painful connections: densification versus fibrosis of fascia", Lecture at Fascia Research Summer School, Ulm, Germany.

Vleeming A. (2012), "The thoracolumbar fascia: an integrated functional view of the anatomy of the TLF and coupled structures", in R. Schleip, T.W. Findley, L. Chaitow et al., *Fascia: The Tensional Network of the Human Body,* Churchill Livingstone, Edinburgh, ch. 1.7 (pp. 37–44), pp. 37–43.

Chapter 5

Bartley J. (2014), "Nasal influences on breathing", in L. Chaitow, D. Bradley, C. Gilbert et al., *Recognizing and Treating Breathing Disorders,* 2nd edition, Churchill Livingston Elsevier, Edinburgh, ch. 2.3 (pp. 45–50), p. 46.

Bernardi L., Passino C.,Wilmerding V. et al. (2001), "Breathing patterns and cardiovascular autonomic modulation during hypoxia by simulated altitude", *Journal of Hypertension* 19(5): 947–958.

Bradley D. (2014), "Physiotherapy in rehabilitation of breathing pattern disorders", in L. Chaitow, D. Bradley, C. Gilbert et al., *Recognizing and Treating Breathing Disorders,* 2nd edition, Churchill Livingston Elsevier, Edinburgh, p. 188.

Chaitow L., Bradley D., Gilbert C. (2014), *Recognizing and Treating Breathing Disorders,* 2nd edition, Churchill Livingstone, Elsevier, pp. 26, 35–36, 79.

Clifton-Smith T. (2014), "Breathing pattern disorder and the athlete", in L. Chaitow, D. Bradley, C. Gilbert et al., *Recognizing and Treating Breathing Disorders,* 2nd edition, Churchill Livingston Elsevier, pp. 221–222.

Grenier S., McGill S. (2007), "Quantification of lumbar stability by using 2 different abdominal activation strategies", *Archives of Physical Medicine and Rehabilitation* 88: 54–62.

Hemborg B., Moritz U., Lowing H. (1985), "Intra-abdominal pressure and trunk muscle activity during lifting IV. The causal factors of the intra-abdominal pressure rise", *Scandinavian Journal of Rehabilitation Medicine* 17: 25–38.

Hodges P.W. (1999), "Is there a role for the transversus abdominis in lumbo-pelvic stability?", *Manual Therapy* 4(2): 74–86.

Hodges P. (2008), "Transversus abdominis: a different view of the elephant", *British Journal of Sports Medicine* 42: 941–944.

Hodges P.W., Gandevia S.C. (2000), "Activation of the human diaphragm during a repetitive postural task", *Journal of Physiology* 522: 165–175.

Kolár P., Šulc J., Kynčl M. et al. (2012), "Postural function of the diaphragm in persons with and without chronic lower back pain", *Journal of Orthopaedic and Sports Physical Therapy* 42(4): 352–362.

Kolár P., Kobesova A., Valouchova P. et al. (2014), "Dynamic neuromuscular stabilization: assessment methods", in L. Chaitow, D. Bradley, C. Gilbert et al., *Recognizing and Treating Breathing Disorders,* 2nd edition, Churchill Livingston Elsevier, Edinburgh, p. 15.

Lee D. (2011), *The Pelvic Girdle,* 4th edition, Churchill Livingstone Elsevier, Edinburgh, p. 52.

Myers T. (2001), *Anatomy Trains,* Churchill Livingstone Elsevier, Edinburgh, pp. 208–209.

Paoletti S. (2012), "Diaphragmatic structure", in R. Schleip, T.W. Findley, L. Chaitow et al., *Fascia: The Tensional Network of the Human Body,* Churchill Livingstone, Edinburgh, ch. 1.10 (67–75), pp. 68–69.

Paramahansa Hariharanda (1907–2002) http://www.hariharanandakriyayoga.org/english/who_we_are/kriya/Quotes_Hariharananda.htm (accessed April 14, 2015).

Pilates J.H., Miller W.J. (1945), *Return to Life Through Contrology,* republished 1998, Presentation Dynamics Inc. pp. 13, 23.

Rolf I. (1989), *Rolfing: Reestablishing the Natural Alignment and Structural Integration of the Human Body for Vitality and Well-Being,* Healing Arts Press, Rochester, VT, p. 152.

Sweigard L. (1974), *Human Movement Potential: Its Ideokinetic Facilitation,* Harper & Row, New York, p. 187.

Willard F.H.., Vleeming A., Schuenke M.D. et al. (2012), "The thoracolumbar fascia: anatomy, function and clinical considerations", *Journal of Anatomy* 221(6): 507–536.

Chapter 6

Beach P. (2010), *Muscles and Meridians,* Elsevier, Edinburgh, p. 108.

Blakeslee S., Blakeslee M. (2007), *Body Has Mind of Its Own,* Random House, New York, pp. 15–22.

Doidge N. (2007), *The Brain that Changes Itself,* Penguin Group, New York, pp. 48–49.

Kapandji I.A. (1982), *The Physiology of the Joints,* vol. 1, 5th edition, Churchill Livingstone, Edinburgh, pp. 38, 54.

Moore K., Persaud T.V.N, Torchia M.G. (2011), *Before We Are Born: Essentials of Embryology and Birth Defects,* Elsevier Health Sciences, Philadelphia, pp. 240–243.

Myers T. (2001), *Anatomy Trains,* Churchill Livingstone Elsevier, Edinburgh, pp. 139, 185.

Norkin C., Levangie P. (2011), *Joint Structure and Function, A Comprehensive Analysis,* 5th edition, F.A. Davis, Philadelphia, pp. 232–266.

Rumi http://www.allgreatquotes.com/rumi_quotes.shtml (accessed April 14, 2015).

Schoenwolf G., Bleyl S.B., Brauer P.R. et al. (2009), *Larsen's Human Embryology,* 4th edition, Churchill Livingstone, Edinburgh, pp. 619–621.

Stecco C., Stecco A. (2012), "Deep fascia of the shoulder and arms ", in R. Schleip, T.W. Findley, L. Chaitow et al., *Fascia: The Tensional Network of the Human Body,* Churchill Livingstone, Edinburgh, pp. 25–29.

Theodoridis D., Ruston S. (2002). "The effect of shoulder movements on thoracic spine 3D motion", *Clinical Biomechanics* 17(5): 418–421.

Vleeming, Andry (2012), "The thoracolumbar fascia: an integrated functional view of the anatomy of the TLF and coupled structures", in R. Schleip, T.W. Findley, L. Chaitow et al., *Fascia: The Tensional Network of the Human Body,* Churchill Livingstone, Edinburgh, p. 38.

Chapter 7

Abram D. (1996), *The Spell of the Sensuous,* Random House, New York, p. 68.

Agur A., Dalley A.F. (2013), *Grant's Atlas of Anatomy,* 13th edition, Lippincott Williams & Wilkins, Philadelphia, p. 501.

Barral J.-P. (2007), *Study Guide Sampler,* Barral Institute, p. 2. www.barralinstitute.com

Chaitow L., Coughlin P., Findley T.W. et al. (2012), "Fascial palpation", in R. Schleip, T.W. Findley, L. Chaitow et al., *Fascia: The Tensional Network of the Human Body,* Churchill Livingstone, Edinburgh, ch. 6.2 (pp. 269–278), p. 272.

Kapandji I.A. (1999), *The Physiology of the Joints,* vol. 1, *Upper Limb,* Churchill Livingstone, Edinburgh, pp. 82, 85, 106.

Lowen F. (2011), *The Roots and Philosophy of Dynamic Manual Interface,* North Atlantic Books, Berkeley, CA, pp. 29–30, 107, 120.

Norkin C., Levangie P. (2011), *Joint Structure and Function, A Comprehensive Analysis,* 5th edition, F.A. Davis, Philadelphia, p. 306.

Stecco C., Stecco A. (2012), "Deep fascia of the shoulder and arms", in R. Schleip, T.W. Findley, L. Chaitow et al., *Fascia: The Tensional Network of the Human Body,* Churchill Livingstone, Edinburgh, pp. 25–29.

Chapter 8

Barral, J.-P., Mercier P. (2007), *Visceral Manipulation II,* Eastland Press, Seattle.

Breul R. (2012), "The deeper fascia of the neck and ventral torso", in R. Schleip, T.W. Findley, L. Chaitow et al., *Fascia: The Tensional Network of the Human Body,* Churchill Livingstone, Edinburgh, ch. 1.7, pp. 45–52.

DiGiovanna E.L., Schiowitz S., Dowling D.J. (2005), *An Osteopathic Approach to Diagnosis and Treatment,* Lippincott Williams & Wilkins, Philadelphia.

Goffart L., Hafed Z.M., Krauzlis R.J. (2012), "Visual fixation as equilibrium: evidence from the superior colliculis inactivation", *Journal of Neuroscience* 32(31): 10627–10636.

Gray H. (2012), *Gray's Anatomy,* 15th edition, Octopus Publishing Group, London.

Kapandji I.A. (1974), *The Physiology of the Joints,* vol. 3, 2nd edition, Churchill Livingstone, Edinburgh.

Mayoux-Benhamou M.-A., Wybier M., Barbet J. et al. (1992), *Relationship between Force and Cross-sectional Area of Postcervical Muscles in Man: Influence of Variations in the Morphology of the Neck, the Head and Neck Sensory Motor System,* Oxford University Press, Oxford.

Picabia F. (2007), *I Am a Beautiful Monster: Poetry Prose, and Provocation,* trans. Marc Lowenthal, MIT Press, Cambridge, MA, p. 283.

Swartz E., Floyd, R.T., Cendoma M. (2005), "Cervical spine functional anatomy and the biomechanics of injury due to compressive loading", *Journal of Athletic Training* 40(3): 155–161.

Zumpano M.P., Hartwell S., Jagos C.S. (2006), "Soft tissue connection between rectus capitus posterior minor and the posterior atlanto-occipital membrane: a cadaveric study", *Clinical Anatomy* 19(6): 522–527.

Chapter 9

Beach P. (2010), *Muscles and Meridians,* Elsevier, Edinburgh, p. 123.

Blakeslee S., Blakeslee M. (2007), *The Body Has Mind of Its Own,* Random House, New York, pp. 8, 58.

Chaitow L., Bradley D., Gilbert C. (2014), *Recognizing and Treating Breathing Disorders,* 2nd edition, Churchill Livingstone, Edinburgh, p. 8.

Duerden E.G., Laverdure-Dupont D. (2008), "Practice makes cortex", *Journal of Neuroscience* 28(35): 8655–8657.

Ericsson K.A., Charness N., Feltovich P.J. et al. (eds) (2006), *Cambridge Handbook of Expertise and Expert Performance,* Cambridge University Press, New York, pp. 698–699.

Héroux M.E., Walsh L.D., Butler A.A. et al. (2103), "Is this my finger? Proprioceptive illusions of body ownership and representation", *Journal of Physiology* 591(22): 5661–5670.

O Sensei, quoted in W. Palmer (1994), *The Intuitive Body,* North Atlantic Books, Berkeley, CA, p. 41.

Schleip R., Jaeger H. (2012), "Interoception: a new correlate for intricate connections between fascial receptors, emotion, and self recognition", in Robert Schleip, Thomas W. Findley, Leon Chaitow et al., *Fascia: The Tensional Network of the Human Body,* Churchill Livingstone, Edinburgh, ch. 2.4 (pp. 89–94), p. 89.

Southey R. (1837), *The Story of the Three Bears,* Longman, Rees, London.

van der Wal JJ.C. (2012), "Proprioception", in Robert Schleip, Thomas W. Findley, Leon Chaitow et al., *Fascia: The Tensional Network of the Human Body,* Churchill Livingstone, Edinburgh, ch. 2.2 (pp. 81–89), pp. 81–82.

INDEX